TEXTBOOK OF

RECEPTOR PHARMACOLOGY

THIRD EDITION

TEXTBOOK OF

RECEPTOR PHARMACOLOGY

THIRD EDITION

EDITED BY
JOHN C. FOREMAN
TORBEN JOHANSEN
ALASDAIR J. GIBB

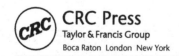

CRC Press
Taylor & Francis Group
Boca Raton London New York

CRC Press is an imprint of the
Taylor & Francis Group, an **informa** business

CRC Press
Taylor & Francis Group
6000 Broken Sound Parkway NW, Suite 300
Boca Raton, FL 33487-2742

First issued in paperback 2021

ISBN 13: 978-1-03-209937-8 (pbk)
ISBN 13: 978-1-4200-5254-1 (hbk)

Library of Congress Cataloging-in-Publication Data

Textbook of receptor pharmacology / editors, John C. Foreman, Torben Johansen, Alasdair J. Gibb. -- 3rd ed.
    p. ; cm.
  Includes bibliographical references and index.
  Summary: "Providing an introduction to the study of drug receptors, the Textbook of receptor pharmacology discusses quantitative descriptions of functional studies with agonists and antagonists; quantitative descriptions of ligands binding to receptors; the molecular structures of drug receptors; and the elements that transport the signal from the activated receptor to the intracellular compartment. This third edition features results from recent research on how the structure of receptors determines the interaction between the receptor and the signal transducer. This edition also offers new information on ligand binding receptor studies that use newly developed techniques"--Provided by publisher.
    ISBN 978-1-4200-5254-1 (hardcover : alk. paper)
  1. Drug receptors. I. Foreman, John C. II. Johansen, Torben. III. Gibb, Alasdair J.
  [DNLM: 1. Receptors, Drug--agonists. 2. Receptors, Drug--antagonists & inhibitors. 3. Radioligand Assay--methods. 4. Receptors, Drug--physiology.
  5. Signal Transduction--physiology. QV 38 T356 2011]

RM301.41.T486 2011
615'.7--dc22
        2010021866

Visit the Taylor & Francis Web site at
http://www.taylorandfrancis.com

and the CRC Press Web site at
http://www.crcpress.com

Contents

SECTION I   Drug-Receptor Interactions

SECTION II   Molecular Structure of Receptors

SECTION III   Ligand-Binding Studies of Receptors

SECTION IV   Transduction of the Receptor Signal

SECTION V   Receptors as Pharmaceutical Targets

Preface

For about five decades, a course in receptor pharmacology has been offered at University College London for undergraduate students in their final year of study for their Bachelor of Science degree in pharmacology. More recently, the course has also been taken by students reading for the Bachelor of Science degree in medicinal chemistry. The students following the course have relied for their reading upon a variety of sources, including original papers, reviews, and various textbooks, but no single text brought together the material included in the course. Beginning in 1993, we organized courses for graduate students and research workers from the pharmaceutical industry from the Nordic and European countries. In many cases, generous financial support from the Danish Research Academy and the Nordic Research Academy made this possible. These courses, too, were based on those for students at University College London, and we are grateful for the constructive criticisms of the many students on all of the courses that have shaped this book.

The first edition of the book provided a single text for the students, and the enthusiasm with which it was received encouraged us to work on further editions. There have been significant steps forward since the first edition of this book, particularly in the molecular biology of receptors. These advances are reflected in the rewritten chapters for the section of the book that deals with molecular biology. The book concentrates on cell membrane receptors themselves, together with their immediate signal transducers: ion channels, heterotrimeric G-proteins, and tyrosine kinases.

The chapter authors have been actively involved in teaching the various courses, and our joint aim has been to provide a logical introduction to the study of drug receptors. Characterization of drug receptors involves a number of different approaches, including: quantitative description of the functional studies with agonists and antagonists, quantitative description of the binding of ligands to receptors, the molecular structure of drug receptors, and the elements that transduce the signal from the activated receptor to the intracellular compartment.

The book is intended as an introductory text on receptor pharmacology but further reading has been provided for those who want to follow up on topics. Some problems are also provided for readers to test their grasp of material in some of the chapters.

John C. Foreman

Torben Johansen

Alasdair J. Gibb

Editors

John C. Foreman, Ph.D., D.Sc., M.B., B.S., F.R.C.P., is emeritus professor of pharmacology at University College London (UCL). After qualifying in medicine, he spent two years as visiting instructor of medicine at Johns Hopkins University School of Medicine in Baltimore, Maryland, before joining the permanent staff at University College London in the Pharmacology Department. He has been a visiting professor at the University of Tasmania and the University of Southern Denmark.

Dr. Foreman's research interests have included the role of bradykinin receptors in the human nasal airway, the control of microvascular circulation in human skin, and the mechanism of activation of dendritic cells. He served two terms as an editor of the *British Journal of Pharmacology* and was an associate editor of *Immunopharmacology*. He has published 170 research papers as well as reviews and contributions to books.

Torben Johansen, M.D., Dr. Med. Sci., is docent of pharmacology, Department of Physiology and Pharmacology, Institute of Medical Biology, Faculty of Health Sciences, University of Southern Denmark. Dr. Johansen obtained his M.D. degree in 1970 from the University of Copenhagen and became a research fellow in the Department of Pharmacology of Odense University in 1970, lecturer in 1972, and senior lecturer in 1974. Since 1990, he has been docent of pharmacology. In 1979, he was a visiting research fellow for three months at the University Department of Clinical Pharmacology, Oxford University, and in 1998 and 2001 he was a visiting research fellow at the Department of Pharmacology, University College London. In 1980, he did his internship in medicine and surgery at Odense University Hospital. He obtained his Dr. Med. Sci. in 1988 from Odense University.

Dr. Johansen is a member of the British Pharmacological Society, the Physiological Society, the Scandinavian Society for Physiology, the Danish Medical Association, the Danish Pharmacological Society, the Danish Society for Clinical Pharmacology, and the Danish Society for Hypertension. He has published 70 research papers in refereed journals. His current major research interests are N-methyl-D-aspartate (NMDA) receptors in the stubstantia nigra in relation to cell death in Parkinson's disease and also ion transport and signaling in mast cells in relation to intracellular pH and volume regulation.

Alasdair J. Gibb, B.Sc., Ph.D., is reader in pharmacology at University College London. He graduated in biochemistry and pharmacology and completed his Ph.D. at the University of Strathclyde, Glasgow, United Kingdom, studying the mechanisms of action of neuromuscular-blocking drugs. After two years of postdoctoral research at the Australian National University in Canberra, he came to the Pharmacology Department at UCL in 1986 to take up a postdoctoral fellowship. Dr. Gibb was appointed lecturer in pharmacology in 1990. He is currently vice dean for teaching in biosciences at UCL. He is one of the coordinators of the Wellcome Trust four-year Ph.D. program in neuroscience at UCL and a lecturer and joint organizer of the International Brain Research Organization (IBRO) Visiting Lecture Team Programme, a UNESCO and Grass Foundation–funded program that delivers neuroscience teaching to postgraduate students in developing countries around the world. He currently leads the General and Advanced Receptor Theory Workshop of the British Pharmacological Society Diploma in Pharmacology and is a course leader on the British Pharmacological Society short course on Translational Pharmacology.

Dr. Gibb is a member of the British Pharmacological Society and the Physiological Society. He is a past member of the Medical Research Council New Investigator Awards Panel, editor and distributing editor of the *Journal of Physiology*, and coordinator of the Ion Channels Special Interest Group of the Physiological Society, and is currently an editor of the *British Journal of Pharmacology*. He has published more than 50 research papers, reviews, and contributions to books. Dr. Gibb's current main research interest is in the pharmacology and function of NMDA receptors.

Contributors

Sir James W. Black, F.R.S.*
Nobel Laureate
James Black Foundation
London, United Kingdom

David A. Brown, F.R.S.
Research Department of Neuroscience,
  Physiology, and Pharmacology
University College London
London, United Kingdom

Jan Egebjerg, Ph.D.
Department for Molecular and Structural Biology
Aarhus University, Aarhus
Discovery Biology Research, Lundbeck A/S
Valby, Denmark

Elisabeth Genot, Ph.D.
Cellular Signalling Group
IECB—INSERM U889
Bordeaux, France

Dennis G. Haylett, Ph.D.
Department of Pharmacology
University College London
London, United Kingdom

Donald H. Jenkinson, Ph.D.
Department of Pharmacology
University College London
London, United Kingdom

IJsbrand Kramer, Ph.D.
Cellular Signalling Group
IECB—INSERM U889
Bordeaux, France

Michel Laguerre, Ph.D.
Molecular Modelling
IECB—CNRS UMR 5144
Bordeaux, France

* During production of the third edition of this book Sir James Black died on March 22, 2010. James Black was a pioneer in the application of careful quantitative pharmacology to the development of new therapeutic agents. He developed the first of the β-blocking drugs, propranolol, to relieve angina pectoris which subsequently became for many years a mainstay in the treatment of high blood pressure. His approach was to take the structure of the natural hormone and then in collaboration with medicinal chemists, make chemical analogues that would be effective antagonists with selective affinity for the receptor of interest, while lacking the agonist efficacy of the natural hormone. He used a similar approach to develop histamine H_2 antagonists for the treatment of stomach and duodenal ulcers. He shared the 1988 Nobel Prize for Physiology or Medicine with George H. Hitchings and Gertrude Elion. β-blockers and H_2-receptor antagonists have benefited millions of patients and often saved lives. By his example, Black made a massive contribution to establishing the importance of receptor pharmacology in drug discovery.

Professor Black graduated in medicine from St. Andrews University in 1946 and, after academic posts at the University of Glasgow, joined ICI as a pharmacologist (1958–1964) where he worked on the development of β-blockers. After working with Smith, Kline and French, where he developed the H_2 antagonists, he became Professor of Pharmacology at University College London (1973–1977), before joining Wellcome as the Director of Therapeutic Research (1978–1984). Since 1984, he was a professor of Analytical Pharmacology at King's College London.

Section I

Drug-Receptor Interactions

1 Classical Approaches to the Study of Drug-Receptor Interactions

Donald H. Jenkinson

CONTENTS

1.1   INTRODUCTION

1.1.1   SOME HISTORY

The term *receptor* is used in pharmacology to denote a class of cellular macromolecules that are concerned directly and specifically in chemical signaling between and within cells. The combination of a hormone, neurotransmitter, or intracellular messenger with its receptor(s) results in a change in cellular activity. Hence a receptor has not only to recognize the particular molecules that activate it but also, when recognition takes place, to alter cell function by causing, for example, a change in membrane permeability, enzyme activity, or gene transcription.

The concept has a long history. Mankind has always been intrigued by the remarkable ability of animals to distinguish different substances by taste and smell. Writing in ~50 B.C., Lucretius (in *De Rerum Natura, Liber IV*) speculated that odors might be conveyed by tiny, invisible "seeds" with distinctive shapes that would have to fit into minute "spaces and passages" in the palate and nostrils. In his words,

> Some of these must be smaller, some greater, they must be three-cornered for some creatures, square for others, many round again, and some of many angles in many ways.

The same principle of complementarity between substances and their recognition sites is implicit in John Locke's prediction in his *Essay Concerning Human Understanding* (1690):

> Did we but know the mechanical affections of the particles of rhubarb, hemlock, opium and a man, as a watchmaker does those of a watch, ... we should be able to tell beforehand that rhubarb will purge, hemlock kill and opium make a man sleep.

(Here, *mechanical affections* could be replaced in today's usage by *chemical affinities*.)

Prescient as they were, these early ideas could be taken further only when, in the early 19th century, it became possible to separate and purify the individual components of materials of plant and animal origin. The simple but powerful technique of fractional crystallization allowed plant alkaloids such as nicotine, atropine, pilocarpine, strychnine, and morphine to be obtained in pure form for the first time. The impact on biology was immediate and far reaching, for these substances proved to be invaluable tools for the unraveling of physiological function. To take a single example, J. N. Langley made brilliant use of the ability of nicotine to first activate and then block nerves originating in the autonomic ganglia. This allowed him to map out the distribution and divisions of the autonomic nervous system.

Langley also studied the actions of atropine and pilocarpine, and in 1878 he published (in the first volume of the *Journal of Physiology*, which he founded) an account of the interactions between pilocarpine (which causes salivation) and atropine (which blocks this action of pilocarpine). Confirming and extending the pioneering work of Heidenhain and Luchsinger, Langley showed that the inhibitory action of atropine could be overcome by increasing the dose of pilocarpine. Moreover, the restored response to pilocarpine could in turn be abolished by further atropine. Commenting on these results, Langley wrote,

> We may, I think, without too much rashness, assume that there is some substance or substances in the nerve endings or [salivary] gland cells with which both atropine and pilocarpine are capable of forming compounds. On this assumption, then, the atropine or pilocarpine compounds are formed according to some law of which their relative mass and chemical affinity for the substance are factors.

If we replace *mass* with *concentration*, the second sentence can serve as well today as when it was written, though the nature of the law that Langley had inferred must exist was not to be formulated (in a pharmacological context) until almost 60 years later. It is considered in Section 1.5.2.

J. N. Langley maintained an interest in the action of plant alkaloids throughout his life. From work with nicotine (which can contract skeletal muscle) and curare (which abolishes this action of nicotine, and also blocks the response of the muscle to nerve stimulation, as first shown by Claude Bernard), he was able to infer in 1905 that the muscle must possess a "receptive substance":

> Since in the normal state both nicotine and curari abolish the effect of nerve stimulation, but do not prevent contraction from being obtained by direct stimulation of the muscle or by a further adequate injection of nicotine, it may be inferred that neither the poison nor the nervous impulse act directly on the contractile substance of the muscle but on some accessory substance.
>
> Since this accessory substance is the recipient of stimuli which it transfers to the contractile material, we may speak of it as the receptive substance of the muscle.

At the same time, Paul Ehrlich, working in Frankfurt, was reaching similar conclusions, though from evidence of a quite different kind. He was the first to make a thorough and systematic study of the relationship between the chemical structure of organic molecules and their biological actions. This was put to good use in collaboration with the organic chemist Alfred Bertheim. Together, they prepared and tested more than 600 organometallic compounds incorporating mercury and arsenic. Among the outcomes was the introduction into medicine of drugs such as salvarsan that were toxic to pathogenic microorganisms responsible for, for example, syphilis, at doses that had relatively minor side effects in man. Ehrlich also investigated the selective staining of cells by dyes, as well as the remarkably powerful and specific actions of bacterial toxins. All these studies convinced him that biologically active molecules had to become bound in order to be effective, and after the fashion of the time he expressed this neatly in Latin: *Corpora non agunt nisi fixata.*[*]

In Ehrlich's words (Collected papers, Vol. III, Chemotherapy)

> When the poisons and the organs sensitive to it do not come into contact, or when sensitiveness of the organs does not exist, there can be no action.
>
> If we assume that those peculiarities of the toxin which cause their distribution are localized in a special group of the toxin molecules and the power of the organs and tissues to react with the toxin are localized in a special group of the protoplasm, we arrive at the basis of my side chain theory. The distributive groups of the toxin I call the "haptophore group" and the corresponding chemical organs of the protoplasm the "receptor"..... Toxic actions can only occur when receptors fitted to anchor the toxins are present.

---

[*] Literally: Entities do not act unless attached.

Today, it is accepted that Langley and Ehrlich deserve comparable recognition for the introduction of the receptor concept.[*] In the same years, biochemists studying the relationship between substrate concentration and enzyme velocity had also come to think that enzyme molecules must possess an *active site* that discriminates between different substrates and inhibitors. As often happens, different strands of evidence had converged to point to a single conclusion.

Finally, a note on the two ways in which present-day pharmacologists and biochemists use the term *receptor*. The first, as in the opening sentences of this section, is to refer to the entire macromolecule, often with several subunits, that carries the binding site(s) for the agonist. This usage has become common as advances in molecular biology have revealed the amino acid sequences and structures of more and more signaling macromolecules. But pharmacologists still sometimes employ the term *receptor* when they have in mind only the particular regions of the macromolecule that are concerned in the binding of agonist and antagonist molecules. Hence *receptor occupancy* is often used as convenient shorthand for the fraction of the binding sites occupied by a ligand.[†]

1.2   MODELING THE RELATIONSHIP BETWEEN AGONIST CONCENTRATION AND TISSUE RESPONSE

With the concept of the receptor established, pharmacologists turned their attention to understanding the quantitative relationship between drug concentration and the response of a tissue. This entailed, first, finding out how the fraction of binding sites occupied and activated by agonist molecules varies with agonist concentration and, second, understanding the dependence of the magnitude of the observed response on the extent of receptor activation.

Though the first question can now often be studied directly using techniques described in later chapters, this was not an option for the early pharmacologists. Also, the only responses that could then be measured (e.g., the contraction of an intact piece of smooth muscle, or a change in the rate of the heartbeat) were indirect, in the sense that many cellular events lay between the initial step (activation of the receptors) and the observed response. For these reasons, the early workers had no choice but to devise ingenious indirect approaches, several of which are still important. These are based on *modeling* (i.e., making particular assumptions about) the two relationships identified above, and then comparing the predictions of the models with the actual behavior of isolated tissues. This will now be illustrated.

1.2.1   RELATIONSHIP BETWEEN LIGAND CONCENTRATION AND RECEPTOR OCCUPANCY

We begin with the simplest possible representation of the combination of a ligand, A, with its binding site on a receptor, R:

$$A + R \underset{k_{-1}}{\overset{k_{+1}}{\rightleftharpoons}} AR \tag{1.1}$$

Here, binding is regarded as a bimolecular reaction and k_{+1} and k_{-1} are respectively the *association rate constant* ($M^{-1} s^{-1}$) and the *dissociation rate constant* (s^{-1}).

The law of mass action states that the rate of a reaction is proportional to the product of the concentrations of the reactants. We will apply it to this simple scheme, making the assumption that equilibrium has been reached so that the rate at which AR is formed from A and R is equal to the rate at which AR dissociates. This gives

$$k_{+1}[A][R] = k_{-1}[AR]$$

---

[*] For a fuller account, see Prüll, Maehle, and Halliwell (2009).

[†] *Ligand* here means a small molecule that binds to a specific site (or sites) on a receptor macromolecule. The term *drug* is often used in this context, especially in the older literature.

where [R] and [AR] denote the concentrations of receptors in which the binding sites for A are free and occupied, respectively.

It may well seem odd to refer to receptor *concentrations* in this context when receptors can often move only in the plane of the membrane (and then perhaps to no more than a limited extent, since many kinds of receptors are anchored). However, the model can be formulated just as well, or better, in terms of the proportions of a population of binding sites that are either free or occupied by a ligand. If we define p_R as the proportion free,[*] equal to $[R]/[R]_T$, where $[R]_T$ represents the total concentration of receptors, and p_{AR} as $[AR]/[R]_T$, we have

$$k_{+1}[A]\, p_R = k_{-1}\, p_{AR}$$

Because for now we are concerned only with equilibrium conditions and not with the rate at which equilibrium is reached, we can combine k_{+1} and k_{-1} to form a new constant, K_A, $= k_{-1}/k_{+1}$, which has the unit of concentration. K_A is an *equilibrium dissociation constant* (see Appendix 1.2.1), though this is often abbreviated to either *equilibrium constant* or *dissociation constant*. Replacing k_{+1} and k_{-1} gives

$$[A]\, p_R = K_A\, p_{AR}$$

Because the binding site is either free or occupied, we can write

$$p_R + p_{AR} = 1$$

Substituting for p_R

$$\frac{K_A}{[A]} p_{AR} + p_{AR} = 1$$

Hence,[†]

$$p_{AR} = \frac{[A]}{K_A + [A]} \tag{1.2}$$

This is the important *Hill–Langmuir equation*. A. V. Hill was the first (in 1909) to apply the law of mass action to the relationship between ligand concentration and receptor occupancy at equilibrium, and to the rate at which this equilibrium is approached.[‡] The physical chemist I. Langmuir showed a few years later that a similar equation (the *Langmuir adsorption isotherm*) applies to the adsorption of gases at a surface (e.g., of a metal or of charcoal).

In deriving Equation (1.2), we have assumed that the concentration of the ligand A does not change as ligand receptor complexes are formed. In effect, the ligand is considered to be present in such excess that it is scarcely depleted by combination of a little of it with the receptors; thus [A] can be regarded as constant.

The relationship between p_{AR} and [A] predicted by Equation (1.2) is illustrated in Figure 1.1. The concentration of A has been plotted using a linear (left) and a logarithmic scale (right). The value of

---

[*] p_R can be also be defined as N_R/N where N_R is the number of receptors in which the binding sites are free of A and N is their total number. Similarly, p_{AR} is given by N_{AR}/N, where N_{AR} is the number of receptors in which the binding site is occupied by A. These terms are used when we come to discuss the action of irreversible antagonists (Section 1.6.4).

[†] If you find this difficult, see Appendix 1.2.2 at the end of this section.

[‡] Hill had been an undergraduate student in the Department of Physiology at Cambridge, where J. N. Langley suggested to him that this would be useful to examine in relation to finding whether the rate at which an agonist acts on an isolated tissue is determined by diffusion of the agonist or by its combination with the receptor. See Colquhoun (2006) for a fuller account.

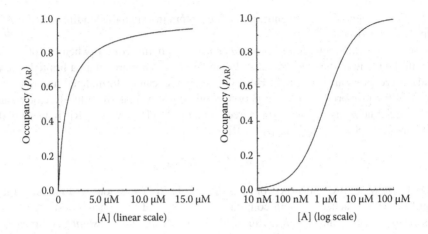

FIGURE 1.1   The relationship between binding-site occupancy and ligand concentration ([A]; linear scale, left; log scale, right), as predicted by the Hill–Langmuir equation. K_A has been set to 1 μM for both curves.

K_A has been taken to be 1 μM. Note from Equation (1.2) that when $[A] = K_A$, $p_{AR} = 0.5$; that is, half of the receptors are occupied.

With the logarithmic scale, the slope of the line initially increases: The curve has the form of an elongated S and hence is said to be *sigmoidal*. In contrast, with a linear (arithmetic) scale for [A], there is no sigmoidicity: The slope declines as [A] increases, and the curve forms part of a rectangular hyperbola.

Equation (1.2) can be rearranged to

$$\frac{p_{AR}}{1 - p_{AR}} = \frac{[A]}{K_A}$$

Takings logs, we have

$$\log\left(\frac{p_{AR}}{1 - p_{AR}}\right) = \log[A] - \log K_A$$

Hence a plot of $\log(p_{AR}/(1 - p_{AR}))$ against $\log[A]$ should give a straight line with a slope of unity. Such a graph is described as a *Hill plot*, again after A. V. Hill, who was the first to employ it, and is often used when p_{AR} is measured directly with a radiolabeled ligand (see Chapter 5). In practice, the slope of the line is not always unity, or even constant, as will be discussed. It is referred to as the *Hill coefficient* (n_H): The term *Hill slope* is also used.

1.2.2   RELATIONSHIP BETWEEN RECEPTOR OCCUPANCY AND TISSUE RESPONSE

This is the second of the two questions identified at the start of Section 1.2, where it was noted that the earliest pharmacologists had no choice but to use indirect methods in their attempts to account for the relationship between the concentration of a drug and the tissue response that it elicits. In the absence at that time of any means of obtaining direct evidence on the point, A. V. Hill and A. J. Clark explored the consequences of assuming (1) that the law of mass action applies, so that Equation (1.2) (derived above) holds, and (2) that the response of the tissue is linearly related to receptor occupancy. Clark went further and made the *tentative* assumption that the relationship might be one of direct proportionality (though he was well aware that this was almost certainly an oversimplification, as we now know it usually is).

Should there be direct proportionality, and using y to denote the response of a tissue (expressed as a percentage of the maximum response attainable with a large concentration of the agonist), the relationship between occupancy[*] and response becomes

$$\frac{y}{100} = p_{AR} \tag{1.3}$$

Combining this with Equation (1.2) gives an expression that predicts the relationship between the concentration of the agonist and the response that it elicits:

$$\frac{y}{100} = \frac{[A]}{K_A + [A]} \tag{1.4}$$

This is often rearranged to

$$\frac{y}{100 - y} = \frac{[A]}{K_A} \tag{1.5}$$

Taking logs,

$$\log\left(\frac{y}{100 - y}\right) = \log\,[A] - \log\,K_A$$

One approach to testing the applicability of this expression (and so of Equation 1.4) is to measure a series of responses (y) to different concentrations of A and then plot log ($y/(100 - y)$) against log [A]. If Equation (1.4) holds, a straight line with a slope of unity should be obtained. Also, were all the underlying assumptions to be correct, the value of the intercept of the line on the abscissa (i.e., when the response is half-maximal) would give an estimate of K_A. A. J. Clark was the first to explore this using the responses of isolated tissues, and Figure 1.2 illustrates some of his findings. Figure 1.2a shows that Equation (1.4) provides a reasonably good fit to the experimental values. Also, Clark's values for the slopes of the Hill plots in Figure 1.2b are quite close to unity (0.9 for the frog ventricle, 0.8 for the rectus abdominis[†]).

While these findings are in keeping with the simple model that has been outlined, *they do not amount to proof that it is correct*. Also, later studies with a variety of tissues have shown that many concentration-response relationships cannot be fitted by Equation (1.4). For example, the Hill coefficient is almost always greater than unity for responses mediated by ligand-gated ion channels (see Appendix 1.2.3 and also Chapter 6). What is more, it is now known that in many tissues the maximal response (e.g., contraction of intestinal smooth muscle) can occur when an agonist such as acetylcholine occupies less than a tenth of the available receptors, rather than all of them as postulated in Equation (1.3). By the same token, when an agonist is applied at the concentration (usually termed the $[A]_{50}$ or EC_{50}) needed to give a half-maximal response, receptor occupancy may be as little as 1% in some tissues,[‡] rather than the 50% to be expected were the response to be directly proportional to occupancy. An additional complication is that many tissues contain enzymes (e.g., cholinesterase) or uptake processes (e.g., for noradrenaline) for which agonists are substrates. Because of this, the agonist concentration in the inner regions of an isolated tissue may be much less than that applied in the external solution.

---

[*] Note that no distinction is made here between occupied and activated receptors: It is tacitly assumed that all the receptors occupied by agonist molecules are in an active state, hence contributing to the initiation of the observed tissue response. As we shall see in the following sections, this is a crucial oversimplification.

[†] These experiments have been reanalyzed by Colquhoun (2006).

[‡] For evidence on this, see Section 1.6 on irreversible antagonists.

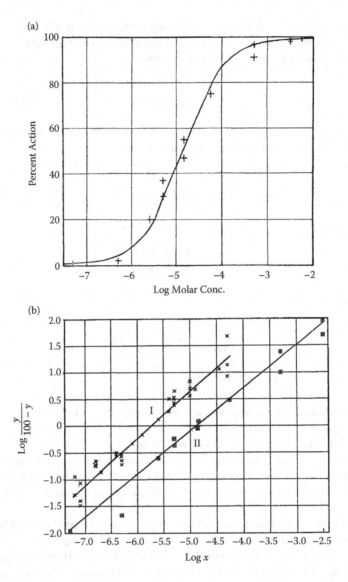

FIGURE 1.2 Upper: Concentration-response relationship for the action of acetylcholine in causing contraction of the frog rectus abdominis muscle. The curve has been drawn using Equation (1.4). Lower: Hill plots for the action of acetylcholine on frog ventricle (curve I) and rectus abdominis (curve II). (Adapted from Clark, A. J., *J. Physiol.*, 61, 530–547, 1926.)

For all these reasons, pharmacologists have had to abandon (sometimes rather reluctantly and belatedly) not only their attempts to explain the shapes of the dose-response curves of complex tissues in terms of the simple models first explored by Clark and by Hill, but also the hope that the value of the concentration of an agonist that gives a half-maximal response might provide even an approximate estimate of K_A. Nevertheless, as Clark's work showed, the relationship between the concentration of an agonist and the response of a tissue commonly has the same general form shown in Figure 1.1. In keeping with this, concentration-response curves can often be described *empirically*, and at least to a first approximation, by the simple expression

$$y = y_{max} \frac{[A]^{n_H}}{[A]_{50}^{n_H} + [A]^{n_H}} \tag{1.6}$$

This is usually described as the *Hill equation* (see also Appendix 1.2.3). Here n_H is again the *Hill coefficient* and y and y_{max} are respectively the observed response and the maximum response to a large concentration of the agonist, A. $[A]_{50}$ is the concentration of A at which y is half maximal. Because it is a constant for a given concentration-response relationship, it is sometimes denoted by K. While this is algebraically neater (and was the symbol used by Hill), it should be remembered that K in this context does not necessarily correspond to an equilibrium constant. Employing $[A]_{50}$ rather than K in Equation (1.6) helps to remind us that the relationship between $[A]$ and response is here being *described* rather than *explained* in terms of a model of receptor action. The difference is important.

1.2.3 THE DISTINCTION BETWEEN AGONIST BINDING AND RECEPTOR ACTIVATION

To end, we return to models of receptor action and to a further limitation of the early attempts to account for the shapes of concentration-response curves. As already noted, the simple concepts expressed in Equations (1.3) and (1.4) do not distinguish between the *occupation* and the *activation* of a receptor by an agonist. This distinction, it is now appreciated, is crucial to the understanding of the action of agonists and partial agonists. Indeed all contemporary accounts of receptor activation take as their starting point a mechanism of the following kind[*]:

$$\underset{inactive}{\overset{vacant}{A+R}} \quad \overset{K_A}{\rightleftharpoons} \quad \underset{inactive}{\overset{occupied}{AR}} \quad \overset{E}{\rightleftharpoons} \quad \underset{active}{\overset{occupied}{AR^*}} \tag{1.7}$$

Here the occupied receptors can exist in two forms, one of which is inactive (AR) and the other active (AR*) in the sense that its formation leads to a tissue response. AR and AR* can interconvert (often described as isomerization), and at equilibrium the receptors will be distributed between the R, AR, and AR* conditions.[†] The position of the equilibrium between AR and AR*, and hence the magnitude of the maximum response of the tissue, will depend on the value of the equilibrium constant E[‡]. Suppose that a very large concentration of the agonist A is applied, so that all the binding sites are occupied, that is, the receptors are in either the AR or the AR* state. If the position of the equilibrium strongly favors AR, with few active (AR*) receptors, the response will be relatively small. The reverse would apply for a very effective agonist. This will be explained in greater detail in Sections 1.4.3 through 1.4.7, where we will also look into the quantitative relationship between agonist concentration and the fraction of receptors in the active state.

APPENDICES TO SECTION 1.2

APPENDIX 1.2.1 EQUILIBRIUM, DISSOCIATION, AND AFFINITY CONSTANTS

Confusingly, the terms *equilibrium*, *dissociation*, and *affinity constant* are all in current use to express the position of the equilibrium between a ligand and its receptors. The choice arises because the ratio of the rate constants k_{-1} and k_{+1} can be expressed either way. In this chapter we take K_A to be k_{-1}/k_{+1}, and it is then strictly an *equilibrium dissociation constant*, often abbreviated to either *dissociation constant* or *equilibrium constant*. The inverse ratio, k_{+1}/k_{-1}, gives the *association equilibrium constant*, which is usually referred to as the *affinity constant*.

---

[*] This will be described as the del Castillo–Katz scheme since it was first applied to receptor action by J. del Castillo and B. Katz (University College London) in 1957 (see also Section 1.4.3).

[†] The scheme is readily extended to include the possibility that some of the receptors may be active even in the absence of an agonist (see Section 1.4.7).

[‡] This constant is sometimes denoted by L or by K_2. E has been chosen for this introductory account because of the relation to efficacy and also because it is the term used in a seminal review by Colquhoun (1998) on binding, efficacy, and the effects thereon of receptor mutations.

TABLE 1.1
Some Terms and Symbols

	Abbreviation	Unit
Equilibrium dissociation constant	K_A	M
Affinity constant	K'_A	M^{-1}
Normalized concentration	$\cent_A$	—

One way to reduce the risk of confusion is to express ligand concentrations in terms of K_A. This *normalized* concentration is defined as $[A]/K_A$, and will be denoted here by the symbol $\cent_A$. We can therefore write the Hill–Langmuir equation in three different, though equivalent, ways:

$$p_{AR} = \frac{[A]}{K_A + [A]} = \frac{K'_A [A]}{1 + K'_A [A]} = \frac{\cent_A}{1 + \cent_A}$$

where the terms are as shown in Table 1.1.

APPENDIX 1.2.2   STEP-BY-STEP DERIVATION OF THE HILL–LANGMUIR EQUATION

We start with the two key equations given in Section 1.2.1:

$$[A]\, p_R = K_A\, p_{AR} \tag{A.1}$$

$$p_R + p_{AR} = 1 \tag{A.2}$$

From Equation (A.1),

$$p_R = \frac{K_A}{[A]}\, p_{AR} \tag{A.3}$$

Remember, if $ax = by$ then $x = (b/a)y$.

Next, use Equation (A.3) to replace p_R in Equation (A.2). This is done because we wish to find p_{AR}.

$$\frac{K_A}{[A]}\, p_{AR} + p_{AR} = 1$$

$$p_{AR}\left(\frac{K_A}{[A]} + 1\right) = 1$$

Remember, $ax + x = x\,(a + 1)$.

$$p_{AR}\left(\frac{K_A + [A]}{[A]}\right) = 1$$

Remember, $(s/t) + 1 = (s + t)/t$.

$$p_{AR} = \frac{[A]}{K_A + [A]}$$

Remember, if $x(u/v) = 1$, then $x = v/u$.

The Hill–Langmuir equation may be rearranged by cross-multiplying

$$p_{AR}\, K_A + p_{AR}\, [A] = [A]$$

For cross multiplication, if $a/b = c/d$ then $(a \times d) = (c \times b)$. Remember, $y = x/(a + x)$ is the same as $(y/1) = x/(a + x)$, which is ready for cross-multiplication.

$$p_{AR} K_A = [A] (1 - p_{AR})$$

$$\frac{p_{AR}}{1 - p_{AR}} = \frac{[A]}{K_A}$$

Taking logs,

$$\log\left(\frac{p_{AR}}{1 - p_{AR}}\right) = \log[A] - \log K_A$$

Remember, $\log(a/b) = \log a - \log b$.

APPENDIX 1.2.3 THE HILL EQUATION AND THE HILL PLOT

In some of his earliest work, published in 1910, A. V. Hill examined how the binding of oxygen to hemoglobin varied with the oxygen partial pressure. He found that the relationship between the two could be described by the following equation:

$$y = \frac{K'x^n}{1 + K'x^n}$$

Here, y is the fractional binding, x is the partial pressure of O_2, K' is an affinity constant, and n is a number which in Hill's work varied from 1.5 to 3.2.

This equation can also be written as

$$y = \frac{x^n}{K_e + x^n} \tag{1.8a}$$

where $K_e = 1/K'$, and as

$$y = \frac{x^n}{K^n + x^n} \tag{1.8b}$$

This variant is convenient because K has the same units as x, and moreover is the value of x for which y is half maximal.

Equation (1.8b) can be rearranged and expressed logarithmically as:

$$\log\left(\frac{y}{1 - y}\right) = n \log x - n \log K$$

Hence a Hill plot (see earlier) should give a straight line of slope n.

Hill plots are often used in pharmacology, when y may be either the fractional response of a tissue or the amount of a ligand bound to its binding site, expressed as a fraction of the maximum binding, and x is the concentration. It is sometimes found (especially when tissue responses are measured) that the Hill coefficient differs markedly from unity. What might this mean?

One of the earliest explanations to be considered was that n molecules of ligand might bind simultaneously to a single binding site, R:

$$nA + R \rightleftharpoons A_nR$$

This would lead to the following expression for the proportion of binding sites occupied by A:

$$p_{A_nR} = \frac{[A]^n}{K + [A]^n}$$

where K is an equilibrium constant. Hence the Hill plot would be a straight line with a slope of n. However, this model is quite unlikely to apply. Extreme conditions aside, there are few examples of chemical reactions in which three or more molecules (e.g., two of A and one of R) combine simultaneously. Another explanation has to be sought. One possibility arises when the tissue response measured is indirect, in the sense that a sequence of cellular events links receptor activation to the response that is finally observed. The Hill coefficient may not then be unity (or even a constant) because of a nonlinear and variable relation between the proportion of receptors activated and one or more of the events that follow.

Even when it is possible to observe receptor activation directly, the Hill coefficient may still not be unity. This has been studied in detail for ligand-gated ion channels such as the nicotinic receptor for acetylcholine. Here the activity of individual receptors can be followed as it occurs by measuring the tiny flows of electrical current through the ion channel that is intrinsic to the receptor (see Figure 1.9 and also Chapter 6). On determining the relationship between this response and agonist concentration, the Hill coefficient is found to be greater than unity (characteristically 1.3–2.0) and to change with agonist concentration. The explanation is to be found in the structure of this class of receptor. Each receptor macromolecule is composed of several (often five) subunits of which usually two carry binding sites for the agonist. Both of these sites have to be occupied for the receptor to become activated, at least in its normal mode. The scheme introduced in Section 1.2.3 has then to be elaborated:

$$A + R \rightleftharpoons AR + A \rightleftharpoons A_2R \rightleftharpoons A_2R^* \tag{1.9}$$

Suppose that the two sites are identical (an oversimplification) and that the binding of the first molecule of agonist does not affect the affinity of the site that remains vacant. The equilibrium dissociation constant for each site is denoted by K_A and the equilibrium constant for the isomerization between A_2R and A_2R^* by E, so that $[A_2R^*] = E[A_2R]$.

The proportion of receptors in the active state (A_2R^*) is then given by

$$p_{A_2R^*} = \frac{E[A]^2}{(K_A + [A])^2 + E[A]^2} \tag{1.10}$$

This predicts a nonlinear Hill plot. Its slope will vary with [A] according to

$$n_H = \frac{2(K_A + [A])}{K_A + 2[A]}$$

When [A] is small in relation to K_A, n_H approximates to 2. However, as [A] is increased, n_H tends towards unity.

On the same scheme, the amount of A that is bound (expressed as a fraction, p_{bound}, of the maximum binding when [A] is very large, so that all the sites are occupied) is given by

$$p_{bound} = \frac{[A](K_A + [A]) + E[A]^2}{(K_A + [A])^2 + E[A]^2} \tag{1.11}$$

The Hill plot for binding would again be nonlinear with a Hill coefficient given by

$$n_H = \frac{(K_A + [A])^2 + E[A](2K_A + [A])}{(K_A + [A])\{K_A + (1+E)[A]\}} \tag{1.12}$$

This approximates to unity if [A] is either very large or very small. In between, n_H may be as much as 2 for very large values of E. It is perhaps surprising that this should be so even though the affinities for the first and the second binding steps have been taken to be the same, provided only that there is some isomerization of the receptor to the active form. This is because isomerization increases the total amount of binding by displacing the equilibria shown in Equation (1.9) to the right, that is, toward the bound forms of the receptor.

We now consider what would happen if the binding of the first molecule of agonist altered the affinity of the second identical site. The equilibrium dissociation constants for the first and second bindings will be denoted by $K_{A(1)}$ and $K_{A(2)}$, respectively, and E is defined as before.

The proportion of receptors in the active state (A_2R^*) is then given by

$$P_{A_2R^*} = \frac{E[A]^2}{K_{A(1)}K_{A(2)} + 2K_{A(2)}[A] + (1+E)[A]^2} \tag{1.13}$$

and the Hill coefficient n_H would be

$$n_H = 1 + \frac{K_{A(1)}K_{A(2)}}{K_{A(1)}K_{A(2)} + (K_{A(1)} + K_{A(2)})[A]}$$

These relationships are discussed further in Chapter 6 (see Equations 6.4 and 6.5).

On the same scheme, the amount of A that is bound is given by

$$p_{bound} = \frac{K_{A(2)}[A] + (1+E)[A]^2}{K_{A(1)}K_{A(2)} + 2K_{A(2)}[A] + (1+E)[A]^2} \tag{1.14}$$

The Hill plot would again be nonlinear with the Hill coefficient given by

$$n_H = \frac{K_{A(1)}K_{A(2)} + (1+E)[A](2K_{A(1)} + [A])}{(K_{A(1)} + [A])\{K_{A(2)} + (1+E)[A]\}} \tag{1.15}$$

This approximates to unity if [A] is either very large or very small. In between, n_H may be greater (up to 2) or less than 1, depending on the magnitude of E and on the relative values of $K_{A(1)}$ and $K_{A(2)}$. If, for simplicity, we set E to 0, and if $K_{A(2)}$ is less than $K_{A(1)}$, then $n_H > 1$ and there is said to be positive cooperativity. Negative cooperativity occurs when $K_{A(2)} > K_{A(1)}$ and n_H is then < 1. This is discussed further in Chapter 5, where plots of Equations (1.14) and (1.15) are shown (Figure 5.3) for widely ranging values of the ratio of $K_{A(1)}$ to $K_{A(2)}$, and with E taken to be zero.

APPENDIX 1.2.4   LOGITS, THE LOGISTIC EQUATION, AND THEIR RELATION TO THE HILL PLOT AND EQUATION

The *logit transformation* of a variable p is defined as

$$\text{logit}\,[p] = \log_e\left(\frac{p}{1-p}\right)$$

Hence, the Hill plot can be regarded as a plot of logit (p) against the logarithm of concentration (though it is more usual to employ logs to base 10 than to base e).

It is worth noting the distinction between the *Hill equation* and the *logistic equation*, which was first formulated in the 19th century as a means of describing the time-course of population increase. It is defined by the expression

$$p = \frac{1}{1 + e^{-(a+bx)}} \qquad (1.16)$$

This rearranges to

$$\frac{p}{1-p} = e^{a+bx}$$

Hence

$$\text{logit}\,[p] = \log_e\left(\frac{p}{1-p}\right) = a + bx$$

If we redefine a as $-\log_e K$, and x as $\log_e z$, then

$$p = \frac{z^b}{K + z^b} \qquad (1.17)$$

which is a form of the Hill equation (see Equation 1.8a). However, note that Equation (1.17) has been obtained from Equation (1.16) only by transforming one of the variables. It follows that the terms *logistic equation* (or *curve*) and *Hill equation* (or *curve*) should not be regarded as interchangeable. To illustrate the distinction, if the independent variable in each equation is set to zero, the dependent variable becomes $1/(1 + e^{-a})$ in Equation (1.16) as compared with zero in Equation (1.17).

1.3 THE TIME COURSE OF CHANGES IN RECEPTOR OCCUPANCY

1.3.1 INTRODUCTION

At first glance, the simplest approach to finding how quickly a drug combines with its receptors is to measure the rate at which an isolated tissue responds to it. But there are two immediate problems. The first is that the relationship between the effect on a tissue and the proportion of receptors occupied by the drug is often not known, and cannot be assumed to be simple, as we have already seen. A half-maximal tissue response only rarely corresponds to half-maximal receptor occupation. We can take as an example the action of the neuromuscular blocking agent tubocurarine on the contractions that result from stimulation of the motor nerve supply to skeletal muscle *in vitro*. The rat phrenic nerve-diaphragm preparation is often used in such experiments. Because neuromuscular transmission normally has a large safety margin, the contractile response to nerve stimulation begins to fall only when tubocurarine has occupied on average more than 80% of the binding sites on the nicotinic acetylcholine receptors located on the superficial muscle fibers. So when the twitch of the whole muscle has fallen to half its initial amplitude, receptor occupancy by tubocurarine in the surface fibers is much greater than 50%.

The second problem is that the rate at which a drug acts on an isolated tissue is often determined by the diffusion of drug molecules through the tissue rather than by their combination with the receptors. Again taking as our example the action of tubocurarine on the isolated diaphragm, the slow development of the block reflects not the rate of binding to the receptors but rather the failure of neuromuscular transmission in an increasing number of individual muscle fibers as tubocurarine slowly diffuses between the closely packed fibers into the interior of the preparation. Moreover, as an individual drug molecule passes deeper into the tissue, it may bind and unbind several times (and for different periods) to a variety of sites (including receptors). This repeated binding and dissociation can greatly slow diffusion into and out of the tissue.

For these reasons, kinetic measurements are now usually done with isolated cells (e.g., a single neuron or a muscle fiber) or even a patch of cell membrane held on the tip of a suitable microelectrode. Another approach is to work with a cell membrane preparation and examine directly the rate at which a suitable radioligand (see Chapter 5) combines with, or dissociates from, the receptors that the membrane carries. Our next task is to consider the kinetics of binding under such conditions.

1.3.2 INCREASES IN OCCUPANCY

We continue with the simple model for the combination of a ligand with its binding sites that was introduced in Section 1.2.1 (Equation 1.1). Assuming as before that the law of mass action applies, the rate at which receptor occupancy (p_{AR}) changes with time should be given by the expression:

$$\frac{d(p_{AR})}{dt} = k_{+1}[A]p_R - k_{-1}p_{AR} \tag{1.18}$$

In words, this states that the rate of change of occupancy is simply the difference between the rate at which ligand-receptor complexes are formed and the rate at which they break down.[*]

At first sight, Equation (1.18) looks difficult to handle because there are no less than four variables: p_{AR}, t, [A], and p_R. However, we know that $p_R = (1 - p_{AR})$. Also, we will assume as before that [A] remains constant: that is, that so much A is present in relation to the number of binding sites that the combination of some of it with the sites will not appreciably reduce the overall concentration. Hence only p_{AR} and t remain as variables.

Substituting for p_R, we have

$$\frac{d(p_{AR})}{dt} = k_{+1}[A](1 - p_{AR}) - k_{-1}p_{AR} \tag{1.19}$$

Rearranging terms,

$$\frac{d(p_{AR})}{dt} = k_{+1}[A] - (k_{-1} + k_{+1}[A])p_{AR} \tag{1.20}$$

This still looks rather complicated, so we will drop the subscript from p_{AR} and also make two substitutions for the constants in the equation:

$$a = k_{+1}[A]$$

$$b = k_{-1} + k_{+1}[A]$$

Hence

$$\frac{dp}{dt} = a - bp$$

---

[*] If the reader is new to calculus, or not at ease with it, a slim volume (*Calculus Made Easy*) by Silvanus P. Thompson is strongly recommended.

This can be integrated in order to find how the occupancy changes with time:

$$\int_{p_1}^{p_2} \frac{dp}{a-bp} = \int_{t_1}^{t_2} dt$$

$$\log_e \left(\frac{a-b\,p_2}{a-b\,p_1} \right) = -b(t_2 - t_1)$$

We can now consider how quickly occupancy rises after the ligand is first applied, at time zero $(t_1 = 0)$. Receptor occupancy is initially 0, so that p_1 is 0. Thereafter occupancy increases steadily, and will be denoted $p_{AR}(t)$ at time t:

$$t_1 = 0 \qquad p_1 = 0$$

$$t_2 = t \qquad p_2 = p_{AR}(t)$$

Hence

$$\log_e \left\{ \frac{a - b\,p_{AR}(t)}{a} \right\} = -bt$$

$$\frac{a - b\,p_{AR}(t)}{a} = e^{-bt}$$

$$p_{AR}(t) = \frac{a}{b}(1 - e^{-bt})$$

Replacing a and b by the original terms, we have

$$p_{AR}(t) = \frac{k_{+1}[A]}{k_{-1} + k_{+1}[A]} \left\{ 1 - e^{-(k_{-1}+k_{+1}[A])t} \right\} \qquad (1.21)$$

Recalling that $k_{-1}/k_{+1} = K_A$, we can write

$$p_{AR}(t) = \frac{[A]}{K_A + [A]} \left\{ 1 - e^{-(k_{-1}+k_{+1}[A])t} \right\}$$

When t is very great, the ligand and its binding sites come into equilibrium. The term in large brackets then becomes unity (because $e^{-\infty} = 0$) so that

$$p_{AR}(\infty) = \frac{[A]}{K_A + [A]}$$

We can then write

$$p_{AR}(t) = p_{AR}(\infty) \left\{ 1 - e^{-(k_{-1}+k_{+1}[A])t} \right\} \qquad (1.22)$$

This is the expression we need. It has been plotted in Figure 1.3 for three concentrations of A.

Note how the rate of approach to equilibrium increases as [A] becomes greater. This is because the time course is determined by $(k_{-1} + k_{+1}[A])$. This quantity is sometimes replaced by a single constant, so that Equation (1.22) can be rewritten as either

$$p_{AR}(t) = p_{AR}(\infty)\,(1 - e^{-\lambda t}) \qquad (1.23)$$

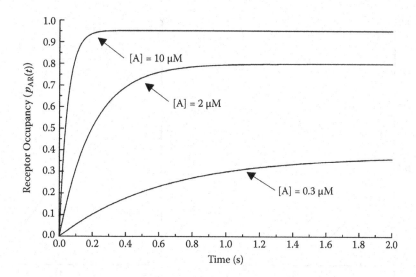

FIGURE 1.3 The predicted time course of the rise in receptor occupancy following the application of a ligand at the three concentrations shown. The curves have been drawn according to Equation (1.22), using a value of 2×10^6 M^{-1} s^{-1} for k_{+1}, and of 1 s^{-1} for k_{-1}.

or

$$p_{AR}(t) = p_{AR}(\infty)(1 - e^{-t/\tau}) \tag{1.24}$$

where

$$\lambda = k_{-1} + k_{+1}[A], = 1/\tau$$

τ (tau) is the *time constant* and has the unit of *time*. λ (lambda) is the *rate constant* which is sometimes written as k_{on} (as in Chapter 5) and has the unit of *time^{-1}*.

1.3.3 FALLS IN OCCUPANCY

Earlier, we had assumed for simplicity that the occupancy was zero when the ligand was first applied. It is straightforward to extend the derivation to predict how the occupancy will change with time even if it is not initially zero. We change the limits of integration to

$$t_1 = 0 \qquad p_1 = p_{AR}(0)$$

$$t_2 = t \qquad p_2 = p_{AR}(t)$$

Here $p_{AR}(0)$ is the occupancy at time zero, and the other terms are as before.

Exactly the same steps then lead to a more general expression to replace Equation (1.22)

$$p_{AR}(t) = p_{AR}(\infty) + \left\{ p_{AR}(0) - p_{AR}(\infty) \right\} e^{-(k_{-1} + k_{+1}[A])t} \tag{1.25}$$

We can use this to examine what would happen if the ligand is rapidly removed. This is equivalent to setting [A] abruptly to zero, at time zero. $p(\infty)$ also becomes zero because eventually all the ligand receptor complexes will dissociate. Equation (1.25) then reduces to

$$p_{AR}(t) = p_{AR}(0) e^{-k_{-1}t} \tag{1.26}$$

This has been plotted in Figure 1.4.

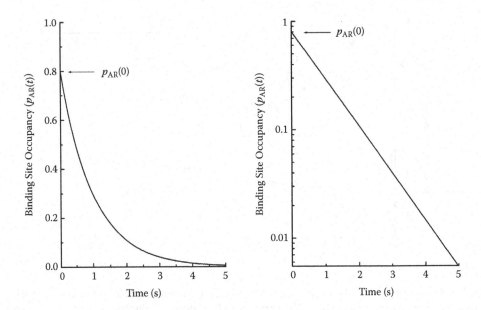

FIGURE 1.4 The predicted time course of the decline in binding site occupancy. The lines have been plotted using Equation (1.26), taking k_{-1} to be 1 s^{-1}, and $p_{AR}(0)$ to be 0.8. A linear scale for $p_{AR}(t)$ has been used on the left, and a logarithmic one on the right.

The time constant, τ, for the decline in occupancy is simply the reciprocal of k_{-1}. A related term is the *half-time* ($t_{1/2}$). This is the time needed for the quantity ($p_{AR}(t)$ in the present example) to reach halfway between the initial and the final value, and is given by

$$t_{1/2} = \frac{0.693}{k_{-1}}$$

For the example illustrated in Figure 1.4, $t_{1/2} = 0.693$ s. Note that τ and $t_{1/2}$ have the unit of *time*, as compared with *time*$^{-1}$ for k_{-1}.

This introductory account assumes that so many binding sites are present that the average number occupied will rise or fall smoothly with time after a change in ligand concentration: Events at single sites have not been considered. When a ligand is abruptly removed, the period for which an individual binding site remains occupied will, of course, vary from site to site, just as do the lifetimes of individual atoms in a sample of an element subject to radioactive decay. It can be shown that the *median* lifetime of the occupancy of individual sites is given by $0.693/k_{-1}$. The *mean* lifetime is $1/k_{-1}$. The introduction of the single channel recording technique has made it possible to obtain direct evidence about the duration of occupancy of individual receptors, and this will be described in Chapter 6.

1.4 PARTIAL AGONISTS

1.4.1 Introduction: Early Concepts

The development of a new drug usually requires the synthesis of a large number of structurally similar compounds. If a set of related agonists of this kind is tested on a particular tissue, they are likely to fall into two categories. Some can elicit a maximal tissue response and are described as *full agonists* in that experimental situation. The others cannot elicit this maximal response, no matter how high their concentration, and are termed *partial agonists*. Examples are given in Table 1.2.

TABLE 1.2
Some Full and Partial Agonists

Partial Agonist	Full Agonist	Acting at:
prenalterol	adrenaline, isoprenaline	β-adrenoceptors
pilocarpine	acetylcholine	muscarinic receptors
impromidine	histamine	histamine H_2 receptors

Figure 1.5 shows concentration response curves that compare the action of the β-adrenoceptor partial agonist prenalterol with that of the full agonist isoprenaline on a range of tissues and responses. In every instance, the maximal response to prenalterol is smaller, though the magnitude of the difference varies greatly. The prenalterol curves are also less steep.

It might be argued that a partial agonist cannot match the response to a full agonist because it fails to combine with all the receptors. This can easily be ruled out by testing the effect of increasing

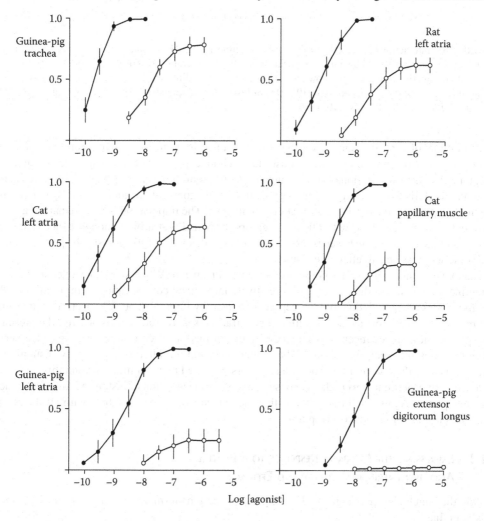

FIGURE 1.5 Comparison of the log concentration-response relationships for β-adrenoceptor mediated actions, on six tissues, of a full and a partial agonist (isoprenaline (•) and prenalterol (o) respectively). The ordinate shows the response as a fraction of the maximal response to isoprenaline. (Adapted from Kenakin, T. P., and Beek, D., *J. Pharmacol. Exp. Ther.*, 213, 406–413, 1980.)

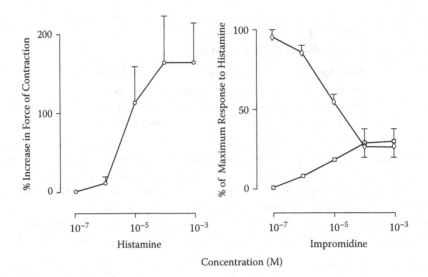

FIGURE 1.6 Interaction between the full agonist histamine and the H_2-receptor partial agonist impromidine on isolated ventricular strips from human myocardium. The concentration-response curve on the left is for histamine alone, and those on the right show the response to impromidine acting either on its own (squares) or in the presence of a constant concentration (100 μM) of histamine (diamonds). (Adapted from English, T. A. H. et al., *Br. J. Pharmacol.*, 89, 335–340, 1986).

concentrations of a partial agonist on the response of a tissue to a fixed concentration of a full agonist. Figure 1.6 (right, upper curve) illustrates such an experiment for two agonists acting at H_2 receptors. As the concentration of the partial agonist impromidine is raised, the response of the tissue gradually falls from the large value seen with the full agonist alone, and eventually reaches the maximal response to the partial agonist acting on its own. The implication is that the partial agonist is perfectly able to combine with all the receptors, provided that a high enough concentration is applied, but the effect on the tissue is less than would be seen with a full agonist. The partial agonist is in some way less able to elicit a response.

The experiment of Figure 1.7 points to the same conclusion. When very low concentrations of histamine are applied in the presence of a relatively large fixed concentration of impromidine, the overall response is mainly due to the receptors occupied by impromidine. However, the concentration-response curves cross as the histamine concentration is increased. This is because the presence of impromidine reduces receptor occupancy by histamine (at all concentrations) and vice versa. When the lines intersect, the effect of the reduction in impromidine occupancy by histamine is exactly offset by the contribution from the receptors occupied by histamine. Beyond this point, the presence of impromidine lowers the response to a given concentration of histamine. In effect, it acts as an antagonist. Again, the implication is that the partial agonist can combine with all the receptors, but is less able to produce a response.

1.4.2 EXPRESSING THE MAXIMAL RESPONSE TO A PARTIAL AGONIST: INTRINSIC ACTIVITY AND EFFICACY

In 1954 the Dutch pharmacologist E. J. Ariëns introduced the term *intrinsic activity,* which is now usually defined as

$$\text{Intrinsic activity} = \frac{\text{maximum response to test agonist}}{\text{maximum response to a full agonist acting through the same receptors}}$$

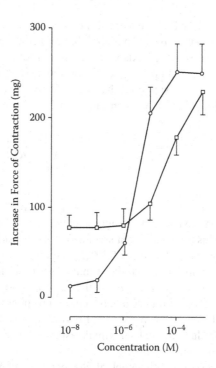

FIGURE 1.7 Log concentration-response curves for histamine applied alone (circles) or in the presence (squares) of a constant concentration of the partial agonist impromidine (10 μM). Tissue and experimental conditions as in Figure 1.6. (Adapted from English, T. A. H. et al., *Br. J. Pharmacol.,* 89, 335–340, 1986.)

For full agonists, the intrinsic activity (often denoted by α) is unity, by definition, as compared with zero for a competitive antagonist. Partial agonists have values between these limits. Note that the definition is entirely descriptive—nothing is assumed about mechanism. Also, 'intrinsic' should not be taken to mean that a given agonist has a characteristic activity, regardless of the experimental circumstances. To the contrary, the intrinsic activity of a partial agonist such as prenalterol can vary greatly not only between tissues, as Figure 1.5 illustrates, but also in a given tissue depending on the experimental conditions (see later). Indeed, the same compound can be a full agonist with one tissue and a partial agonist with another. For this reason, the term *maximal agonist effect* is perhaps preferable to *intrinsic activity.*

Similarly, the finding that a pair of agonists can each elicit the maximal response of a tissue (i.e., they have the same intrinsic activity, unity) should not be taken to imply that they are equally able to activate receptors. Suppose that the tissue has many spare receptors (see Section 1.6.3). One of the agonists might have to occupy 5% of the receptors in order to produce the maximal response, whereas the other might require only 1% occupancy. Evidently the second is more effective, despite both being full agonists. A more subtle measure of the ability of an agonist to activate receptors is clearly needed. It was provided by R. P. Stephenson, who postulated that receptor activation resulted in a *stimulus* or *signal* (S) being communicated to the cells, and that the magnitude of this stimulus was determined by the product of what he termed the *efficacy* (e) of the agonist and the proportion, p, of the receptors that it occupies[*]:

$$S = ep \tag{1.27}$$

---

[*] No distinction is made here between occupied and activated receptors. This is of key importance, as already noted in Section 1.2.3, and is discussed further in the following pages.

An important difference from Ariëns's concept of intrinsic activity is that efficacy, unlike intrinsic activity, has no upper limit—it is always possible that an agonist with a greater efficacy than any existing compound may be discovered. Also, Stephenson's proposal was not linked to any specific assumption about the relationship between receptor occupancy and the response of the tissue. (Ariëns, like A. J. Clark, had initially supposed that there was direct proportionality—an assumption later to be abandoned). According to Stephenson,

$$y = f(S_A) = f(e_A p_{AR}) = f\left(e_A \frac{[A]}{K_A + [A]}\right) \qquad (1.28)$$

Here y is the response of the tissue, and e_A is the efficacy of the agonist, A. $f(S_A)$ means merely "some function of S_A" (i.e., y depends on S_A in some as yet unspecified way). Note that, in keeping with the thinking at the time, Stephenson used the Hill–Langmuir equation to relate agonist concentration, [A], to receptor occupancy (p_{AR}). This most important assumption is reconsidered in the next section.

In order to be able to compare the efficacies of different agonists acting through the same receptors, Stephenson proposed the convention that the stimulus S is unity for a response that is 50% of the maximum attainable with a full agonist. This is the same as postulating that a partial agonist that has to occupy all the receptors to produce a half-maximal response has an efficacy of unity. We can see this from Equation (1.27); if our hypothetical partial agonist has to occupy all the receptors (i.e., $p = 1$) in order to produce the half-maximal response, at which point S too is unity (by Stephenson's convention), then e must also be 1.

R. F. Furchgott later suggested a refinement of Stephenson's concept. Recognizing that the response of a tissue to an agonist is influenced by the number of receptors as well as by the ability of the agonist to activate them, he wrote

$$e = \varepsilon[R]_T$$

Here $[R]_T$ is the total *concentration* of receptors, and ε (epsilon) is the *intrinsic efficacy* (not to be confused with *intrinsic activity*). ε can be regarded as a measure of the contribution of individual receptors to the overall efficacy.

The efficacy of a particular agonist, as defined by Stephenson, can vary between different tissues in the same way as can the intrinsic activity, and for the same reasons. Moreover, the value of both the intrinsic activity and the efficacy of an agonist in a given tissue will depend on the experimental conditions. This is illustrated in Figure 1.8. Relaxations of tracheal muscle in response to the β-adrenoceptor agonists isoprenaline and prenalterol were measured first in the absence (circles) and then in the presence (triangles, squares) of a muscarinic agonist, carbachol, which causes contraction and so tends to oppose β-adrenoceptor-mediated relaxation. Hence greater concentrations of the β-agonists are needed, and the curves shift to the right. With isoprenaline, the maximal response can still be obtained, despite the presence of carbachol at either concentration. The pattern is quite different with prenalterol. Its inability to produce complete relaxation becomes even more evident in the presence of carbachol at 1 μM. Indeed, when administered with 10 μM carbachol, prenalterol causes little or no relaxation: Its intrinsic activity and efficacy (in Stephenson's usage) have become negligible.

In the same way, reducing the number of available receptors (for example, by applying an alkylating agent—see Section 1.6.1) will always diminish the maximal response to a partial agonist. In contrast, the log concentration-response curve for a full agonist may first shift to the right, and the maximal response will become smaller only when there are no longer any spare receptors for that agonist (see also Section 1.6.3). Conversely, increasing the number of receptors (e.g., by upregulation, or by deliberate overexpression of the gene coding for the receptor) will cause the maximal response to a partial agonist to become greater whereas the log concentration-response curve for a full agonist will move to the left.

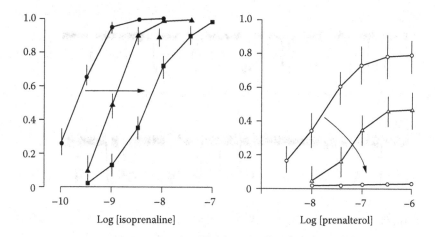

FIGURE 1.8 The effect of carbachol at two concentrations, 1 μM (triangles) and 10 μM (squares), on the relaxations of tracheal smooth muscle caused by a partial agonist, prenalterol, and by a full agonist, isoprenaline. The responses are plotted as a fraction of the maximum relaxation to isoprenaline. (Adapted from Kenakin, T. P., and Beek, D., *J. Pharmacol. Exp. Ther.*, 213, 406–413, 1980.)

1.4.3 The Interpretation of Partial Agonism in Terms of Events at Individual Receptors

The concepts of intrinsic activity and efficacy just outlined are purely descriptive, without reference to mechanism. We turn now to how differences in efficacy might be explained in terms of the molecular events that underlie receptor activation, and we begin by considering some of the experimental evidence that has provided remarkably direct evidence about these events.

Just a year after Stephenson's classical paper of 1956, J. del Castillo and B. Katz published an electrophysiological study of the interactions that occurred when pairs of agonists with related structures were applied simultaneously to the nicotinic receptors at the endplate region of skeletal muscle. Their findings could be best explained in terms of a model for receptor activation that has already been briefly introduced in Section 1.2.3 (see, in particular Equation 1.7). On this scheme, the occupied receptor can isomerize between an active and an inactive state. This is very different from the classical model of Hill, Clark, and Gaddum, in which no distinction was made between the *occupation* and the *activation* of a receptor by an agonist.

Direct evidence for this mechanism was to come from the introduction by E. Neher and B. Sakmann in 1976 of the single channel recording technique. This allowed the minute electrical currents passing through the ion channel intrinsic to the nicotinic receptor, and other ligand-gated ion channels, to be measured directly and as they occurred. It now became possible to study the activity of individual receptors *in situ* and in real time (see Chapter 6). It was soon shown that for a wide range of nicotinic agonists, these currents had exactly the same amplitude. This is illustrated for four such agonists in Figure 1.9. What differed between agonists was the fraction of time for which the current flowed (i.e., for which the channels were open). This is just what would be expected on the del Castillo–Katz scheme if the active state (AR*) of the occupied receptor is the same (*in terms of the flow of ions through the open channel*) for different agonists. With a weak partial agonist, the receptor is in the AR* state for only a small fraction of the time, even if all the binding sites are occupied.

The next questions to be considered are, first, the relationship between agonist concentration and response and, second, the interpretation of efficacy (both in the particular sense introduced by Stephenson and in more general terms) in the context of the model proposed by del Castillo and Katz.

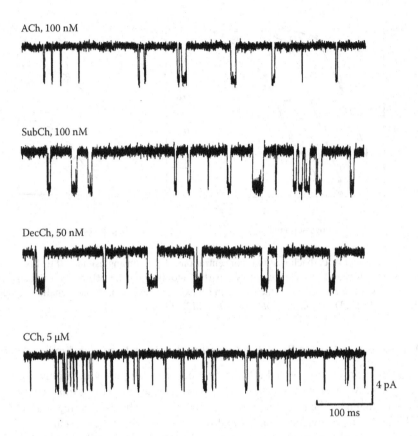

FIGURE 1.9   Records of the electrical currents (downward deflections) that flow through single ligand-gated ion channels in the junctional region of frog skeletal muscle. The currents arise from brief transitions of individual nicotinic receptors to an active (channel open) state in response to the presence of various agonists (ACh = acetylcholine; SubCh = suberyldicholine; DecCh = the dicholine ester of decan-1,10-dicarboxylic acid; CCh = carbamylcholine). (Adapted from Colquhoun, D., and Sakmann, B., *J. Physiol.*, 369, 501–557, 1985.)

1.4.4   THE DEL CASTILLO–KATZ MECHANISM: THE RELATIONSHIP BETWEEN AGONIST CONCENTRATION AND THE FRACTION OF RECEPTORS IN AN ACTIVE FORM

Our initial task is to apply the law of mass action to derive a relationship between the concentration of agonist and the proportion of receptors that are in the active form at equilibrium. This proportion will be denoted by p_{AR^*}.

As in all the derivations in this chapter, only three steps are needed. The first is to apply the law of mass action to each of the equilibria that exist. The second is to write an equation that expresses the fact that the fractions of receptors in each condition that can be distinguished must add up to 1 (the conservation rule). In the del Castillo–Katz scheme in its simplest form (see Equation 1.7 in Section 1.2.3) there are three such conditions: R (vacant and inactive), AR (inactive though A is bound), and AR* (bound and active). The corresponding fractions of receptors in these conditions[*] are p_R, p_{AR}, and p_{AR^*}.

---

[*] The term *state* rather than *condition* is often used in this context. However, the latter seems preferable in an introductory account. This is because the del Castillo–Katz mechanism is often described as a two-state model of receptor action, meaning here that the occupied receptor exists in two distinct (albeit interconvertible) forms, AR and AR*, whereas three conditions of the receptor (R, AR, and AR*) have to be distinguished when applying the law of mass action to the binding of the ligand, A.

Applying the law of mass action to each of the two equilibria gives

$$[A]p_R = K_A p_{AR} \tag{1.29}$$

$$p_{AR^*} = E\, p_{AR} \tag{1.30}$$

where K_A and E are the equilibrium constants indicated in Equation (1.7).

Also,

$$p_R + p_{AR} + p_{AR^*} = 1 \tag{1.31}$$

We can now take the third and last step. What we wish to know is p_{AR^*}, so we use Equations (1.29) and (1.30) to substitute for p_R and p_{AR} in Equation (1.31), obtaining:

$$\frac{K_A}{E[A]}p_{AR^*} + \frac{1}{E}p_{AR^*} + p_{AR^*} = 1$$

$$\therefore \quad p_{AR^*} = \frac{E[A]}{K_A + (1+E)[A]} \tag{1.32}$$

This is the expression we require. Though it has the same general form as the Hill–Langmuir equation, there are two important differences to note.

1. As [A] is increased, p_{AR^*} tends not to unity but to

$$\frac{E}{1+E}$$

Thus the value of E will determine the maximal response to A. Only if E is very large in relation to one, will almost all of the receptors be active. This is illustrated in Figure 1.10, which plots Equation (1.32) for a range of values of E.

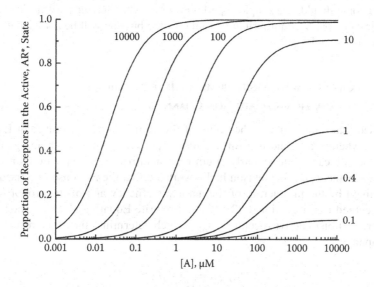

FIGURE 1.10 The relationship between p_{AR^*} and [A] predicted by Equation (1.32) for a range of values of E (given with each line). Note that as E rises above 10, the curves move to the left even though the value of K_A, the equilibrium dissociation constant for the initial combination of A with its binding site, is 200 μM for each curve.

2. Equation (1.32) gives the proportion of *active* receptors (p_{AR*}), rather than *occupied* receptors ($p_{occ} = p_{AR} + p_{AR*}$). To obtain the occupancy, we can use Equation (1.30) to express p_{AR} in terms of p_{AR*}:

$$p_{occ} = p_{AR} + p_{AR*} = \left(\frac{1+E}{E}\right) p_{AR*} \tag{1.33}$$

$$= \frac{(1+E)[A]}{K_A + (1+E)[A]}$$

$$= \frac{[A]}{\dfrac{K_A}{1+E} + [A]} \tag{1.34}$$

This can be rewritten as

$$p_{occ} = \frac{[A]}{K_{eff} + [A]} \tag{1.35}$$

where K_{eff}, the effective equilibrium dissociation constant* is defined as

$$K_{eff} = \frac{K_A}{1+E} \tag{1.36}$$

Because K_{eff} applies to a scheme that involves more than one equilibrium (see Equation 1.7), it is referred to as a *macroscopic equilibrium constant*, to distinguish it from the *microscopic equilibrium constants* (K_A and E) that describe the individual equilibria.

It also follows that if the relationship between the concentration of an agonist and the proportion of receptors that it occupies is measured directly, for example, using a radioligand binding method, the outcome should be a simple hyperbolic curve. Although the curve is describable by the Hill–Langmuir equation, the equilibrium constant for the binding will be not K_A but K_{eff}, which is determined by both E and K_A.

1.4.5 THE DEL CASTILLO–KATZ MECHANISM: THE INTERPRETATION OF EFFICACY FOR LIGAND-GATED ION CHANNELS

It is easy to see that, qualitatively, the value of the equilibrium constant E in Equation (1.7) will determine whether a ligand is a full agonist, a partial agonist, or an antagonist. We next consider whether we can relate an early attempt to quantify the efficacy of agonists to the del Castillo–Katz scheme. R. P. Stephenson had postulated that the response of a tissue to an agonist is determined by the product, S, of the agonist's efficacy and of the proportion of receptors that it occupied (see Equation 1.27). We can rewrite Equation (1.33) to show the relation between the proportion of active receptors, p_{AR*} (which determines the tissue response) and total receptor occupancy:

$$p_{AR*} = \frac{E}{1+E} p_{occ} \tag{1.37}$$

---

* It is easily shown that K_{eff} is also the $[A]_{50}$ for the action of an agonist on this mechanism.

From this we can see that the term $E/(1 + E)$ is equivalent, if only in a formal sense, to Stephenson's efficacy. If an agonist is applied at a very high concentration, so that all the receptors are occupied, the proportion in the active state is $E/(1 + E)$. If this agonist is also very effective, that is, if E is $\gg 1$, the proportion of active receptors becomes close to unity, the upper limit.

Consider next a hypothetical partial agonist which, even when occupying all the receptors ($p_{occ} = 1$), causes only half of them to be in the active form (i.e., $p_{AR} = p_{AR^*} = 0.5$). From Equation (1.37), we can see that E must be unity for this agonist. On Stephenson's scheme, such an agonist would have an efficacy of unity provided that the response measured is a direct indication of the proportion of activated receptors. Promising though this might seem, we cannot take the analogy between Stephenson's formulation and the del Castillo–Katz scheme much further. This is because it is now clear that *efficacy* and *affinity* are not separable quantities in the way that Stephenson had envisaged. To emphasize the point, the proportion of the binding sites occupied by an agonist depends on the value of E as well as of K_A, as we have seen (Equation 1.34). Also, not all of the occupied receptors are active, as Stephenson and the other early workers had assumed them to be.

The realization that the ability of an agonist to activate a receptor is best expressed in terms of the del Castillo–Katz model has made it of the greatest interest to measure the rate constants (two each for K_A and E, at the simplest) that determine not only the values of K_A and E but also the kinetics of agonist action. The single channel recording technique allows this to be achieved for ligand-gated ion channels. This is described in Chapter 6. Note, however, the complication that such receptors generally carry more than one binding site for the agonist, so that the simple scheme just considered (Equation 1.7) has to be elaborated (see Equation 1.9 in Appendix 1.2.3, and also Chapter 6).

Another difficulty encountered in such work, and one that has to be considered in any study of the relationship between the concentration of an agonist and its action, is the occurrence of *desensitization*. The response falls despite the continued presence of the agonist. Several factors can contribute. One that has been identified in work with ligand-gated ion channels is that receptors occupied by an agonist, and in the active state (AR*), may isomerise to an inactive, desensitized, state, AR_D. This can be represented as:

$$A + R \underset{\text{(inactive)}}{\overset{K_A}{\rightleftharpoons}} AR \underset{\text{(inactive)}}{\overset{E}{\rightleftharpoons}} AR^* \underset{\text{(inactive)}}{\overset{K_D}{\rightleftharpoons}} AR_D$$

As explained in Chapter 6, quantitative studies of desensitization at ligand-gated ion channels have shown that even this scheme is an oversimplification, and it is necessary to include the possibility that the receptor can exist in a desensitized state even when no ligand is bound.

Desensitization can occur in other ways. With G-protein coupled receptors (GPCRs), it can result from phosphorylation of the receptor by one or more protein kinases[*] that become active following the application of an agonist (see Chapter 2). This is sometimes followed by the loss of receptors from the cell surface. An agonist-induced reduction in the number of functional receptors over a relatively long time period is described as downregulation. Receptor upregulation can also occur, for example, following the prolonged administration of antagonists *in vivo*.

Returning to ligand-gated ion channels, recent work suggests that although the del Castillo–Katz model remains the starting point for discussions of receptor mechanisms, the functioning of at least some varieties of this class of receptor has previously unsuspected and revealing subtleties. For example, a subset of receptors that respond to AMPA (α-amino-3-hydroxy-5-methyl-4-isoxazole propionate) show a single channel conductance that varies somewhat with both the nature and the concentration of the agonist applied. Moreover, intermediate pre-open "flip" states between resting and activated receptors have been identified. Though these features have only begun to become accessible to experimental study, their exploration is already throwing new light on receptor function.

---

[*] Some of which are specific for particular receptors (e.g., β-adrenergic receptor kinase [βARK], also referred to as GRK2).

1.4.6 THE INTERPRETATION OF EFFICACY FOR RECEPTORS ACTING THROUGH G-PROTEINS

Some of the most revealing studies of partial agonism (including Stephenson's classical work) have been done with tissues in which GTP-binding proteins (see Chapters 2 and 7) provide the link between receptor activation and the initiation of the response. In contrast to the situation with fast receptors with intrinsic ion channels (see above), it is not yet possible to observe the activity of individual GPCRs (with the potential exception of some that are linked to potassium channels). However, enough is known to show that the mechanisms are complex. The interpretation of differences in efficacy for agonists acting at such receptors is correspondingly less certain.

An early model for the action of such receptors was as follows:

$$A + R \xrightleftharpoons{K_A} AR$$

$$AR + G \xrightleftharpoons{K_{ARG}} ARG^*$$

Here the agonist-receptor complex (AR) combines with a G-protein (G) to form a ternary complex (ARG*) that can initiate further cellular events, such as the activation of adenylate cyclase. However, this simple scheme (the ternary complex model) was not in keeping with what was already known about the importance of isomerization in receptor activation (see Sections 1.2.3 and 1.4.3), and it also failed to account for findings that were soon to come from studies of mutated receptors. In all current models of GPCRs, receptor activation by isomerization is assumed to occur so that the model becomes

$$A + R \xrightleftharpoons{K_A} AR \xrightleftharpoons{E} AR^*$$

$$AR^* + G \xrightleftharpoons{K_{ARG}} AR^*G^* \tag{1.38}$$

Here, combination of the activated receptor (AR*) with the G-protein causes the latter to enter an active state (G*) that can initiate a tissue response through, for example, adenylate cyclase, phospholipase C, or the opening or closing of ion channels. On this scheme, what will determine whether a particular agonist can produce a full or only a limited response? Suppose that a high concentration of the agonist is applied, so that all the receptors are occupied. They will then be distributed between the AR, AR*, and AR*G* conditions, of which AR*G* alone leads to a response. The values of both E and K_{ARG} will then influence how much AR*G* is formed, and hence whether the agonist in question is partial or otherwise. In principle, each of these two equilibrium constants could vary from agonist to agonist. By analogy with (most) ligand-gated ion channels, it is tempting to suppose that only E is agonist dependent and that the affinity of the active, AR*, state of the receptor for the G-protein is the same for all agonists. However, there is now evidence that this is so. Note that, in any case, the magnitude of the response may also depend on the availability of the G-protein. If there is very little, only a correspondingly small amount of AR*G* can be formed, regardless of the concentration of agonist and the number of receptors. Similarly, if there are few receptors in relation to the total quantity of G-protein, that too will limit the formation of AR*G*. Thus the maximum response to an agonist is influenced by tissue factors as well as by K_A, E, and K_{ARG}. This can be shown more formally by applying the law of mass action to the three equilibria shown in Equation (1.38). The outcome, with some further discussion, is given in Appendix 1.4.2.

Complicated though these schemes might seem, they are in reality oversimplifications (see Chapter 2). Factors that have not been considered include:

1. The likelihood that some receptors are coupled to G-protein even in the absence of agonist.
2. The activated receptor combines with the G-protein in its G_{GDP} form, with the consequence that GTP can replace previously bound guanosine diphosphate (GDP). The extent to which this can occur will be influenced by the local concentration of GTP.

3. The heterotrimeric structure of the G-protein. Following activation by GTP binding, the trimer dissociates into its α and βγ subunits, each of which may elicit cell responses.
4. The cyclical nature of G-protein activation. The α-subunit can hydrolyze the GTP that is bound to it, thereby allowing the heterotrimer to reform. The lifetime of individual αGTP subunits will vary (cf. the lifetimes of open ion channels).
5. The presence in many cells of more than one type of G-protein, each with characteristic cellular actions.
6. The finding that some GPCRs are constitutively active (see Section 1.4.7).
7. Several GPCRs exist as dimers and some can form heteromers with other GPCRs.
8. The function of GPCRs is modulated by accessory proteins described collectively as regulators of G-protein signaling (RGS) (see Chapter 2).

In principle, these features could be built into formal models of receptor activation though the large number of disposable parameters makes testing difficult and the exercise is likely to be unrewarding. Some at least of the rate and equilibrium constants need to be known beforehand. One experimental tactic is to alter the relative proportions of receptors and G-protein, and then find whether the efficacy of agonists changes in the way to be expected from the models. The discovery that some receptors are constitutively active has provided another approach as well as additional information about receptor function, as we shall now see.

1.4.7 Constitutively Active Receptors, Inverse Agonists

The del Castillo–Katz scheme (in common of course with the simpler model explored by Hill, Clark, and Gaddum) supposes that the receptors are inactive in the absence of agonist. It is now known that this is not always so: Several types of receptors are constitutively active. Examples include mutated receptors responsible for several genetically determined diseases. Thus, hyperthyroidism can result from mutations that cause the receptors for thyrotropin (TSH) to be active even in the absence of the hormone. Also, receptor variants that are constitutively active have been created in the laboratory by site-directed mutagenesis. Finally, deliberate overexpression of receptors by receptor gene transfection of cell lines and even laboratory animals has revealed that many wild-type receptors also show some activity in the absence of agonist. What might the mechanism be? The most likely possibility, and one that is in keeping with what has been learned about how ion channels work, is that such receptors can isomerize spontaneously to and from an active form:

$$R \rightleftharpoons R^*$$
$$\text{(inactive)} \qquad \text{(active)}$$

In principle, both forms could combine with agonist, or indeed with any ligand, L, with affinity (see Figure 1.11).

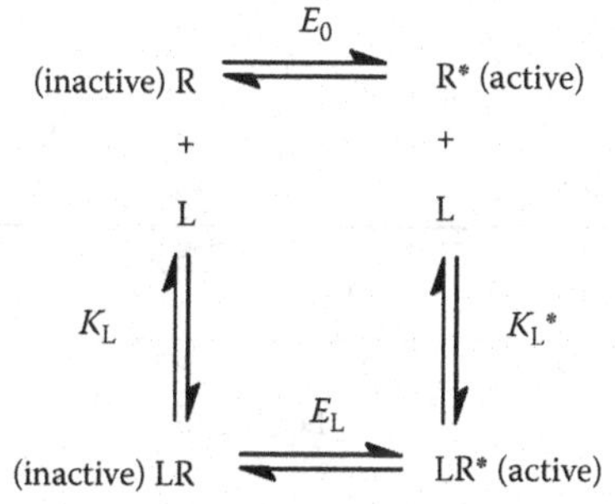

FIGURE 1.11 A model to show the influence of a ligand, L, on the equilibrium between the active and inactive forms of a constitutively active receptor, R. Note that if L, R, and LR are in equilibrium, and likewise L, R*, and LR*, then the same must hold for LR and LR* (see Appendix 1.6.2 for a further explanation).

Suppose that L combines only with the inactive, R, form. Then the presence of L, by promoting the formation of LR at the expense of the other species, will *reduce* the proportion of receptors in the active, R*, state. L is said to be an *inverse agonist* or *negative antagonist* and to possess *negative efficacy*. If, in contrast, L combines with the R* form alone, it will act as a *conventional* or *positive* agonist of very high intrinsic efficacy.

Exploring the scheme further, a partial agonist will bind to both R and R*, but with some preferential affinity for one or other of the two states. If the preference is for R, the ligand will be a *partial inverse agonist* as its presence will reduce the number of receptors in the active state, though not to zero.

As shown in the "Solutions to Problems" at the end of this chapter (see the solution to Problem 1.4), applying the law of mass action to the scheme of Figure 1.11 provides an expression for the fraction of receptors in the active state (i.e., $p_{R*} + p_{LR*}$) at equilibrium:

$$p_{\text{active}} = \frac{E_0}{E_0 + \left(\dfrac{1 + \dfrac{[L]}{K_L}}{1 + \dfrac{[L]}{K_L^*}}\right)} \tag{1.39}$$

Here the equilibrium constant E_0 is defined by p_{R*}/p_R, K_L by $[L]\, p_R / p_{LR}$, and K_L^* by $[L]\, p_{R*}/p_{LR*}$. Figure 1.12 plots this relationship for three hypothetical ligands that differ in their relative affinities for the active and the inactive states of the receptor. The ratio of K_L to K_L^* has been expressed by α. When $\alpha = 0.1$, the ligand is an inverse agonist, whereas when $\alpha = 100$, it is a conventional agonist. In the third example, with a ligand that shows no selectivity between the active and inactive forms of the receptor ($\alpha = 1$), the proportion of active receptors remains unchanged as [L], and therefore receptor occupancy is increased.

Such a ligand will, however, reduce the action of either a conventional or an inverse agonist, and so in effect is an antagonist. More precisely, it is a neutral competitive antagonist. If large numbers of competitive antagonists of the same pharmacological class (e.g., β-adrenoceptor blockers) are carefully tested on a tissue or cell line showing constitutive activity, some will be found to cause a

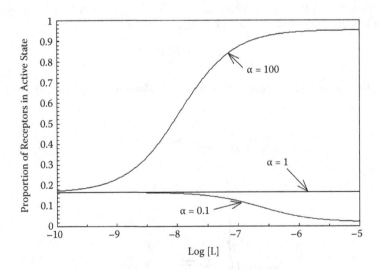

FIGURE 1.12 The relationship between the total fraction of receptors in the active state ($p_{R*} + p_{AR*}$) and ligand concentration ([L]) for a constitutively active receptor. The curve has been drawn according to Equation (1.39), using the following values: $E_0 = 0.2$, $K_L = 200$ nM, $\alpha\ (= K_L / K_L^*) = 0.1$, 1, and 100, as shown. Note that on this model some of the receptors (a fraction given by $E_0/(1 + E_0)$, = 0.167) are active in the absence of ligand.

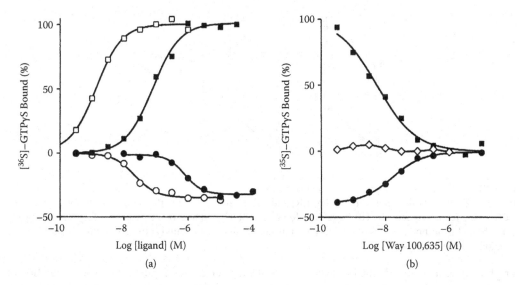

FIGURE 1.13 The effects of a conventional agonist, an inverse agonist, and a neutral antagonist on the activity of a constitutively active G-protein coupled $5HT_{1A}$ receptor. The panel on the left shows the log concentration response curves for the conventional agonist (open squares) and the inverse agonist (open circles). The closed symbols show how the curves change when the antagonist (WAY 100,635 at 10 nM) is included in the incubation fluid. Note the parallel, and similar, shift in the lines. The right hand panel illustrates the effects of a wide range of concentrations of the same antagonist applied on its own (open symbols) or in the presence of a high concentration of either the conventional agonist (closed squares) or the inverse agonist (closed circles). Note that the antagonist by itself causes little change, showing that it has no preference for the active or inactive forms of the receptor. In keeping with this, high concentrations of the antagonist abolish the response to both types of agonist (the curves converge). (Adapted from Newman-Tancredi, A. et al., *Br. J. Pharmacol.*, 120, 737–739, 1997.)

small increase in basal activity. They are in effect weak conventional partial agonists. Others will reduce the basal activity and so may be inverse agonists with what could be a substantial degree of negative efficacy.* Few of the set can be expected to have exactly the same affinity for the active and the inactive forms of the receptor and so be neutral antagonists. However, some compounds of this kind have been identified, and Figure 1.13 illustrates the effect of one on the response to both a conventional and an inverse agonist acting on $5HT_{1A}$ receptors expressed in a cell line.

As with the experiments of Figure 1.13, constitutive activity is often investigated in cultured cell lines that do not normally express the receptor to be examined but have been forced to by transfection with the gene coding for either the native receptor or a mutated variant of it. The number of receptors per cell (receptor density) may then be much larger than in cells that express the receptors naturally. While overexpression of this kind has the great advantage that small degrees of constitutive activity can be detected and studied, it is worth noting that constitutive activity is often much less striking *in situ* than in transfected cells. Hence the partial agonist action (conventional or inverse) of an antagonist may be much less marked, or even negligible, when it is studied in an intact tissue. Simple competitive antagonism, as described in Section 1.5, may then be observed.

Nevertheless, the evidence that some receptors have sufficient constitutive activity to influence cell function *in vivo* even in the absence of agonist makes it necessary to extend the simple models already considered for the activation of GPCRs. In principle, the receptor can now exist in no less than eight different conditions (R, R*, LR, LR*, RG, R*G, LRG, LR*G), and this is best represented

---

* Though the possibility that the depression in basal activity may have some other explanation, e.g., an inhibitory action on one or more of the events that follow receptor activation, must not be overlooked.

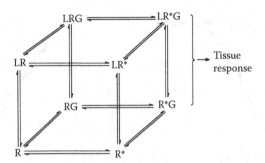

FIGURE 1.14 An elaboration of the model shown in Figure 1.11, which is reproduced as the front face of the cube. Each of its four elements (R, R*, LR, and LR*) can combine with a G-protein to form RG, R*G, LRG, and LR*G, respectively. Of these, only R*G and LR*G lead to a tissue response. The top face of the cube shows ligand-bound states of the receptor. Further details can be found at the end of this chapter (see the solution to Problem 1.5).

graphically as a cube with one of the conditions at each vertex (see Figure 1.14). The calculation of the proportions of activated and occupied receptors is straightforward, if lengthy (see the answer to Problem 1.5 at the end of the chapter). Finding the proportion in the active form is more difficult if the supply of G-protein is limited, but can be done using numerical methods.

1.4.8 Attempting to Estimate the Efficacy of a Partial Agonist from the End Response of a Complex Tissue

Though observations of receptor function at the molecular level (e.g., single channel recording; changes in receptor fluorescence following the binding of a ligand) are becoming increasingly practicable, it still often happens that the only available measure of receptor activation is the response of an intact tissue. This could be the contraction or relaxation of a piece of smooth muscle, secretion by a gland, or a change in heartbeat. How can the action of a partial agonist best be characterized in such a situation? Clearly, the maximal agonist activity (the so-called intrinsic activity, see Section 1.4.2) and the concentration of agonist that produces half the maximal response that that agonist can elicit are invaluable descriptive measures. As we have already seen, R. P. Stephenson took matters further by supposing that the response to an agonist is determined by the product of the agonist's efficacy and the proportion of receptors occupied (see Equation 1.27). He also described experimental methods that promised to allow the efficacies of agonists acting on intact tissues to be compared. These procedures were later extended by others and quite widely applied for a time. An example is given in the passage on irreversible antagonists (Section 1.6.4).

However, as already discussed, it is now certain that the occupancy and the activation of a receptor by an agonist are not equivalent, and hence that Stephenson's use of the Hill–Langmuir equation to relate agonist concentration to receptor occupancy in Equation (1.27) is an oversimplification. Our final task in this account of partial agonism is to reexamine the results of whole-tissue measurements of Stephenson's efficacy in the light of the new knowledge about how receptors function.

A first step is to recast Stephenson's equations in terms of total receptor occupancy (p_{occ}, i.e., occupied but inactive plus occupied and active). Taking this course, and assuming that the del Castillo–Katz mechanism applies in its simplest form (Equation 1.7), we can write

$$S = e_A^* \, p_{occ(A)} = e_A^* \frac{[A]}{K_{eff} + [A]} \tag{1.40}$$

where K_{eff} is defined as in Section 1.4.4 (Equation 1.36). Before going further, it has to be made clear that this modification of Stephenson's scheme departs fundamentally from his original concept that efficacy and affinity can be regarded as separable and potentially independent quantities. To emphasize the point, the symbol e^* rather than e is used. We have already seen in the last section that the macroscopic equilibrium dissociation constant K_{eff} is determined not only by the value of K_A but also by E, which is directly related to efficacy. In the same vein, both the efficacy and the macroscopic affinity of an agonist acting through a GPCR depend on tissue factors such as the relative and absolute quantities of G protein and receptors, as well as on the microscopic equilibrium constants.

With these reservations in mind, no more than a brief mention is needed of three approaches that were used in past years to assess the efficacy of a partial agonist acting on an intact tissue. Each will be analyzed in two ways with the details given in Tables 1.3 and 1.4. The first is of historical interest only and is based on Stephenson's original formulation, as expressed in Equation (1.27) (Section 1.4.2) and with receptor occupancy given by the Hill–Langmuir equation in its simplest form (which we have already seen to be inadequate for agonists). The second analysis defines receptor occupancy as all the receptors that are occupied, active plus inactive.

The first two of the three methods presuppose that the measurements are made with a tissue that has a large receptor reserve. It is also assumed that a full agonist is available that can evoke a maximal response when occupying only a small fraction of the receptors.

TABLE 1.3

Method 1 (Section 1.4.8) Proposed for the Determination of the Efficacy of a Partial Agonist Acting on an Intact Tissue

Analysis following Stephenson's formulation of efficacy, and using his assumptions and terms	Analysis based on redefining the stimulus as the product of efficacy (e^*) and the total receptor occupancy by the agonist (i.e., p_{occ})
For a half-maximal response, $S = 1$ (by Stephenson's convention) and $p_{AR} \approx [A]_1/K_A$. This approximation holds because if A occupies few receptors (i.e., $[A] \ll K_A$), then	For a half-maximal response, $S = 1$ (by Stephenson's convention) and $p_{occ(A)} \approx [A]_1/K_{eff(A)}$. This approximation holds because if A occupies few receptors, then
$$\frac{[A]}{K_A+[A]} \approx \frac{[A]}{K_A}$$	$$\frac{[A]}{K_{eff(A)}+[A]} \approx \frac{[A]}{K_{eff(A)}}$$
Hence, recalling that $S_A = e_A\, p_{AR}$, we have	Hence, recalling the redefinition of S_A as $e^*_A\, p_{occ(A)}$, we have
$$1 = e_A \frac{[A]_1}{K_A} \qquad (1.44)$$	$$1 = e^*_A \frac{[A]_1}{K_{eff(A)}} \qquad (1.46)$$
When the partial agonist P occupies all the binding sites in order to produce its maximal response, $p_{PR} = 1$. Hence, the stimulus (S_P) attributable to P is simply e_P. Assuming that the same tissue response, whether elicited by A or by P, corresponds to the same value of S, we can write	When the partial agonist occupies all the receptors in order to produce its maximal response, $p_{occ(P)} = 1$. Hence the stimulus (S_P) attributable to P is e^*_P. Assuming that the same tissue response corresponds to the same value of S, we can write
$$S_P = S_A$$	$$S_P = S_A$$
$$\therefore\ e_P = e_A \frac{[A]_2}{K_A} \qquad (1.45)$$	$$\therefore\ e^*_P = e^*_A \frac{[A]_2}{K_{eff(A)}} \qquad (1.47)$$
Dividing Equation (1.45) by (1.44), we obtain	Dividing Equation (1.47) by (1.46), we obtain
$$e_P = \frac{[A]_2}{[A]_1}$$	$$e^*_P = \frac{[A]_2}{[A]_1}$$

TABLE 1.4
Method 2 (Section 1.4.8) Proposed for the Determination of the Efficacy of a Partial Agonist Acting on an Intact Tissue

Analysis following Stephenson's formulation of efficacy	Analysis based on redefining the stimulus as the product of efficacy (e*) and the total receptor occupancy by the agonist, as before
Just as before, we assume that S_A equals S_P for the same magnitude of response. Therefore	We again assume that S_A equals S_P, for the same magnitude of response. Therefore

$$e_A \frac{[A]}{K_A+[A]} = e_P \frac{[P]}{K_P+[P]}$$

$$e_A^* \frac{[A]}{K_{eff(A)}+[A]} = e_P^* \frac{[P]}{K_{eff(P)}+[P]}$$

If A occupies few receptors (so that $[A] \ll K_A$—see method 1), we can write

If A occupies few receptors (so that $[A] \ll K_{eff(A)}$—see method 1), we can write

$$e_A \frac{[A]}{K_A} \approx e_P \frac{[P]}{K_P+[P]}$$

$$\Rightarrow \frac{1}{e_A} \frac{K_A}{[A]} = \frac{1}{e_P} \frac{K_P}{[P]} + \frac{1}{e_P}$$

$$\Rightarrow \frac{1}{[A]} = \frac{e_A K_P}{e_P K_A} \frac{1}{[P]} + \frac{e_A}{e_P K_A}$$

$$e_A^* \frac{[A]}{K_{eff(A)}} \approx e_P^* \frac{[P]}{K_{eff(P)}+[P]}$$

$$\Rightarrow \frac{1}{e_A^*} \frac{K_{eff(A)}}{[A]} = \frac{1}{e_P^*} \frac{K_{eff(P)}}{[P]} + \frac{1}{e_P^*}$$

$$\Rightarrow \frac{1}{[A]} = \frac{e_A^* K_{eff(P)}}{e_P^* K_{eff(A)}} \frac{1}{[P]} + \frac{e_A^*}{e_P^* K_{eff(A)}}$$

Hence a plot of $1/[A]$ against $1/[P]$ should provide a straight line of slope $e_A K_P/e_P K_A$ and intercept $e_A/e_P K_A$. The ratio of the slope to the intercept should give an estimate of K_P. If the partial agonist can produce a response equal to or greater than 50% of that to the full agonist, the value of e_P can then be calculated by using K_P to work out the proportion of receptors occupied by the partial agonist when it elicits the half-maximal response: The reciprocal of this occupancy gives e_P (since S is then unity, by definition). If, however, the partial agonist can produce only a small response, then Method 1 can be applied to estimate e_P.

Hence a plot of $1/[A]$ against $1/[P]$ should provide a straight line of slope $e_A^* K_{eff(P)} / e_P^* K_{eff(A)}$ and intercept $e_A^* / e_P^* K_{eff(A)}$. The ratio of the slope to the intercept should give an estimate of $K_{eff(P)}$. The value of e_P^* can then be calculated as described on the left for e_P.

Method 1: Concentration-response curves are constructed for the full agonist (A) and for the partial agonist [P] whose efficacy is to be determined (Figure 1.15). Two concentrations are read off the curve for the full agonist. The first, $[A]_1$, causes a half maximal response. The second, $[A]_2$, elicits the same response as the maximum seen with the partial agonist. Then the efficacy of the partial agonist is given by the ratio of $[A]_2$ to $[A]_1$ (see Table 1.3).

Method 2: Exactly the same measurements and assumptions are made as before (see again Figure 1.15). From the concentration-response curves for the full and the partial agonist, the values of [A] and [P] that elicit the same response are read off, for several levels of response. A plot of $1/[A]$ against $1/[P]$ is constructed and should yield a straight line from which the efficacy of the partial agonist could be obtained were the underlying assumptions to be correct (see Table 1.4).

Method 3: This is more general than the other two in the sense that it is also applicable to full agonists, at least in principle. Suppose that we had some reliable means of determining the equilibrium dissociation constant for the combination of the agonist with its receptors. One procedure that has been used in the past is Furchgott's irreversible antagonist method,

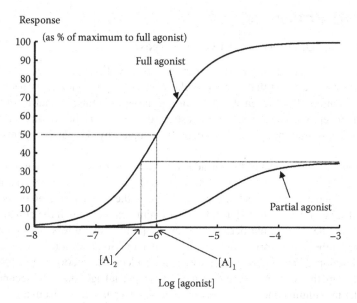

FIGURE 1.15 Estimating the efficacy of a partial agonist by comparing its concentration-response curve with that for a full agonist. See text for further detail.

described in Section 1.6.4. We can then apply the appropriate occupancy relationship to calculate the proportion of receptors occupied at the concentration of agonist that produces a half-maximal response. Because on Stephenson's convention S is then unity, the reciprocal of this occupancy gives the value of e (from Equation 1.27). This is the basis of Furchgott's estimate of the efficacy of histamine acting on isolated guinea-pig ileum (see Figure 1.24 in Section 1.6.3).

Clearly this method stands or falls by the validity of the procedures used to measure the equilibrium dissociation constant and to relate agonist concentration to occupancy. We shall see in Section 1.6.4 that Furchgott's irreversible antagonist method provides an estimate not, as was first thought, of the microscopic equilibrium constant, K_A, but rather of the macroscopic equilibrium constant, K_{eff}. Hence, receptor occupancies calculated from it using the Hill–Langmuir equation will be of *total* occupancy, active plus inactive. It follows that efficacies calculated in this way are to be regarded as defined by Equation (1.40), and not Equation (1.28) as formulated by Stephenson.

Are the efficacy values obtained in these ways useful? They are certainly no substitute for measurements, if these can be made, of the microscopic equilibrium constants that govern the proportion of receptors in the occupied and active forms. Also, because e^* is influenced by tissue factors (e.g., $[G]_T$, $[R]_T$ as well as E and K_{ARG} for GPCRs), a particular value can result from several combinations of these variables: E, the isomerization equilibrium constant for the formation of active receptors, is not the only determinant. Hence the value of e^* (or of e) cannot be used as a reliable measure of E. Comparison of e^* values for different agonists acting on a particular tissue is more informative because tissue-dependent factors such as $[G]_T$ and $[R]_T$ are the same. The ratio of e^* for two agonists should then give an estimate of the inverse ratio of the total receptor occupancies needed to elicit a certain response. However, the key question of how these occupied receptors are distributed between the active and inactive states remains unanswered in the absence of other kinds of evidence. Despite the historical importance of Stephenson's concept, we have to conclude that numerical estimates of efficacy, as originally defined, and based on measuring the responses of intact tissues, are of little more than descriptive value.

APPENDICES TO SECTION 1.4

APPENDIX 1.4.1   THE DEFINITION OF A PARTIAL AGONIST

The term *partial agonist* has come to be used in two slightly different senses. The first, as in this account, is to refer to an agonist that in a particular tissue or organism, under specified conditions, cannot elicit as great an effect (even when applied in large amounts) as can a full agonist acting through the same receptors. The second, more restricted, usage adds the condition that the response is submaximal because not enough of the receptors occupied by the partial agonist convert to an active form.

The distinction can be illustrated by considering the action of decamethonium on the nicotinic receptors of skeletal muscle. Like acetylcholine, decamethonium opens the ion channels intrinsic to these receptors, so increasing the electrical conductance of the endplate region of the muscle fibers. However, even at very high concentrations, decamethonium cannot match the conductance increase caused by acetylcholine. This is not because decamethonium is much less able to cause the receptors to isomerize to the active form. Rather, the smaller maximal response is attributable mainly to an additional action of decamethonium, which is to block the nicotinic receptor ion channel. Hence, though decamethonium might not be regarded as a partial agonist in the second sense defined above, the smaller maximum conductance response makes it a partial agonist in the broader meaning of the term.

APPENDIX 1.4.2   EXPRESSIONS FOR THE FRACTION OF G-PROTEIN COUPLED RECEPTORS IN THE ACTIVE FORM

Application of the law of mass action to each of the three equilibria shown in Equation (1.38), and the use of the conservation rule (see earlier) leads to the following expression[*] for $p_{AR^*G^*}$:

$$p_{AR^*G^*} = \frac{E[G]_T[A]}{K_A K_{ARG} + \left\{E[G]_T + K_{ARG}(1+E)\right\}[A]} \tag{1.41}$$

Though this looks complicated, it still predicts a simple hyperbolic relationship (as with the Hill–Langmuir equation) between agonist concentration and the proportion of receptors in the state (AR*G*) that leads to a response. If a very large concentration of A is applied, so that all the receptors are occupied, the value of $p_{AR^*G^*}$ asymptotes to

$$\frac{E[G]_T}{E[G]_T + K_{ARG}(1+E)}$$

Thus the intrinsic efficacy[†] of an agonist is influenced by both K_{ARG} and $[G]_T$ as well as of course by E.

In deriving Equation (1.41), it has been assumed that the concentration of G does not fall as a consequence of the formation of AR*G*. This would be so if the total concentration of G, $[G]_T$, greatly exceeds the concentration of receptors ($[R]_T$), so that the concentration of G could be regarded as a constant, approximately equal to $[G]_T$.

---

[*] This is derived in the "Solutions to Problems"; see the solution to Problem 1.3.

[†] This term has increasingly come to be employed (as here) in a rather different sense to that introduced by R. F. Furchgott (Section 1.4.2). On this newer usage, intrinsic efficacy indicates the maximum receptor activation (often expressed as the fraction of receptors in the active state) that can be achieved by an agonist acting through a mechanism that can be formulated and studied at the molecular level. The intention of this redefinition is to focus on the agonist and the receptor, and its immediate transduction mechanism (e.g., the opening of an ion channel, coupling to a G-protein), rather than on the cellular events that follow. (See also Neubig et al., 2003.)

But can we really regard [G] as constant? Suppose instead that $[R]_T \gg [G]_T$, rather than the reverse. Then Equation (1.41) has to be replaced by

$$p_{AR^*G^*} = \frac{E[G]_T[A]}{K_A K_{ARG} + \{E[R]_T + K_{ARG}(1+E)\}[A]} \tag{1.42}$$

The maximum value of $p_{AR^*G^*}$ would now be

$$\frac{E[G]_T}{E[R]_T + K_{ARG}(1+E)}$$

so that the intrinsic efficacy of the agonist would be influenced by $[R]_T$ as well as by K_{ARG} and $[G]_T$.

Clearly, it would be best to avoid the need to have to make any assumptions about either the constancy of [G] or the relative magnitudes of $[R]_T$ and $[G]_T$. This can be done for the scheme of Equation (1.38), with the outcome that the concentration of AR*G* is obtainable from the roots of a quadratic equation

$$[AR^*G^*]^2 - (Q + [G]_T + [R]_T)[AR^*G^*] + [R]_T[G]_T = 0 \tag{1.43}$$

where

$$Q = K_{ARG}\left\{1 + \frac{1}{E}\left(1 + \frac{K_A}{[A]}\right)\right\}$$

This predicts a nonhyperbolic relationship between [AR*G*] and [A], as well as between binding and [A]. In general, the intrinsic efficacy is determined by E and K_{ARG} as well as by $[R]_T$ and $[G]_T$.

1.5 INHIBITORY ACTIONS AT RECEPTORS: SURMOUNTABLE ANTAGONISM

1.5.1 OVERVIEW OF DRUG ANTAGONISM

Many of the most useful drugs are antagonists, i.e., substances that reduce the action of another agent that is often an endogenous agonist (e.g., a hormone, neurotransmitter, or autacoid). Though the most common mechanism is simple competition, antagonism can occur in a variety of ways.

1.5.1.1 Mechanisms Not Involving the Receptor Macromolecule through Which the Agonist Acts

1. *Chemical antagonism*—The antagonist combines directly with the substance being antagonized. Receptors are not involved. For example, the chelating agent EDTA (ethyl-enediaminetetraacetic acid) can be used to treat poisoning by lead (a less toxic chelate is formed and excreted).
2. *Functional antagonism*—This involves cellular sites other than that for the agonist and can take several forms.

In *physiological antagonism*, the action of an agonist is countered by a second agonist, which exerts an opposing biological effect. Each acts through its own receptors. For example, adrenaline relaxes bronchial smooth muscle, thus reducing the bronchocon-striction caused by histamine and the cysteinyl-leukotrienes.

In *indirect antagonism*, the antagonist acts at another downstream receptor that links the action of the agonist to the final response observed. For example, β-adrenoceptor blockers such as propranolol reduce the rise in heart rate caused by indirectly acting sympathomimetic amines such as tyramine. This is because tyramine acts by releasing noradrenaline from noradrenergic nerve endings, and the released noradrenaline acts on β-adrenoceptors to increase heart rate:

tyramine $\rightarrow$ release of noradrenaline $\rightarrow$ β adrenoceptor activation $\rightarrow$ response

A third possibility is that the antagonist interferes with other postreceptor events that contribute to the tissue response. Calcium channel blockers such as verapamil block the influx of calcium needed for maintained smooth muscle contraction, and so reduce the contractile response to acetylcholine.

3. *Pharmacokinetic antagonism*—Here the "antagonist" effectively lowers the concentration of the active drug at its site of action. For example, repeated administration of phenobarbitone induces an increase in the activity of hepatic enzymes that inactivate the anticoagulant drug warfarin. Hence if phenobarbitone and warfarin are given together, the plasma concentration of warfarin is reduced, so that it becomes less active.

1.5.1.2 Mechanisms Involving the Receptor Macromolecule

1. *The binding of agonist and antagonist is mutually exclusive.* This may be because the agonist and antagonist compete for the same binding site, or combine with adjacent sites that overlap. A third possibility is that different sites are involved but they interact in such a way that agonist and antagonist molecules cannot be bound to the receptor macromolecule at the same time.

   This type of antagonism has two main variants:
   a. The agonist and antagonist form only short-lasting combinations with the binding sites, so that equilibrium between agonist, antagonist, and sites can be reached during the presence of the agonist. The interaction between the antagonist and the binding site is freely reversible. Hence the blocking action can always be surmounted by increasing the concentration of agonist, which will then occupy a higher proportion of the binding sites. This is described as *reversible competitive antagonism* (see Section 1.5.2). For example: Atropine competitively blocks the action of acetylcholine on all muscarinic receptors.
   b. The antagonist combines irreversibly (or effectively so within the time scale of the agonist application) with the binding site for the agonist. When enough receptors have been irreversibly blocked in this way, the antagonism is *insurmountable* (i.e., no amount of agonist can elicit a full response because too few unblocked receptors are left). For example: Phenoxybenzamine forms a covalent bond at or near the agonist binding sites on α-adrenoceptors, resulting in insurmountable antagonism. Note that most pharmacologists now describe this as *irreversible competitive antagonism*, which is the term used in this account; others have regarded it as *noncompetitive*.

2. *The agonist and the antagonist can be bound at the same time to different regions of the receptor macromolecule.* This is noncompetitive antagonism. It is also referred to as allotopic or allosteric antagonism (*allotopic* means different place, in contrast to *syntopic*, meaning same place; for a note on allosteric, see Appendix 1.6.1). In principle, noncompetitive antagonists can be either reversible or irreversible. An example of the former is the action of hexamethonium, which reversibly reduces the response to acetylcholine acting on the nicotinic receptors of sympathetic ganglion cells by blocking the receptor's intrinsic ion channel. In principle, this form of antagonism is insurmountable. Note that in the past the term *noncompetitive* was sometimes extended to forms of antagonism that do not involve the agonist receptor macromolecule (see, e.g., indirect antagonism in Section 1.5.1.1).

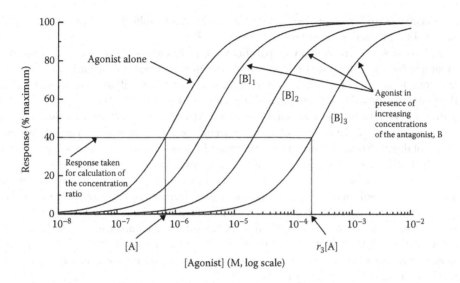

FIGURE 1.16 The predicted effect of three concentrations of a reversible competitive antagonist, B, on the log concentration-response relationship for an agonist. The calculation of the concentration ratio (r_3) for the highest concentration of antagonist, $[B]_3$, is illustrated.

1.5.2 Reversible Competitive Antagonism

We start by examining how a reversible competitive antagonist (for example, atropine) alters the concentration-response relationship for the action of an agonist (for example, acetylcholine). It is found experimentally that the presence of such an antagonist causes the log concentration-response curve for the agonist to be shifted to the right, often without a change in slope or maximal response. The antagonism is *surmountable*, commonly over a wide range of antagonist concentrations. This is illustrated in Figure 1.16.

The extent of the shift is best expressed as a concentration ratio.* This is defined as the factor by which the agonist concentration must be increased to restore a given response in the presence of the antagonist. The calculation of the concentration ratio is done as follows. First, a certain magnitude of response is selected. This is often 50% of the maximum attainable, but in principle any value would do.† In the illustration, 40% has been taken. In the absence of antagonist, this response is elicited by a concentration [A] of agonist. When the antagonist is present, the agonist concentration has to be increased by a factor r, that is, to r[A]. Thus, for antagonist concentration $[B]_3$ in Figure 1.16, the concentration ratio is r_3 (= (r_3 [A])/[A]).

The negative logarithm of the concentration of antagonist that causes a concentration ratio of x is commonly denoted by pA_x. This term was introduced by H. O. Schild as an empirical measure of the activity of an antagonist. The value most often quoted is pA_2, where

$$pA_2 = -\log [B]_{r=2}$$

To illustrate this notation we consider the ability of atropine to block the muscarinic receptors for acetylcholine. The presence of atropine at a concentration of only 1 nM makes it necessary to

---

* The term *dose ratio* is also used.

† Though clearly it is sensible to avoid the extreme ends of the range. The concentration ratio can also be estimated by using a least squares minimization procedure to fit the Hill equation (Sections 1.2.2 and 1.2.4.3), or some other suitable function, to each of the concentration-response curves. This also allows the parallelism of the curves to be assessed. A further possibility is to fit all the curves (i.e., with and without antagonist) simultaneously by assuming that the Gaddum equation holds (see below), and by making use of the Hill equation, or another function, to relate receptor activation to the measured tissue response.

double the acetylcholine concentration needed to elicit a given submaximal response of a tissue. Hence $pA_2 = 9$ for this action of atropine $(-\log (10^{-9}) = 9)$.

We next look at why there should be a parallel shift in the curves, and at the same time we will derive a simple but most important relationship between the amount of the shift, as expressed by the concentration ratio, and the concentration of the antagonist. We will assume for simplicity that when the tissue is exposed to the agonist and the antagonist at the same time, the two drugs come into equilibrium with the binding sites on the receptor. At a given moment an individual site may be occupied by either an agonist or an antagonist molecule, or it may be vacant. The relative proportions of the total population of binding sites occupied by agonist and antagonist are governed, just as Langley had surmised (see Section 1.1.1), by the concentrations of agonist and antagonist, and by the affinities of the sites for each. Because the agonist and the antagonist bind reversibly, raising the agonist concentration will increase the proportion of sites occupied by the agonist, at the expense of antagonist occupancy. Hence the response will become greater.

The law of mass action was first applied to competitive antagonism by Clark, Gaddum, and Schild at a time before the importance of receptor activation by isomerization was established. It was assumed therefore that the equilibrium between agonist, antagonist, and their common binding site could be represented quite simply by the reactions

$$A + R \rightleftharpoons AR$$

$$B + R \rightleftharpoons BR$$

As shown in Table 1.5 (left hand column), application of the law of mass action to these simultaneous equilibria leads to the following expression for the proportion of the binding sites occupied by agonist:

$$p_{AR} = \frac{[A]}{K_A\left(1 + \dfrac{[B]}{K_B}\right) + [A]} \tag{1.48}$$

Here K_A and K_B are the equilibrium dissociation constants for the binding of agonist and antagonist, respectively. This is the *Gaddum equation*, after J. H. Gaddum, who was the first to derive it in the context of competitive antagonism. Note that if [B] is set to zero, we have the Hill–Langmuir equation (Section 1.2.1).

If instead we take as our starting point the del Castillo–Katz mechanism for receptor activation (see Equation 1.7), three equilibria need to be considered:

$$A + R \xrightleftharpoons{K_A} AR \xrightleftharpoons{E} AR^*$$

$$B + R \xrightleftharpoons{K_B} BR$$

Applying the law of mass action, (see Table 1.5, right column), we obtain an expression for the proportion of receptors in the active state:

$$p_{AR^*} = \frac{E[A]}{K_A\left(1 + \dfrac{[B]}{K_B}\right) + (1 + E)[A]} \tag{1.49}$$

Here K_A and E are as defined in Section 1.2.3 and K_B is as before the equilibrium dissociation constant for the combination of the antagonist with the binding site. If [B] is set to zero, we have Equation (1.32).

Equations (1.48) and (1.49) embody the law that Langley had concluded must relate the amounts of the "compounds" he postulated to the concentrations of the agonist and antagonist (see Section 1.1). However, in order to apply these expressions to the practical problem of understanding how a

TABLE 1.5
Application of the Law of Mass Action to Reversible Competitive Antagonism

Classical analysis of competitive antagonism, following Gaddum and Schild	Competitive antagonism on the del Castillo–Katz scheme for receptor activation (see Section 1.2.3, Equation 1.7)
We begin by assuming that both the agonist (A) and the antagonist (B) combine with their binding site according to the law of mass action, and in a way that can be represented by the two equilibria	Receptor isomerization to the active form occurs when the binding site is occupied by A but not by the antagonist B:

$$A + R \rightleftharpoons AR$$

$$B + R \rightleftharpoons BR$$

$$A + R \xrightarrow{K_A} AR \xrightarrow{E} AR^*$$

$$B + R \xrightarrow{K_B} BR$$

| Our first task is to work out how the proportion of receptors occupied by the agonist varies with the concentrations of the agonist and the antagonist. Equilibrium is assumed. Applying the law of mass action gives: | Applying the law of mass action to each of the three equilibria, we have |

$$[A][R] = K_A[AR]$$

$$[B][R] = K_B[BR]$$

$$[A][R] = K_A[AR]$$

$$[AR^*] = E[AR]$$

$$[B][R] = K_B[BR]$$

where K_B is the equilibrium dissociation constant for the combination of B with the binding site and K_A and E are as previously defined.

As in Section 1.2.1, these equations can be rewritten in terms of the proportions of binding sites that are free (p_R) or occupied by either A (p_{AR}) or B (p_{BR}):

$$[A] p_R = K_A p_{AR} \tag{1.52}$$

$$[B] p_R = K_B p_{BR} \tag{1.53}$$

These equations can be rewritten in terms of the fractions of receptors in different conditions:

$$[A] p_R = K_A p_{AR}$$

$$p_{AR^*} = E p_{AR}$$

$$[B] p_R = K_B p_{BR}$$

An individual site is either vacant or occupied by an agonist or an antagonist molecule. Hence

$$p_R + p_{AR} + p_{BR} = 1 \tag{1.54}$$

Adding up the fractions of receptors, we have:

$$p_R + p_{AR} + p_{AR^*} + p_{BR} = 1$$

What we need to know is p_{AR}, so we use Equations (1.52) and (1.53) to substitute for p_R and p_{BR} in Equation (1.54):

Substituting to obtain p_{AR^*} gives

$$\frac{K_A}{[A]} \cdot p_{AR} + p_{AR} + \frac{[B]}{K_B} \frac{K_A}{[A]} \cdot p_{AR} = 1$$

$$\frac{K_A}{E[A]} p_{AR^*} + \frac{p_{AR^*}}{E} + p_{AR^*} + \frac{[B]}{K_B} \frac{K_A}{E[A]} p_{AR^*} = 1$$

Hence

$$\Rightarrow p_{AR} = \frac{[A]}{K_A \left(1 + \dfrac{[B]}{K_B}\right) + [A]}$$

$$p_{AR^*} = \frac{E[A]}{K_A \left(1 + \dfrac{[B]}{K_B}\right) + (1 + E)[A]}$$

competitive antagonist will affect the response to the agonist, we need to make some assumptions about the relationship between the response and the proportion of active receptors. Gaddum and Schild recognized that the best way to proceed was to assume that the same response (say 30% of the maximum attainable) corresponded to the same receptor activation by agonist whether the agonist was acting alone or at a higher concentration in the presence of the competitive antagonist.

It is then unnecessary to know the exact form of the relationship between receptor activation and response. This was a most important advance, however obvious it might seem on looking back.

We can now consider an experiment in which the same submaximal response is elicited first by a concentration [A] of agonist acting alone and then by a greater concentration (r[A]) applied in the presence of the antagonist. r is the concentration ratio, as already defined. Since p_{AR*} is assumed to be the same in the two situations, we can write, from Equation (1.49)*,

$$\frac{E[A]}{K_A + (1+E)[A]} = \frac{Er[A]}{K_A \left(1 + \dfrac{[B]}{K_B}\right) + (1+E)r[A]}$$

Here the left- and right-hand sides refer to, respectively, the fraction of receptors in the active state when A is applied first on its own and then in the presence of the antagonist at concentration [B].

Dividing each term on the right side by r, we have

$$\frac{E[A]}{K_A + (1+E)[A]} = \frac{E[A]}{K_A \left(\dfrac{1 + \dfrac{[B]}{K_B}}{r}\right) + (1+E)[A]}$$

If the expressions on the left and right are to take the same value, the following identity must hold:

$$\frac{1 + \dfrac{[B]}{K_B}}{r} = 1$$

Hence

$$r - 1 = \frac{[B]}{K_B} \tag{1.50}$$

This is the *Schild equation*, which was first stated and applied to the study of competitive antagonism by H. O. Schild in 1949. It is probably the most important single quantitative relationship in pharmacology and has been shown to apply to the action of many competitive antagonists over a wide range of concentrations. Though originally derived on the basis of the simple scheme for receptor activation described in Sections 1.2.1 and 1.2.2, it holds equally for the del Castillo–Katz scheme, as we have just shown, as well as for more complex models in which the receptor is constitutively active.

One of the predictions of the Schild equation is that a reversible competitive antagonist should cause a parallel shift in the log agonist concentration response curve (as illustrated in Figure 1.16; see also Figure 1.18). This is because if the equation holds, the concentration ratio, r, is determined only by the values of [B] and of K_B, regardless of the concentration and even the identity of the agonist (provided that it acts through the same receptors as the antagonist). With a logarithmic scale, a constant value of r corresponds to a constant separation of the concentration-response curves, that is, parallelism (because $\log(r[A]) - \log[A] = \log r + \log[A] - \log[A], = \log r$, whatever the value of [A]).

Probably the most important application of the Schild equation is that it provides a way of estimating the equilibrium dissociation constant for the combination of an antagonist with its binding site. A series of agonist concentration-response curves is established, first without and then with increasing concentrations of antagonist present, and tested for parallelism. If this condition is met, the value of ($r - 1$) is plotted against the antagonist concentration, [B]. This should give a straight line of slope equal to the reciprocal of K_B.

---

* We assume here that the del Castillo–Katz model applies. Use of the Gaddum equation, based on the simpler scheme explored by Hill and by Clark, leads to exactly the same conclusions, as the reader can easily show by following the same steps but starting with Equation (1.48) rather than Equation (1.49).

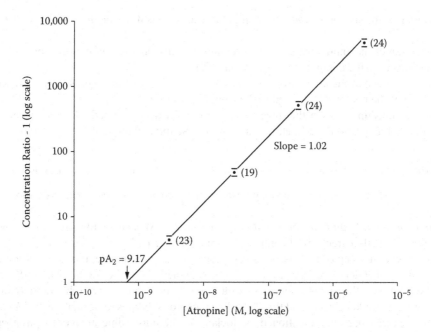

FIGURE 1.17 Schild plot for the action of atropine in antagonizing the action of acetylcholine on guinea-pig ileum. Each point gives the mean ± the standard error of the mean of the number of observations shown.

More usually, both $(r-1)$ and [B] are plotted on logarithmic scales (the *Schild plot*). The outcome should be a straight line with a slope of unity, and the intercept on the *x*-axis provides an estimate of $\log K_B$. The basis for these statements can be seen by expressing the Schild equation in logarithmic form:

$$\log(r-1) = \log[B] - \log K_B \qquad (1.51)$$

A Schild plot (based on the results of a student class experiment on the effect of atropine on the contractile response of guinea-pig ileum to acetylcholine) is shown in Figure 1.17. Note that the line is straight, and its slope close to unity, as Equation (1.51) predicts.

How might the value of pA_2 be interpreted in these terms? *If the Schild equation is obeyed*, pA_2 then gives an estimate of $-\log K_B$, because (from Equation 1.51)

$$\log(2-1) = \log(1) = 0 = \log[B]_{r=2} - \log K_B$$

$$\therefore -\log[B]_{r=2}, = pA_2, = -\log K_B$$

The term pK_B is often used[*] to denote $-\log K_B$.

---

[*] The distinction between pK_B and pA_2 is subtle but can be important. pA_2, as Schild defined it, is an empirical index of the action of an antagonist: It can be measured whether or not the predictions of the Schild equation have been met. Thus the intercept of a Schild plot on the abscissa gives an estimate of pA_2 even if the slope of the line is not unity. If, however, the line is adequately defined experimentally and is straight (but with a slope that is not precisely unity, though not differing significantly from it), it is common, and appropriate, to constrain the slope to unity. The intercept on the abscissa now provides an estimate not of pA_2 but of pK_B, as defined above. pK_B and pA_2 coincide only if the slope is exactly unity, and there are no complicating factors. If the slope of the Schild plot differs significantly from unity, so that the Schild equation does not hold, K_B cannot be estimated. A common misunderstanding is to suppose that Schild defined pA_2 as $-\log K_B$ for a competitive antagonist. As already noted, his definition was more general than this and without reference to theory.

To summarize to this point, reversible competitive antagonism has the following characteristics:

1. The action of the antagonist can be overcome by a sufficient increase in the concentration of agonist (i.e., the antagonism is surmountable).
2. In the presence of the antagonist, the curve relating the log of the agonist concentration to the size of the response is shifted to the right in a parallel fashion.
3. The relationship between the magnitude of the shift (as expressed by the concentration ratio) and the antagonist concentration obeys the Schild equation.

1.5.3 PRACTICAL APPLICATIONS OF STUDIES OF REVERSIBLE COMPETITIVE ANTAGONISM

The quantitative study of competitive antagonism by the methods just described has important uses.

1. *The identification and characterization of receptors*—Measuring the value of K_B for the action of a well-characterized competitive antagonist can allow the identification of a particular type of receptor in a tissue or cell preparation. For example, if a tissue is found to respond to acetylcholine, and if the response is antagonized by atropine with a pK_B value of about 9, then the receptor involved is likely to be muscarinic. Preferably more than one antagonist should be used, and this can allow receptor subtypes to be identified. For example, if the response just mentioned is blocked by the muscarinic antagonist pirenzepine with a pK_B of 7.9–8.5, whereas the corresponding value for the antagonist himbacine is found to be 7.0–7.2, then the receptor is very probably of the M_1 subtype.
2. *The assessment of new competitive antagonists*—The procedures developed by Gaddum and Schild have been invaluable for the development of new competitive antagonists. Examples include the H_2-receptor antagonists such as cimetidine, which reduce gastric acid secretion (see below), and the $5HT_3$-receptor antagonists such as ondansetron, which can control the nausea and vomiting caused by cytotoxic drugs. These competitive antagonists, and others, were discovered by careful examination of the relationship between chemical structure and biological activity, as assessed by the methods of Gaddum and Schild. Having a reliable measure of the change in affinity that results from modifying the chemical structure of a potential drug provides the medicinal chemist with a powerful tool with which to discover compounds with greater activity and selectivity.
3. *The classification of agonists*—At first sight, this may seem a surprising application of a method developed primarily for the study of antagonists. However, recall that only the *ratio* of agonist concentrations appears in the Schild equation, not the actual values of the concentrations. It follows that for a given competitive antagonist acting at a fixed concentration, the concentration ratio should be the same for all agonists acting through the receptors at which the antagonist acts. So it is possible to test if a new agonist acts at a given receptor by examining whether the concentration ratio is the same for the novel agonist as it is for a well-characterized agonist known to act at that receptor. Figure 1.18, from the work of Arunlakshana and Schild, illustrates the approach. It can be seen that the competitive antagonist diphenhydramine, which acts at H_1-receptors, caused exactly the same shift (i.e., the same concentration ratio) of the log concentration-response curve for pyridylethylamine as for histamine. This strongly suggested that pyridylethylamine was acting through the same receptors as histamine, even though it is almost 100 times less active as an agonist.

The application of these principles is well illustrated by the classical work of J. W. Black and his colleagues, which led to the discovery of the first competitive antagonists acting at the H_2-receptors for histamine. Although the objective was to develop compounds that would reduce gastric acid secretion in disease, much of the work was done not with secretory tissue but with two isolated

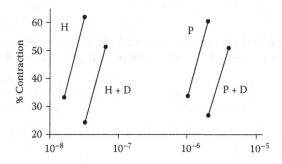

FIGURE 1.18 Responses of guinea-pig ileum to histamine (H) and pyridylethylamine (P) in the absence and presence of diphenhydramine (D, at 3.3 ng/ml.). The equal shift in the lines (from H to H+D, and from P to P+D) suggests that the two agonists act on the same receptor. (Adapted from Arunlakshana, O., and Schild, H. O., *Br. J. Pharmacol.*, 14, 48–58, 1959.)

tissue preparations, guinea-pig atria and rat uterus. These could be used because they were shown to possess histamine receptors of the same kind (H_2) as concerned in gastric acid secretion. Also, their responses to histamine (increased rate of beating of the atria; relaxation of the rat uterus) were more easily measured than was gastric secretion. This allowed large numbers of compounds to be tested.

The successful outcome included the synthesis of burimamide, the first H_2-receptor antagonist to be tested in man. Table 1.6 compares its ability to antagonize the actions of three agonists on guinea-pig atria: histamine, 4-methylhistamine, and 2-methylhistamine. The K_B values are almost the same, despite the varying potencies of the agonists. This suggested that all three agonists were acting through the same receptors (see item 3 in the list above).

Table 1.7 shows that the value of K_B for blockade by burimamide of the action of histamine on the rat uterus is similar to that for the guinea-pig atria, as would be expected were the receptors in the two tissues to be the same (see item 1 in the list above). In contrast, when burimamide was tested for its inhibitory action against the H_1-mediated contractile action of histamine on guinea-pig ileum, it was found to be approximately 40-fold less active (as judged by the apparent K_B value). Moreover, the characteristics of the inhibition no longer conformed to the predictions of competitive antagonism. Thus, the slope of the Schild plot, at 1.32, was significantly greater than unity. Further, when burimamide was tested against carbachol (carbamoyl choline), which also contracts the guinea-pig ileum (though through muscarinic rather than H_1 receptors), the slope was similarly divergent, and the apparent K_B value was of the same order. This suggested that the burimamide's inhibition of the response of the ileum to the two agonists was more likely to have resulted from a

TABLE 1.6

Comparison of the Antagonism by Burimamide of the Actions of Histamine and Two Related Agonists on Guinea-Pig Atria

Agonist	EC_{50} on guinea-pig atria (μM)	Equilibrium dissociation constant (K_B) for the blocking action of burimamide (μM)
histamine	1.1	7.8
4-methylhistamine	3.1	7.2
2-methylhistamine	19.8	6.9

Source: Black, J. W. et al., *Nature*, 236, 385–390, 1972.

TABLE 1.7
Comparison of the Ability of Burimamide to Block the Actions of Histamine on Guinea-Pig (G.-P.) Ileum and Atrium, and on Rat Uterus

Tissue	Agonist	n_s (slope of Schild plot)	Apparent equilibrium dissociation constant (K_B) for the blocking action of burimamide
G.-P. atrium (H_2)	histamine	0.98	7.8 μm
rat uterus (H_2)	histamine	0.96	6.6 μm
G.-P. ileum (H_1)	histamine	1.32	288 μm
G.-P. ileum	carbachol	1.44	174 μm

Source: Black, J. W. et al., *Nature*, 236, 385–390, 1972.

nonspecific depression of the tissue rather than from weak competitive antagonism at both H_1 and muscarinic receptors.

1.5.4 COMPLICATIONS IN THE STUDY OF REVERSIBLE COMPETITIVE ANTAGONISM

Though the predictions of competitive antagonism are often fulfilled over a wide range of agonist and antagonist concentrations, divergences sometimes occur and much can be learned from them. Two examples follow.

1.5.4.1 Example 1

Figure 1.19 shows two Schild plots, one of which (open circles) is far from the expected straight line of unit slope. Both sets of experiments were done with a smooth muscle preparation, the isolated

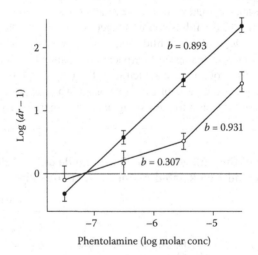

FIGURE 1.19 Schild plots for the antagonism of noradrenaline by phentolamine, studied in the isolated nictitating membrane of the cat. The values plotted are the means (± S.E.) for four or five experiments. Closed circles, denervated nictitating membrane; open circles, normal membrane; *b* indicates the slope. The slope values for normal membrane were calculated for the three lowest concentrations and the two highest concentrations of phentolamine. (From Furchgott, R. F., *Handbook of Experimental Pharmacology*. Vol. 23, 1972, pp. 283–335; based on the results of Langer, S. Z., and Trendelenburg, U., *J. Pharmacol. Exp. Ther.*, 167, 117–142, 1969. With permission.)

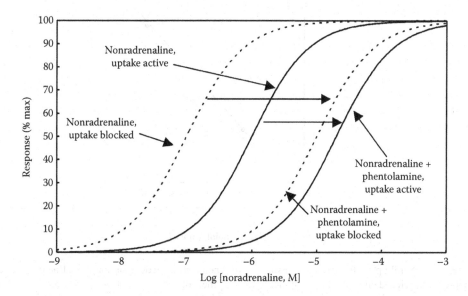

FIGURE 1.20 Hypothetical concentration-response curves to illustrate how the uptake$_1$ process can influence the study of the antagonism of noradrenaline by phentolamine. The two full lines show the response to noradrenaline, first in the absence and then in the presence of phentolamine. If the experiment is repeated, but with the uptake process blocked, the dotted lines would be obtained. Noradrenaline has become more active, and phentolamine now causes a greater shift (compare the lengths of the two horizontal arrows), as explained in the text.

nictitating membrane of the cat's eye. This tissue receives a dense noradrenergic innervation and contracts in response to noradrenaline, which was the agonist used. The adrenoceptors concerned are of the α-subtype and can be blocked by the reversible competitive antagonist phentolamine. In accounting for the nonlinear Schild plot, the key observation was that when the experiments were repeated, but with a nictitating membrane that had previously been denervated (i.e., the adrenergic nerve supply had been cut and allowed to degenerate), the concentration ratios became larger and the Schild plot became linear, with a slope near to unity.

This suggested an explanation in terms of the presence in the normal but not the denervated muscle of the neuronal uptake mechanism (uptake$_1$) for noradrenaline. This uptake process can be so effective that when noradrenaline is added to the bathing fluid, the concentration attained in the interior of the preparation may be much less than that applied. As noradrenaline diffuses in, some of it is taken up by the adrenergic nerves, so that a concentration gradient is maintained. In keeping with this, blockade of uptake$_1$ (for example, by cocaine) can greatly potentiate the action of noradrenaline. This is illustrated schematically in Figure 1.20. The left-most full line shows the control concentration-response curve for an adrenergically innervated tissue. The dotted line (extreme left) represents the consequence of blocking the uptake process: Much lower concentrations of noradrenaline are now sufficient to elicit a given response.[*] The full line on the right shows the displacement of the control curve caused by the application of phentolamine, and the dotted line just to its left depicts the effect of blocking uptake when phentolamine is present. Note that this dotted line is closer to the full line than is seen with the pair of curves on the left. This is because the influence of uptake (which is a saturable process) on the local concentration of noradrenaline will be proportionately smaller when a large noradrenaline concentration is applied, as

---

[*] The curves in Figure 1.20 are stylized: The leftward displacement due to the blockade of noradrenaline uptake would not be expected to be exactly parallel.

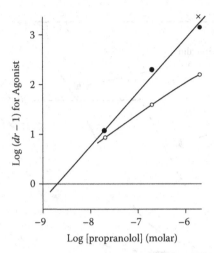

FIGURE 1.21   Schild plots for the antagonism by propranolol of the actions of noradrenaline (open circles) and isoprenaline (closed circles) on the contractile force of the isolated atrium of the guinea-pig. The x shows the value obtained with noradrenaline as agonist, but in the presence of cocaine (20 μM). (Adapted from Furchgott, R. F., *Handbook of Experimental Pharmacology*, Vol. 23, 1972, 283–335; based on the results of Blinks, J. R., *Ann. N.Y. Acad. Sci.*, 139, 673–685, 1967.)

is required to restore the response in the presence of phentolamine. Hence the concentration ratio will be greater if uptake$_1$ is absent, as it is in the chronically denervated tissue.

1.5.4.2   Example 2

Figure 1.21, like Figure 1.19, shows two Schild plots, one of which (open circles) departs greatly from the expected behavior. The deviation occurs when noradrenaline is the agonist, and again it can be accounted for in terms of the reduction in local concentration caused by the uptake$_1$ process (the tissue used—the atrium of the guinea-pig—has a dense adrenergic innervation). The other agonist used, isoprenaline, is not subject to uptake$_1$. Accordingly, the Schild plot with isoprenaline is linear with a slope close to unity. In keeping with this explanation (and with the prediction that the concentration ratio should be the same for different agonists, provided that they act through the same receptors—see Section 1.5.3), blockade of uptake$_1$ by the inclusion of cocaine in the bathing fluid causes the concentration ratio for noradrenaline to increase to the same value as seen with isoprenaline as agonist.

Deviations from the expected behavior will also be seen if the antagonist has additional actions at the concentrations examined. An example is provided by the ability of the reversible competitive antagonist tubocurarine to block the ion channels that open when nicotinic receptors are activated. This is described in Chapter 6, as are the complications introduced by the presence on such ligand-gated ion channels of two agonist binding sites that may or may not have equal affinities for the antagonist. Nonlinear Schild plots can arise in many other ways. One cause is failure to allow sufficient time for the antagonist to reach equilibrium with the receptors. As discussed in Section 1.3.2, the rate at which a ligand equilibrates with its binding sites becomes slower at lower concentrations (see Figure 1.3). Hence, if the exposure is too short, the concentration ratio will be disproportionately low at such concentrations, and the Schild plot will be steeper in this region than predicted (see also Wyllie and Chen, 2007). Nonlinear Schild plots can also result when the response of a tissue is mediated by more than one receptor with different affinities for the antagonist. These complications, and several others, have been described by T. P. Kenakin, whose detailed account of the analysis of competitive antagonism is recommended (see Chapter 6 in Kenakin, 2009).

1.6   INHIBITORY ACTIONS AT RECEPTORS: INSURMOUNTABLE ANTAGONISM

1.6.1   IRREVERSIBLE COMPETITIVE ANTAGONISM

In this form of drug antagonism, the antagonist forms a relatively long-lasting or even irreversible combination with either the agonist binding site or a region related to it in such a way that agonist and antagonist molecules cannot be bound at the same time. The key point is that the dissociation of the antagonist from its binding site is very slow *in relation to the duration of the agonist application.* This is an important qualification because the rate of dissociation can vary greatly from antagonist to antagonist. For some, hours or even days may be needed so that there is no appreciable fall in occupancy during the 60 seconds or so for which the agonist might be applied. Others may dissociate more quickly and the surmountability of the block will then depend on how long the agonist is present and also on how well the response to the agonist is maintained in the tissue under study.

Under physiological conditions, a naturally occurring agonist (e.g., a neurotransmitter) may be present for a very brief time indeed—only a millisecond or less for acetylcholine released from the motor nerve endings on skeletal muscle. This is unlikely to be long enough to allow an appreciable fall in receptor occupancy by a competitive antagonist such as tubocurarine, which would therefore be effectively irreversible *on this time scale.* If, however, the interaction between acetylcholine and tubocurarine is studied in the classical pharmacological manner, in which both agents are applied for enough time for equilibrium to be reached, the blocking action then shows all the characteristics of reversible competitive antagonism (albeit with the additional feature that tubocurarine also blocks open ion channels).

An example of an irreversible antagonist with a very long action (usually many hours) is *phenoxybenzamine*, which blocks α-adrenoceptors and, less potently, H₁-histamine and muscarinic receptors. Its structure is shown below. Also illustrated is *benzilylcholine mustard*, a highly active and selective irreversible blocker of muscarinic receptors.

phenoxybenzamine   benzilylcholine mustard

Both compounds are β-*haloalkylamines*, that is, they contain the grouping

where X is a halogen atom. Once in aqueous solution, such agents cyclize to form an unstable ethyleneiminium* ion (Figure 1.22). Because an ionic bond can now be formed, this ion is likely to have a greater affinity than the parent molecule for the binding site on the receptor. After the ethyleneiminium ion has docked with the site, there are two main possibilities. One is merely that the ion dissociates from the site, unchanged. The other is that the ethyleneiminium ring in the docked compound opens to create a reactive intermediate, with the consequence that a covalent bond between the drug molecule and the binding site can be formed. In effect, the receptor becomes alkylated,[†] as illustrated in Figure 1.22.

---

* Other terms used are *ethyleneimmonium* and *aziridinium ion.*
[†] One possibility is via the formation of a reactive carbonium ion: $R_1R_2NCH_2CH_2^+$.

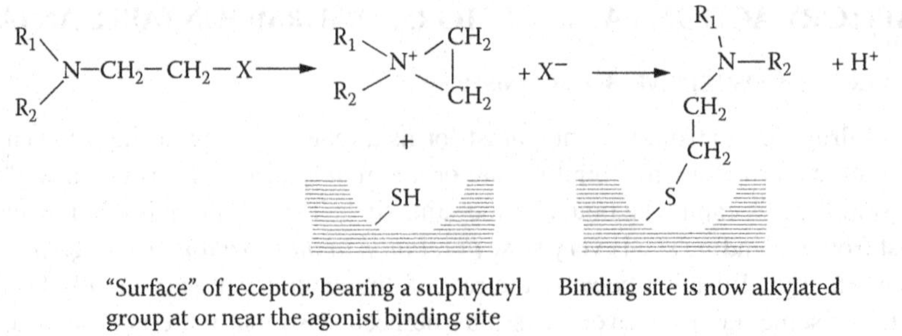

"Surface" of receptor, bearing a sulphydryl   Binding site is now alkylated
group at or near the agonist binding site

FIGURE 1.22   Alkylation of a receptor by a β-haloalkylamine.

Groups that can be alkylated in this way include –SH, –OH, =NH and –COOH. However, not all irreversible antagonists act by forming a covalent bond. Some may "fit" the binding site so closely that the combined strength of the other kinds of intermolecular interaction (ionic, hydrophobic, Van der Waals, hydrogen bonds) that come into play approaches that of a covalent link.

1.6.2   SOME APPLICATIONS OF IRREVERSIBLE ANTAGONISTS

1.6.2.1   Labeling Receptors

Alkylation of the kind illustrated in Figure 1.22, but using a radiolabeled ligand, provides a means of labeling the binding site(s) of receptor macromolecules.[*] The tissue is exposed to the labeled antagonist for long enough to allow combination with most of the receptors. It is then washed with ligand-free solution so that unbound or loosely bound antagonist can diffuse away, leaving (ideally) only the receptors covalently labeled. A related approach is to use a photo-affinity label. This is a compound that has not only affinity for the receptor but also the property of breaking down to form a reactive intermediate following absorption of light energy of the appropriate wavelength. Light sensitivity of this kind can often be achieved by attaching an azido group ($–N_3$) to a drug molecule. The resulting photo-affinity label is allowed to equilibrate with a tissue or membrane preparation, which is then exposed to intense light. The outcome (for an azide) is the formation of a highly reactive nitrene that can combine with immediately adjacent structures (including, it is hoped, the binding regions of the receptor), to form a covalent bond, thus "tagging" the binding site(s).[†] This can provide a first step toward receptor isolation.

1.6.2.2   Counting Receptors

If the antagonist can be radiolabeled, the same general procedure may be used to estimate the number of receptors in an intact tissue, provided that the specific activity (i.e., the radioactivity expressed in terms of the quantity of material) of the ligand is known. An early example was the application of ^{125}I- or ^{131}I-labeled α-bungarotoxin to determine the number of nicotinic receptors at the end-plate region of skeletal muscle. This revealed that the muscular weakness that characterizes myasthenia gravis, a disease affecting the transmission of impulses from motor nerves to skeletal muscle, results from a reduction in the number of nicotinic receptors. A variant of the technique, using α-bungarotoxin labeled with a fluorescent group, allows these receptors to be visualized by light microscopy.

1.6.2.3   Receptor Protection Experiments

The rate at which an irreversible antagonist inactivates receptors will be reduced by the simultaneous presence of a reversible agonist or competitive antagonist that acts at the same binding site. The

---

[*] As well as β-haloalkylamines, substances with haloalkyl groups attached to carbons bonded to oxygen can be used. An interesting example is bromoacetylcholine, which acts as a tethered agonist acting on nicotinic receptors.

[†] Some drugs are intrinsically photolabile. Examples include tubocurarine and chlorpromazine, both of which have been used to label the binding regions of receptors.

reversible agent, by occupying sites, lowers the number irreversibly blocked within a given period: the receptors are said to be protected. This can be a useful tool for the characterization of drugs as well as of receptors. For example, R. F. Furchgott (who introduced the method) tested the ability of three agonists (noradrenaline, adrenaline, and isoprenaline) to protect against the alkylating agent dibenamine (a phenoxybenzamine-like compound) applied to rabbit aortic strips. Each agonist protected the response to the other two. Thus, after the tissue had been exposed to dibenamine in the presence of a large concentration of noradrenaline, followed by a drug-free washing period, adrenaline and isoprenaline as well as noradrenaline were still able to cause contraction. The same exposure to dibenamine on its own abolished the response to the subsequent application of each of the same agonists. This provided evidence that all three agonists caused contraction by acting at a common receptor (now well established to be the α-adrenoceptor subtype), which was uncertain at the time.

Another example of receptor protection, but using a competitive antagonist rather than an agonist, is provided by the ability of tubocurarine to slow the onset of the blocking action of α-bungarotoxin at the neuromuscular junction. Note that the degree of receptor protection will depend not only on the relative concentrations and affinities of the reversible and irreversible antagonists, but also on how long they are allowed to interact with the receptors, as described in Chapter 5. Given enough time, a completely irreversible antagonist will come to occupy all the binding sites even in the presence of a high concentration of a reversible ligand.

1.6.3 Effect of an Irreversible Competitive Antagonist on the Response to an Agonist

A long enough exposure of a tissue to an irreversible antagonist results in *insurmountable antagonism*—the response cannot be fully restored by increasing the concentration of agonist, applied for the usual period. This is because an individual binding site, once firmly occupied by antagonist, is "out of play," in contrast to the dynamic equilibrium between agonist and antagonist that is characteristic of reversible competitive antagonism. Hence it is usual in work with irreversible antagonists that form covalent bonds to apply the compound for just long enough for it to occupy the required fraction of the binding sites, and then to wash the tissue with drug-free solution so that unbound antagonist can diffuse away. The change in the response to the agonist can now be studied. The results of experiments of this kind are illustrated in Figures 1.23 and 1.24.

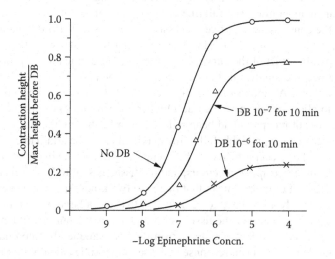

FIGURE 1.23 Effect of a 10-min exposure to two concentrations of a phenoxybenzamine-like compound, dibenamine (DB), on the contractile response of a strip of rabbit aorta to adrenaline (epinephrine). (Adapted from Furchgott, R. F., *Adv. Drug Res.*, 3, 21–55, 1966.)

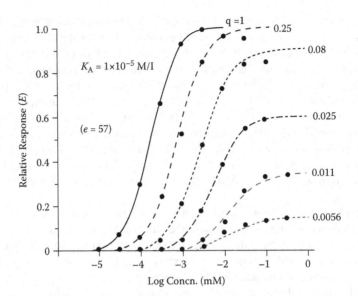

FIGURE 1.24 The effect of progressive receptor blockade by dibenamine on the response of guinea-pig ileum to histamine. Five successive exposures to 1 μM dibenamine, each for 10 min, were used, and the response to histamine was tested after each exposure. The results were analyzed as described in Section 1.6.4, and the value of q listed for each curve gives an estimate of the fraction of receptors remaining unblocked. The dashed curves were constructed from the original, pre-dibenamine, curve by inserting these estimates of q, and also the value of K_A shown, into the equations set out in Section 1.6.4 (which see, together with the related discussion). (Adapted from Furchgott, R. F., *Adv. Drug Res.*, 3, 21–55, 1966; based on data obtained by Ariëns, E. J. et al., *Arch. Int. Pharmacodynamie*, 127, 459–478, 1960.)

The family of concentration-response curves in Figure 1.23 shows the effect of an alkylating agent on the contractile response of rabbit aorta to adrenaline. Note the reduction in the maximal response, the departure from parallelism, and also the fact that the exposure times as well as the concentration of the antagonist have been given for each curve.

Figure 1.24 shows the influence of the same irreversible antagonist on the contractile response of the guinea-pig ileum to histamine. The full line is the control concentration-response curve, and the dotted lines show the consequences of five successive exposures to 1 μM dibenamine, with testing of histamine after each exposure. A striking feature is that the first application of the antagonist caused an almost parallel shift of the curve. Only after further applications of dibenamine did the maximal response become smaller in the expected way (compare Figure 1.23). The most likely explanation is as follows. Although the first application of dibenamine blocked many receptors, enough remained to allow histamine (albeit at a higher concentration) to produce a full response. Only when the number of receptors had been reduced even further by the subsequent applications of dibenamine was there an appreciable fall in the maximal response attainable. The implication is that in this tissue not all the receptors have to be occupied by histamine in order to elicit a maximal response. There are, in effect, *spare receptors*, and the tissue is said to have a *receptor reserve* for this agonist. This does not of course mean that there are two kinds, spare and used—the receptors do not differ. However, only a few need to be activated to cause a large or even maximal response. This can occur when the response of the tissue is limited not by the number of active receptors but one or more of the events that follow receptor activation. For example, the maximal shortening of a piece of smooth muscle may occur in response to a rise in cytosolic calcium that is much less than can be elicited by activating all the receptors.

The situation is different with a partial agonist (see Section 1.4.1). Inactivation of any of the receptors by, for example, phenoxybenzamine will now reduce the maximal response to the partial agonist, without the initial parallel shift in the log concentration-response curve that would be seen (e.g. Figure 1.24) with a full agonist if the tissue has a substantial receptor reserve.

The existence of a receptor reserve in many tissues carries the implication that the value of the $[A]_{50}$ for a full agonist cannot give even an approximate estimate of the equilibrium dissociation constant for the combination of the agonist with its binding sites: As already mentioned, when the response is half maximal, only a small fraction of the receptors may be occupied rather than the 50% envisaged in Clark's tentative assumption of direct proportionality between occupancy and response. So pharmacologists have had to look for other approaches to determining the affinities of receptors for full agonists. Our next task is to evaluate a method based on the availability of irreversible competitive antagonists.

1.6.4 CAN AN IRREVERSIBLE COMPETITIVE ANTAGONIST BE USED TO FIND THE AFFINITY OF AN AGONIST?

The characteristic effects of an irreversible antagonist on the shape and position of an agonist concentration-response relationship (see Figure 1.24) suggested a possible way to estimate the equilibrium dissociation constant for an agonist. R. F. Furchgott was the first to explore it in detail. The experimental procedure is to compare the concentrations of agonist needed to produce a selected response (say 40% of the maximum) before and after the tissue has been exposed to the irreversible antagonist. In the fresh tissue, this response is elicited by a concentration that we represent by $[A]$; after the antagonist has acted, this has to be increased to $[A]'$. The fraction of receptors left free after the application of antagonist will be denoted by q. (If only 10% of the receptors remained unblocked, q would be 0.1). We now ask what relationship would hold between $[A]$, $[A]'$, and q. This will be approached in two ways. First (see the left column of Table 1.8) we follow Furchgott in taking as our starting point the simplest possible model for agonist action, that of Hill and Clark (see Sections 1.2.1 and 1.2.2). Although we have already seen that this scheme is deficient in failing to distinguish between the occupation and the activation of receptors, it is included for historical interest. The second approach (set out in the right column of Table 1.8) is based on a more realistic, if still basic, representation of receptor activation. This is the del Castillo–Katz model (see Section 1.2.3 and Sections 1.4.4 through 1.4.6). The application of Furchgott's method to G-protein coupled receptors is considered briefly in the "Solutions to Problems" section (see the answer to Problem 1.3).

Applying the analysis set out in the left column of Table 1.8 to the results of Figure 1.24, Furchgott estimated K_A to be 10 μM for the combination of histamine with its receptors. He used this figure, and the values of q obtained as just described, to construct the dashed curves in the illustration. These lie close to the experimental points, which is certainly in keeping with the predictions of the approach taken. Equally certainly, this does not prove that the underlying suppositions are correct. One important assumption is that the irreversible antagonist has had no action other than to inactivate the receptors under study. For example, were it to have interfered with one or more of the steps that link receptor activation to the observed response, the approach would be invalid. Furchgott later showed that this was not a complication under the conditions of his experiments.

Continuing with Furchgott's analysis of the experiment of Figure 1.24, we note that in the fresh tissue, the concentration of histamine needed to produce a half-maximal contraction was about 180 nM. The value of K_A was estimated to be 10 μM, as we have seen. Furchgott substituted these figures in the Hill–Langmuir equation to obtain a value for the receptor occupancy needed to elicit half the maximal response. This came to only 0.0177: There is a large receptor reserve. Furchgott's final step was to use this value to obtain an estimate of the efficacy of histamine, in the sense used by Stephenson. Since the response is half maximal, the stimulus as defined by Stephenson is unity, so that (from Equation 1.27) the efficacy is 1/0.0177, = 57, the value given in Figure 1.24 (see also Method 3 in Section 1.4.8).

TABLE 1.8
Example Derivations for Furchgott's Irreversible Method

Classical approach, following Furchgott, and based on the early view that all the receptors occupied by an agonist are activated	Analysis based on the del Castillo–Katz model of receptor activation (see Sections 1.2.3 and 1.4.4)

First we recall one of our two earlier definitions of p_{AR}, the proportion of binding sites occupied by A:

$$p_{AR} = \frac{N_{AR}}{N}$$

Here N_{AR} is the number of receptors in which A occupies its binding site, and N refers to the total number. Hence:

$$N_{AR} = N\frac{[A]}{K_A + [A]}$$

from the Hill–Langmuir equation.

After the irreversible antagonist has acted, N is reduced to qN, and a greater concentration of agonist, $[A]'$, must now be applied in order to achieve the same value of N_{AR} as before:

$$N_{AR} = q\,N\frac{[A]'}{K_A + [A]'}$$

Furchgott then went on to assume that the same (submaximal) response of the tissue before and after the application of antagonist corresponds to the same receptor occupancy by the agonist. Hence he equated

$$N\frac{[A]}{K_A + [A]} = qN\frac{[A]'}{K_A + [A]'}$$

Cancelling N, and inverting, gives

$$\frac{K_A}{[A]} + 1 = \frac{1}{q}\frac{K_A}{[A]'} + \frac{1}{q}$$

$$\frac{1}{[A]} = \frac{1}{q}\frac{1}{[A]'} + \frac{1}{K_A}\left(\frac{1}{q} - 1\right)$$

Hence a plot of $1/[A]$ against $1/[A]'$ should give a straight line with a slope of $1/q$ and an intercept of $(1-q)/q.K_A$. The value of q is obtained from the reciprocal of the slope, and that of K_A from (slope − 1) / intercept.

The fraction of receptors in the active state is defined by

$$p_{AR*} = \frac{N_{AR*}}{N}$$

Here N_{AR*} is the number of receptors in the active (AR*) form, of a total N. Hence:

$$N_{AR*} = N\frac{E[A]}{K_A + (1+E)[A]}$$

from Equation (1.32).

After the irreversible antagonist has acted, N is reduced to qN, and a greater concentration of agonist, $[A]'$, is needed to achieve the same value of N_{AR*} as before:

$$N_{AR*} = qN\frac{E[A]'}{K_A + (1+E)[A]'}$$

We next assume that the same (submaximal) response of the tissue before and after antagonist corresponds to the same number, N_{AR*}, of activated receptors. So we equate

$$N\frac{E[A]}{K_A + (1+E)[A]} = qN\frac{E[A]'}{K_A + (1+E)[A]'}$$

Cancelling N, and inverting, gives

$$\frac{K_A}{E[A]} + \frac{1+E}{E} = \frac{K_A}{qE[A]'} + \frac{1+E}{Eq}$$

$$\frac{1}{[A]} = \frac{1}{q}\frac{1}{[A]'} + \left(\frac{1+E}{K_A}\right)\left(\frac{1}{q} - 1\right)$$

Hence a plot of $1/[A]$ against $1/[A]'$ should give a straight line with a slope of $1/q$ and an intercept of

$$\left(\frac{1+E}{K_A}\right)\left(\frac{1}{q} - 1\right)$$

The value of q is obtained from the reciprocal of the slope, and that of $K_A/(1+E)$ from (slope − 1) / intercept.

However, the validity of these estimates, and of their interpretation, depends crucially on the appropriateness of the model for receptor activation on which the analysis is based. It is important to appreciate that the satisfactory fit of the *theoretical* (dotted) lines in Figure 1.24 does not allow one to distinguish between the two models (Hill and Clark; del Castillo–Katz) of receptor action that have been used to analyze these results. Both models make exactly the same predictions about the *form* of the relationship between [A], [A]', and q. Also, the interpretation of the value of q is the same on each model. What differs, and this is the key issue, is that accepting the concept that the receptor must isomerize to an active form carries the implication that Furchgott's irreversible antagonist method yields an estimate of the *macroscopic* equilibrium dissociation constant (K_{eff} = $K_A/(1 + E)$ for the simple del Castillo–Katz model; see Section 1.4.4) rather than of the *microscopic* equilibrium constant, K_A, for the initial binding step. Only if E is very small in relation to unity (i.e., were A to be a very weak partial agonist) does K_{eff} approximate to K_A. Note, too, that a direct radioligand binding measurement (in the absence of desensitization and other complications) would also yield an estimate of K_{eff}, and not K_A. Finding K_A requires different kinds of measurements and so far has been achieved only for ligand-gated ion channels where single channel recording allows the binding and activation steps to be distinguished, as explained in Chapter 6.

The realization that Furchgott's irreversible antagonist method estimates K_{eff}* rather than K_A has important implications for the calculation of efficacy as defined by Stephenson. As we have just seen, the experiment of Figure 1.24, as analyzed by Furchgott, had suggested that when histamine caused a half-maximal contraction of guinea-pig ileum, only 1.77% of the receptors were occupied. In the light of the foregoing discussion it is likely that this figure refers to the *total* receptor occupancy by agonist, that is, *occupied but inactive* plus *occupied and active*. Hence the value of 57 (the reciprocal of 0.0177) for the efficacy of histamine shown in Figure 1.24 has to be regarded as based on Equation (1.40) rather than Equation (1.27) as used by Furchgott. The limited usefulness of this modified definition of efficacy, e^*, has already been discussed in Section 1.4.8.

1.6.5 REVERSIBLE NONCOMPETITIVE (ALLOTOPIC) ANTAGONISM

In this variant of insurmountable antagonism, the antagonist acts by combining with a separate inhibitory site on the receptor macromolecule. Agonist and antagonist molecules can be bound at the same time, though the receptor becomes active only when the agonist site alone is occupied (Figure 1.25a). The inhibitory site is described as *secondary*, to distinguish it from the *primary* site with which the agonist combines. The terms *allotopic* and *allosteric* are also applied (see Section 1.5.1.2, item 2, and Appendix 1.6.1 as well as Neubig et al. [2003] for more on these usages).

In the presence of a large enough concentration of an antagonist of this kind, the inhibition will become insurmountable: Too few receptors remain free of antagonist to give a full response, even if all the agonist sites are occupied. The point at which this occurs in a particular tissue will depend on the numbers of spare receptors, just as with an irreversible competitive antagonist (see Section 1.6.3). If a full agonist is used, and the tissue has a large receptor reserve, the initial effect of a reversible noncompetitive antagonist will be to shift the log concentration-response curve to the right. Eventually, when no spare receptors remain, the maximum will be reduced. In contrast, if there is no receptor reserve, the antagonist will depress the maximum from the outset.

To model this form of antagonism, we make the following additional assumptions. (1) Each receptor macromolecule carries only one agonist and one antagonist (inhibitory) site. (2) Occupation of the inhibitory site by the antagonist does not change either the affinity of the other site for the agonist or the equilibrium between the active and the inactive states of the receptor on the del Castillo–Katz scheme. However, if the antagonist is bound, no response ensues even if the receptor has isomerized to the active form (i.e., BAR* in Figure 1.25b is inactive). (3) The affinity for the antagonist is not affected by the binding of the agonist or by receptor isomerization.

The proportion of the inhibitory sites occupied by the antagonist is then simply (cf. Equation 1.2):

$$p_{BR} = \frac{[B]}{K_B + [B]}$$

---

* See Equation (1.36) and also the worked answer to Problem 1.3 in the "Solutions to Problems."

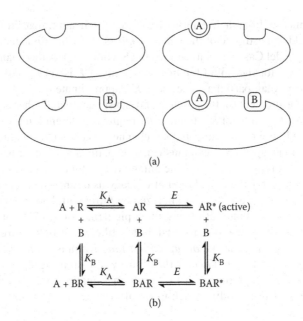

(a)

(b)

FIGURE 1.25 Noncompetitive (allotopic) antagonism. (a) A stylized receptor carries two sites. One can combine only with agonist A and the other only with antagonist B. Four conditions are possible, of which one alone can be active (agonist site occupied, antagonist site empty—top right). (b) An extension of the del Castillo–Katz scheme to this model. Only AR* leads to a response.

The proportion free of antagonist is

$$1 - p_{BR}$$

$$= \frac{K_B}{K_B + [B]}$$

On these rather extensive and not entirely realistic assumptions,[*] the fraction of the receptors in the isomerized state (AR* + BAR*) is unaffected by the presence of B and is given by Equation (1.32). However, only some of these isomerized receptors are free of antagonist and so able to initiate a response. To obtain the proportion (p_{active}) in this condition we simply multiply the fraction in the isomerized state by the fraction free of antagonist:

$$p_{active} = \left(\frac{E[A]}{K_A + (1+E)[A]} \right) \left(\frac{K_B}{K_B + [B]} \right) \tag{1.55}$$

Figure 1.26 shows log concentration-response curves drawn according to this expression. In Figure 1.26a, the response has been assumed to be directly proportional to p_{active}: there are no spare receptors. In Figure 1.26b, many spare receptors have been assumed to be present, and accordingly the application of a relatively low concentration of the antagonist causes an almost parallel shift before the maximum is reduced.

The initial near-parallel displacement of the curves in Figure 1.26b raises the question of whether the Schild equation would be obeyed under these conditions. If we consider the two concentrations of agonist ([A] and r[A] respectively, where r is the concentration ratio) that give equal responses before and during the action of the antagonist, and repeat the derivation set out in Section 1.5.2

---

[*] A more plausible model follows (Section 1.6.6).

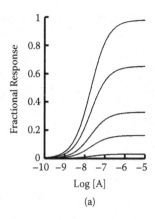 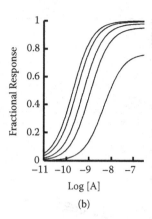

(a)   (b)

FIGURE 1.26 The effect of a reversible allotopic (noncompetitive) antagonist on the response to an agonist, (a) Each of the sets of curves has been constructed using Equation (1.55) and shows the effect of four concentrations of the antagonist (5, 20, 50, and 300 μM). K_A, K_B, and E have been taken to be 1 μM, 10 μM, and 50, respectively. For (a), the response has been assumed to be directly proportional to the fraction of receptors in the active state. (b) Has been constructed using the same values, but now assuming the presence of a large receptor reserve. This has been modeled by supposing that the relationship between the response, y, and the proportion of active receptors is given by $y = \dfrac{1.01 \times p_{\text{active}}}{0.01 + p_{\text{active}}}$, so that a half-maximal response occurs when just under 1% of the receptors are activated.

(though using Equation 1.55 rather than 1.49) we find that the expression equivalent to the Schild equation is

$$r - 1 = \frac{[\text{B}]}{K_\text{B}}\left(1 + \frac{r[\text{A}]}{K_\text{eff}}\right)$$

Here K_{eff} is as defined in Section 1.4.4. If $r[\text{A}]/K_{\text{eff}} \ll 1$ (i.e., if the proportion of receptors occupied by the agonist remains small even when the agonist concentration has been increased to overcome the effect of the reversible noncompetitive antagonist) this expression approximates to

$$r - 1 = \frac{[\text{B}]}{K_\text{B}}$$

Hence the Schild equation *would* apply, albeit over a limited range of concentrations that is determined by the receptor reserve. Moreover, the value of K_B obtained under such conditions will provide an estimate of the equilibrium dissociation constant for the combination of the antagonist with its binding sites.

A corollary is that a demonstration that the Schild equation holds over a small range of concentrations cannot be taken as proof that the action of an antagonist is competitive. Clearly, as wide as practicable a range of antagonist concentrations should be tested, especially if there is evidence for the presence of spare receptors.

1.6.5.1 Open Channel Block

Studies of ligand-gated ion channels have brought to light an interesting and important variant of reversible allotopic antagonism. It has been found that some antagonists block only those channels that are open, by entering and occluding the channel itself. In effect, the antagonist combines only with activated receptors. Examples include the block of neuronal nicotinic receptors by hexamethonium, and of NMDA receptors by dizocilpine (MK801).

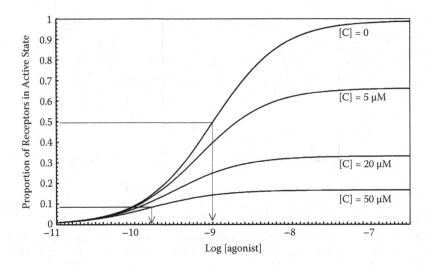

FIGURE 1.27 Curves drawn using Equation (1.57) to illustrate the effect of three concentrations of an open channel blocker, C, on the response to an agonist acting on a ligand-gated ion channel. Values of 100 nM, 100, and 10 μM were taken for K_A, E, and K_C respectively. The vertical arrows show the concentrations of agonist causing a half-maximal response in the absence and presence of C at 50 μM.

Such antagonists cause a characteristic change in the log concentration-response curve for an agonist. In contrast to what is seen with the other kinds of antagonism so far considered, the value of $[A]_{50}$ will become *smaller* rather than larger in the presence of the antagonist. This is illustrated in Figure 1.27, and is best understood in terms of the del Castillo–Katz mechanism. Incorporating the possibility that an antagonist, C, is present that combines specifically with active receptors, we have

$$\underset{\text{(inactive)}}{A+R} \rightleftharpoons \underset{\text{(inactive)}}{AR} \rightleftharpoons \underset{\text{(active)}}{AR^*} + C \rightleftharpoons \underset{\text{(inactive)}}{AR^*C} \qquad (1.56)$$

Hence there are four conditions of the receptor, R, AR, AR*, and AR*C, of which only one, AR*, is active. This scheme predicts that at equilibrium the proportion of active receptors is given by

$$p_{AR^*} = \frac{E[A]}{K_A + \left\{1 + E\left(1 + \frac{[C]}{K_C}\right)\right\}[A]} \qquad (1.57)$$

where K_c is the equilibrium dissociation constant for the combination of C with the activated receptor, AR*. This equation has been used to draw the curves shown in Figure 1.27. Note how $[A]_{50}$ decreases as the antagonist concentration is increased. This is because combination of the antagonist with AR* causes a rightward shift in the positions of the other equilibria expressed in Equation (1.56). The dependence of $[A]_{50}$ on the concentration of the blocker is given by

$$[A]_{50} = \frac{K_A}{1 + E\left(1 + \dfrac{[C]}{K_C}\right)}.$$

Note, too, that the curves plotted in Figure 1.27 converge at low agonist concentrations. The antagonist becomes less effective when the response is small, because there are fewer receptors in the AR* form available to combine with C. Again, in contrast to the other kinds of antagonism that have been described, there is no initial parallel displacement of the curves (even if there are many spare receptors) and the Schild equation is never obeyed.

Some antagonists combine the ability to block open ion channels with a competitive action at or near the agonist binding site. A well-characterized example is the nicotinic blocker tubocurarine (see Chapter 6). Agonists may also be open channel blockers, so limiting the maximal response that they can elicit. Such agents (e.g., decamethonium) may therefore behave as partial agonists when tested on an intact tissue.[*]

1.6.5.2   Co-Agonists, Allotopic Activators

The schemes illustrated in Figure 1.25 assumes that the secondary, allotopic, site is inhibitory. But there are other possibilities. It is now known that some agonists (e.g., glutamate) may be effective only in the presence of another ligand (e.g., glycine in the case of the NMDA receptors for glutamate) that binds to its own site on the receptor macromolecule. Glutamate is then referred to as the *primary agonist* and glycine as a *co-agonist*. In principle, antagonists can act by competing with either the primary agonist or the co-agonist: Both modes of antagonism have been observed.

A related possibility is that an agonist may act by combining with a secondary rather than the primary site. This too has been described, and such an agonist is termed an *allotopic* or *allosteric activator.*

1.6.6   A More General Model for the Action of Agonists, Co-Agonists, and Antagonists

The realization that many receptors show some degree of constitutive activity, that is, they can isomerize to the active state even in the absence of agonist, suggests a more general and at the same time more physically realistic model for the action of allotopic agonists and antagonists. It is illustrated in Figure 1.28 and can be regarded as a straightforward extension of the scheme for constitutive activity introduced in Section 1.4.7 (see Figure 1.11). Two ligands, A and B, can bind to different sites on the receptor so that in principle both can be present at the same time, as in the cartoon of Figure 1.25, which was the starting point for our discussion of noncompetitive antagonism. The scheme in Figure 1.28 covers a wider range of possibilities and also has the merit that it suggests a molecular mechanism not only for noncompetitive antagonism but also, as we shall see, for several

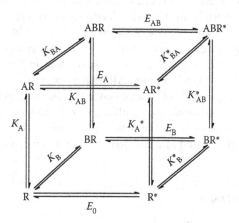

FIGURE 1.28   An extension to two ligands, A and B, of the scheme for the constitutive activity shown in Figure 1.11, which is reproduced as the front face of the cube. We suppose that A and B combine with separate sites on the receptor macromolecule, R, so that both can be bound at the same time (top edge of the rear face of the cube). Active and inactive states of the receptor are represented by the right- and left-side faces, respectively.

---

[*] As discussed in Appendix 1.4.1 (Section 1.4), the characterization of a substance as a partial agonist need not presuppose a particular mechanism for the agonist's inability to elicit a maximal effect.

other patterns of drug action. The underlying concept is that any substance that combines with an accessory (allotopic, allosteric) site can be expected to alter the equilibrium between the active and inactive states of the receptor, and therefore affect agonist action and, more generally, the fraction of receptors in the active form.

Four limiting cases of the general scheme will be considered. Each supposes that A is a conventional, positive agonist, that is, its presence increases the proportion of active receptors because of its preferential affinity for the active form.

1. The ligand B has a much greater affinity for the inactive (R, AR) than the active states (R*, AR*) of the receptor. Little BR* or ABR* is formed. In the presence of large concentrations of both A and B, most of the receptors will be in the inactive, ABR condition (top left rear vertex of the cube). B then acts as a noncompetitive antagonist (see Figure 1.29a).
2. The equilibrium dissociation constants that determine the formation of ABR and ABR* are so large (i.e., the corresponding affinities are so small) that the quantities of these doubly liganded forms are negligible. In effect, the binding of A and B is mutually exclusive. If in addition the affinity of B for the active form of the receptor is very low, B will then act as a competitive antagonist* (see Figure 1.29b).
3. B binds mainly to the active states of the receptor (R* and AR*) and in such a way that the resulting complexes (BR* and ABR*) are inactive. The predicted curves are shown in Figure 1.29c. Open channel block (see Section 1.6.5.1) provides an example (compare Figure 1.27).
4. Though A binds to R and to R*, the position of the equilibrium between A, R, and R* is now assumed to be such that little AR* is formed in the absence of B. However, if B is also present, many of the receptors enter the active ABR* configuration. Under these circumstances, B acts as a co-agonist for A: full activation requires the simultaneous presence of A and B (see Figure 1.29d).

Here (Figure 1.29a) the second ligand, B, has been assumed to have a high preferential affinity for the inactive forms of the receptor. The outcome closely mimics classical noncompetitive antagonism. In Figure 1.29b, the two ligands A and B have been assumed to combine with the receptor in an almost mutually exclusive manner. In effect, A and B are in competition and the model then predicts that increasing concentrations of B cause a near-parallel shift in the curves. In Figure 1.29c, B is assumed to combine mainly with the active forms of the receptor to form complexes (BR*, ABR*) that are inactive. An example is the action of an open channel blocker. Note the convergence of the curves at low agonist concentrations (contrast with the pattern expected for noncompetitive antagonism, Figure 1.29a and Figure 1.26). For the simulation in Figure 1.29d, the equilibrium constant for isomerization between AR and the AR* has been set so that few of the receptors are in the active state even in the presence of a large concentration of A on its own. However, with B also present at increasing concentrations, the equilibria shown in Figure 1.28 are shifted toward the active forms so that the maximum response to A rises to a point at which almost all of the receptors can be activated. In effect, B is acting as a co-agonist. Note that it causes little receptor activation when [A] is small.

APPENDICES TO SECTION 1.6

APPENDIX 1.6.1   A NOTE ON THE TERM *ALLOSTERIC*

Allosteric has come to be used in receptor pharmacology in at least three different senses, making the concept difficult, certainly for beginners and probably for most. The main usages are as follows:

---

* Here, *competitive* is defined as in Section 1.5.1.2 to include the possibility that A and B may combine with different binding sites that interact in such a way (very strong negative cooperativity) that if A is present, B cannot be, and vice versa.

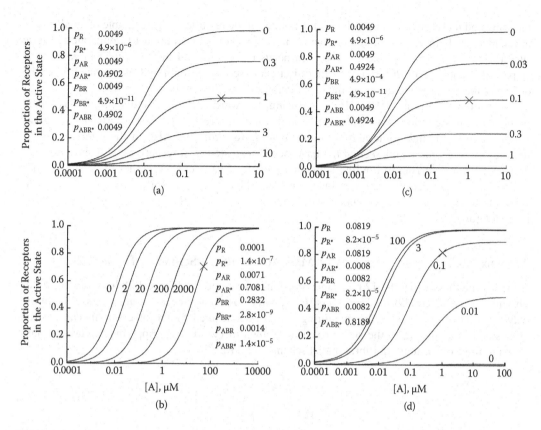

FIGURE 1.29 The effect of a second ligand on the relationship between agonist concentration ([A]) and the proportion of active receptors, as predicted by the scheme shown in Figure 1.28. Each panel illustrates the effect of the additional ligand, B, at the four concentrations (μM) indicated by the number given with each line. For panels (a), (b), and (c), but not (d), the agonist has been assumed to have a high intrinsic efficacy so that almost all of the receptors can be activated by it. An additional assumption throughout is that the constitutive activity of the receptor is low, so that in the absence of ligands, few of the receptors are active. The columns of numbers given with each panel show the fraction of receptors in each condition at the particular concentration of A indicated by X on one of the curves. The values of the equilibrium constants used in the simulations are listed in Table 1.10. See text for further explanation.

1. To denote *either* a binding site other than that for the endogenous agonist *or* a ligand that acts by combining with this other site. For example, the *allosteric antagonist* gallamine influences the activation of muscarinic receptors by binding to a distinct region (an *allosteric site*) of the receptor macromolecule. Some authors have extended this by describing the agonist site as *orthosteric*. Allosteric antagonism can be regarded as a form of noncompetitive antagonism as defined and discussed in this chapter.
2. To describe the all-or-none transition between distinct conformational states of enzymes or receptors—an *allosteric transition*. In keeping with this usage, the constant that describes the position of the equilibrium between the states (e.g., E_0 in the schemes of Figures 1.11 and 1.28) is sometimes described as the *allosteric constant*.
3. To indicate the mechanism whereby the position of the equilibrium between two or more distinct but interconvertible forms of the receptor changes in the presence of a ligand (agonist or antagonist) for which the affinity of the forms is different.

Though each of these usages is self-consistent and can be justified, it is easy to see that *allosteric*, if unqualified, can mean different things to different people. For example, the activation of the nicotinic and muscarinic receptors by acetylcholine can be regarded as an example of an allosteric mechanism as defined previously in usage 3. But acetylcholine does not act through an allosteric site, as defined in usage 1. Clearly, the term needs to be qualified in the context in which it is employed (Neubig et al., 2003). For further discussion, see the account by Colquhoun (1998), who describes the origin of the term and the evolution of the way it is used.

In an attempt to reduce the risk of confusion, the words *allotopic* and *syntopic* have been proposed as designations for *different site* and *same site*, respectively. These terms are gaining acceptance, though some authors prefer *ectopic* to *allotopic*. Also in the interest of clarity, the terms *primary* and *secondary* have been suggested as alternatives to orthosteric and allosteric when referring to binding sites on a receptor (see above). Whether these suggestions will become generally adopted remains to be seen. It has been said with good reason (and considerable feeling) that some scientists would rather use their colleague's toothbrush than their nomenclature.

APPENDIX 1.6.2   APPLYING THE LAW OF MASS ACTION TO THE SCHEME OF FIGURE 1.28

A first assumption is that the 12 reversible reactions represented in Figure 1.28 have reached equilibrium. Of the 12 equilibrium constants that specify how many receptors are in each condition, only seven need be known—the remaining five are determined by the others. This can best be understood by returning to the simpler scheme shown in Figure 1.11. Applying the law of mass action to three of the four equilibria in that scheme, we have:

$$p_{R^*} = E_0 p_R$$

$$[L]p_R = K_L p_{LR}$$

$$[L]p_{R^*} = K_L^* p_{LR^*}$$

Hence, for the remaining equilibrium,

$$E_L = \frac{p_{LR^*}}{p_{LR}} = \frac{p_{R^*}}{p_R}\frac{K_L}{K_L^*} = E_0\frac{K_L}{K_L^*}$$

We see from this that the value of the fourth equilibrium constant, that for isomerization between the active and the inactive forms of the occupied receptor, is determined by the other three, E_0, K_L, and K_L^*.

Returning to the scheme of Figure 1.28, and thinking about the choice of the seven constants that need to be specified, there are advantages in separating the seven into three primary and four secondary constants. The primary ones are taken to be E_0, K_A, and K_B, and the others are expressed as multiples of them. The four multipliers required for this are designated *a, b, d,* and *g,* for consistency with previous accounts of this scheme for receptor activation (see e.g., Colquhoun 1998 and the references therein).

Table 1.9 sets out the relationships between the three primary and the nine other equilibrium constants that appear in Figure 1.28. Table 1.10 lists the particular values used to calculate the sets of curves shown in Figure 1.29. Such calculations can be done in several ways, some being better for exposition and others making for easier evaluation with a spreadsheet. The approach that follows is more flexible, though less concise, than an alternative given in the answer to Problem 1.5.

We start by using the law of mass action to enable us to relate the fraction of receptors in each of the various conditions (R*, AR*, BR*, ABR*, AR, etc.) to the fraction (p_R) in the inactive state (R)

TABLE 1.9
Equilibrium Constants That Determine the Position of the Equilibria in Figure 1.28

Equilibrium constant in Figure 1.28	Equilibrium constants expressed in terms of E_0, K_A or K_B	Notes
E_0, K_A, K_B	—	1. The three primary constants.
K_A^*	K_A/a	2. a is the factor by which the affinity of the active form (R*) for A exceeds that of R. It also expresses the increase in the tendency for the receptor to isomerize to the active form when the binding site for A alone is occupied.
K_B^*	K_B/b	3. As above, but for B.
K_{AB}	K_A/g	4. g expresses the ratio of (1) the affinities of BR and R for A and (2) the affinities of AR and R for B. If g is very small, there will be few bi-liganded receptors (ABR, ABR*).
K_{BA}	K_B/g	See 4.
K_{AB}^*	K_A/adg	5. d, with a and g, determines the ratio of the affinities of BR* and R for A.
K_{BA}^*	K_B/bdg	6. d, with b and g, determines the ratio of the affinities of AR* and R for B.
E_A	aE_0	See 2.
E_B	bE_0	See 3.
E_{AB}	$abdE_0$	7. The product of a, b, and d relates the isomerization of ABR to ABR* to that of R to R*.

TABLE 1.10
Values Used in the Simulations Illustrated in Figure 1.29a,b,c,d

Equilibrium constant[1]	Value of multiplier[2]	Panel (a)	Panel (b)	Panel (c)	Panel (d)
	a	100000	100000	100000	10
	b	0.00001	0.00001	0.0001	10
	d	10	10	10000	1000
	g	100	0.0001	10	1
E_0		0.001	0.001	0.001	0.001
K_A		1	1	1	1
K_B		1	1	1	1
K_A^*		0.00001	0.00001	0.00001	0.1
K_B^*		100000	100000	10000	0.1
K_{AB}		0.01	10000	0.1	1
K_{BA}		0.01	10000	0.1	1
K_{AB}^*		0.00000001	0.01	1E–10	0.0001
K_{BA}^*		100	100000000	0.1	0.0001
E_A		100	100	100	0.01
E_B		0.00000001	0.00000001	0.0000001	0.01
E_{AB}		0.01	0.01	100	100

[1]. The units for all the equilibrium dissociation constants listed are µM.

[2]. These multipliers are used to calculate the secondary constants, (e.g., K^*_A, E_A) from the primary ones (E_0, K_A, K_B), as listed in Table 1.9. For example, if $E_0 = 0.001$ and $a = 100000$, then E_A ($= aE_0$) = 100. Similarly, K^*_A ($= K_A/a$) = 1/100000, = 0.00001 µM.

with both binding sites vacant:

$$p_{R*} = E_0 p_R$$

$$p_{AR*} = \frac{[A]}{K_A^*} p_{R*} = E_0 \frac{[A]}{K_A^*} p_R$$

$$p_{BR*} = \frac{[B]}{K_B^*} p_{R*} = E_0 \frac{[B]}{K_B^*} p_R$$

$$p_{ABR*} = \frac{[B]}{K_{BA}^*} p_{AR*} = E_0 \frac{[B]}{K_{BA}^*} \frac{[A]}{K_A^*} p_R$$

$$p_{AR} = \frac{[A]}{K_A} p_R$$

$$p_{BR} = \frac{[B]}{K_B} p_R$$

$$p_{ABR} = \frac{[B]}{K_{BA}} p_{AR} = \frac{[B]}{K_{BA}} \frac{[A]}{K_A} p_R$$

Also,

$$p_{R*} + p_{AR*} + p_{BR*} + p_{ABR*} + p_R + p_{AR} + p_{BR} + p_{ABR} = 1$$

Substituting for p_{R*}, p_{AR*}, and so forth, in this expression, we have

$$p_R \left(E_0 + E_0 \frac{[A]}{K_A^*} + E_0 \frac{[B]}{K_B^*} + E_0 \frac{[B]}{K_{BA}^*} \frac{[A]}{K_A^*} + 1 + \frac{[A]}{K_A} + \frac{[B]}{K_B} + \frac{[B]}{K_{BA}} \frac{[A]}{K_A} \right) = 1$$

Hence,

$$p_R = \frac{1}{E_0 \left(1 + \frac{[A]}{K_A^*} + \frac{[B]}{K_B^*} + \frac{[B]}{K_{BA}^*} \frac{[A]}{K_A^*} \right) + 1 + \frac{[A]}{K_A} + \frac{[B]}{K_B} + \frac{[B]}{K_{BA}} \frac{[A]}{K_A}} \qquad (1.58)$$

This expression, together with the mass law equilibrium equations just listed, can now be used to calculate the proportions of receptors in any condition or combination of conditions. For example, the fraction in the active state is given by

$$p_{active} = p_{R*} + p_{AR*} + p_{BR*} + p_{ABR*}$$

$$= E_0 \left(1 + \frac{[A]}{K_A^*} + \frac{[B]}{K_B^*} + \frac{[B]}{K_{BA}^*} \frac{[A]}{K_A^*} \right) p_R$$

Substituting for p_R using Equation (1.58) provides the final expression relating the fraction of receptors in the active form to the concentrations of A and B:

$$P_{active} = \frac{E_0}{E_0 + \left(\dfrac{1 + \dfrac{[A]}{K_A} + \dfrac{[B]}{K_B} + \dfrac{[B]}{K_{BA}} \dfrac{[A]}{K_A}}{1 + \dfrac{[A]}{K_A^*} + \dfrac{[B]}{K_B^*} + \dfrac{[B]}{K_{BA}^*} \dfrac{[A]}{K_A^*}} \right)} \cdot \qquad (1.59)$$

This has been used to construct the sets of curves in Figure 1.29*.

---

* Though for panel (c), p_{active} is taken to be $p_{R*} + p_{AR*}$, in keeping with the hypothesis that in this instance BR* and ABR* do not contribute to the response.

In the same way, the proportion of receptors in which A occupies its binding site is given by

$$p_{occupied(A)} = p_{AR} + p_{AR*} + p_{ABR} + p_{ABR*}$$

$$= \left(\frac{[A]}{K_A} + E_0 \frac{[A]}{K_A^*} + \frac{[B]}{K_{BA}} \frac{[A]}{K_A} + E_0 \frac{[B]}{K_{BA}^*} \frac{[A]}{K_A^*} \right) p_R$$

Using Equation (1.58) to substitute for p_R, we have

$$p_{occupied(A)} = \frac{\dfrac{[A]}{K_A} + E_0 \dfrac{[A]}{K_A^*} + \dfrac{[B]}{K_{BA}} \dfrac{[A]}{K_A} + E_0 \dfrac{[B]}{K_{BA}^*} \dfrac{[A]}{K_A^*}}{\dfrac{[A]}{K_A} + E_0 \dfrac{[A]}{K_A^*} + \dfrac{[B]}{K_{BA}} \dfrac{[A]}{K_A} + E_0 \dfrac{[B]}{K_{BA}^*} \dfrac{[A]}{K_A^*} + 1 + E_0 \left(1 + \dfrac{[B]}{K_B^*} \right) + \dfrac{[B]}{K_B}}$$

$$= \frac{1}{1 + \left\{ \dfrac{1 + E_0 \left(1 + \dfrac{[B]}{K_B^*} \right) + \dfrac{[B]}{K_B}}{\dfrac{[A]}{K_A} + E_0 \dfrac{[A]}{K_A^*} + \dfrac{[B]}{K_{BA}} \dfrac{[A]}{K_A} + E_0 \dfrac{[B]}{K_{BA}^*} \dfrac{[A]}{K_A^*}} \right\}}$$

Using the relationship $E_0 = \dfrac{K_A^*}{K_A} E_A$,

$$= \frac{[A]}{K_A \left\{ \dfrac{1 + E_0 \left(1 + \dfrac{[B]}{K_B^*} \right) + \dfrac{[B]}{K_B}}{1 + E_A \left(1 + \dfrac{[B]}{K_{BA}^*} \right) + \dfrac{[B]}{K_{BA}}} \right\} + [A]}$$

From this we see that the relation between the concentration of A and the amount of it that is bound should follow the Hill–Langmuir equation. K_{eff}, the macroscopic equilibrium dissociation constant, is given by

$$K_{eff} = \left\{ \frac{1 + E_0 \left(1 + \dfrac{[B]}{K_B^*} \right) + \dfrac{[B]}{K_B}}{1 + E_A \left(1 + \dfrac{[B]}{K_{BA}^*} \right) + \dfrac{[B]}{K_{BA}}} \right\} K_A$$

$$= \left\{ \frac{1 + E_0 + (1 + E_B) \dfrac{[B]}{K_B}}{1 + E_A + (1 + E_{AB}) \dfrac{[B]}{K_{BA}}} \right\} K_A$$

Note that the term in the large brackets can be greater or less than unity, depending on the values of the six constants. Hence the presence of B can either increase or reduce the binding of A.

1.7 CONCLUDING REMARKS

Modeling the action of receptors in the ways outlined in this chapter remains of value because it allows the effects of drugs to be better described, quantified, and analyzed. But it should be kept in mind that the key advances in understanding what receptors are, and how they work, have come not from modeling and equation writing but rather from developments in experimental techniques such as the radioligand binding method, single channel recording, and the procedures of molecular biology that allow the structures of receptors to be determined and then modified in precise ways. These are the subjects of the chapters that follow.

PROBLEMS

PROBLEM 1.1

A competitive antagonist (B) is applied to a tissue and produces a concentration ratio r_B. A second competitive antagonist (C) acting at the same receptors produces a concentration ratio r_C, under identical conditions. The tissue is next exposed to both antagonists together, at the same concentrations as in the separate applications. The concentration ratio is now observed to be r_{B+C}.

What relationship might be expected to hold between r_B, r_C, and r_{B+C}? Assume that the del Castillo–Katz mechanism of receptor activation holds in its simplest form (Equation 1.7).

PROBLEM 1.2

When studying competitive antagonism, it is sometimes necessary to include an uptake inhibitor or a ganglion blocker in all the bathing solutions used. If this compound has in addition some competitive blocking action at the receptor being studied, how will this affect the estimation of the equilibrium dissociation constant for the competitive antagonist?

PROBLEM 1.3

What quantity would Furchgott's irreversible antagonist method (Section 1.6.4) estimate if the occupied receptor, AR, has first to isomerize to a second form, AR*, which then attaches to another entity, such as a G-protein, in order to elicit a response (as in Equation 1.38)? Assume that the G-protein is present in great excess in relation to the receptors.

PROBLEM 1.4

Derive Equation (1.39) (Section 1.4.7), which expresses how the proportion of active receptors varies with the concentration of a ligand that combines with a receptor with constitutive activity.

PROBLEM 1.5

Apply the law of mass action to work out the proportion of receptors in the active form (p_{active}) for the mechanism for receptor activation shown in Figure 1.14. What will be the value of EC_{50} under these circumstances? (Assume that the response measured is directly proportional to p_{active}.)

SOLUTIONS TO PROBLEMS

PROBLEM 1.1

We have three experimental situations to consider (see Figure 1.30): (1) and (2) are straightforward (see Section 1.5.2) whereas (3) breaks new ground.

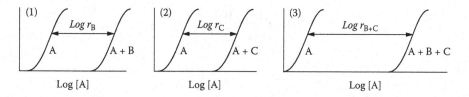

FIGURE 1.30 Schematic Dose-Respose Curves for Problem 1.1.

When B and C are applied together, as in (3) above, and the agonist A is also present, there will be four simultaneous equilibria (at least in principle):

$$A + R \xrightleftharpoons{K_A} AR \xrightleftharpoons{E} AR*$$

$$B + R \xrightleftharpoons{K_B} BR$$

$$C + R \xrightleftharpoons{K_C} CR$$

Applying the law of mass action:

$$[A]p_R = K_A p_{AR}$$

$$p_{AR*} = E p_{AR}$$

$$[B]p_R = K_B p_{BR}$$

$$[C]p_R = K_C p_{CR}$$

Also (see Section 1.5.2),

$$p_R + p_{AR} + p_{AR*} + p_{BR} + p_{CR} = 1$$

From these equations,

$$p_{AR*} = \frac{E[A]}{K_A\left(1 + \dfrac{[B]}{K_B} + \dfrac{[C]}{K_C}\right) + (1 + E)[A]}$$

Hence, equating equal receptor activations by the agonist (at which it is assumed that the responses would also be equal), first in the absence of any antagonist and then in the simultaneous presence of B and C:

$$\frac{E[A]}{K_A + (1 + E)[A]} = \frac{E r_{B+C}[A]}{K_A\left(1 + \dfrac{[B]}{K_B} + \dfrac{[C]}{K_C}\right) + (1 + E)r_{B+C}[A]}$$

$$\frac{E[A]}{K_A + (1 + E)[A]} = \frac{E[A]}{K_A\left(\dfrac{1 + \dfrac{[B]}{K_B} + \dfrac{[C]}{K_C}}{r_{B+C}}\right) + (1 + E)[A]}$$

$$\frac{1+\dfrac{[B]}{K_B}+\dfrac{[C]}{K_C}}{r_{B+C}}=1$$

$$r_{B+C}-1=\frac{[B]}{K_B}+\frac{[C]}{K_C}$$

$$r_{B+C}-1=(r_B-1)+(r_C-1)$$

$$\therefore\quad r_{B+C}=r_B+r_C-1$$

This relationship has often been used to obtain evidence that two antagonists act at the same site. It also applies if we use the Gaddum equation as the starting point rather than expressions based on the del Castillo–Katz mechanism.

PROBLEM 1.2

We will use B to denote the competitive antagonist being investigated and C to represent the substance with some competitive blocking action that is present in all the bathing solutions used in the experiment.

When the control curve is determined, the tissue is exposed to both the agonist A and the substance C at concentrations [A] and [C] respectively. Assuming equilibrium, the proportion of receptors in the active state is then

$$p_{AR*}=\frac{E[A]}{K_A\left(1+\dfrac{[C]}{K_C}\right)+(1+E)[A]}\qquad\text{(see Equation 1.49)}$$

When the competitive antagonist B is also applied, the concentration of A has to be increased by a factor r, the concentration ratio, to restore the same response. The proportion of receptors in the active state is then

$$p_{AR*}=\frac{Er[A]}{K_A\left(1+\dfrac{[B]}{K_B}+\dfrac{[C]}{K_C}\right)+(1+E)r[A]}$$

(see the answer to Problem 1.1).

Assuming that equal responses correspond to equal receptor activations in the two situations (i.e., with and without B present), we can write

$$1+\frac{[C]}{K_C}=\frac{1+\dfrac{[B]}{K_B}+\dfrac{[C]}{K_C}}{r}$$

so that

$$r-1=\frac{[B]}{K_B\left(1+\dfrac{[C]}{K_C}\right)}$$

Hence a Schild plot based on the results of such an experiment will give an estimate not of K_B but of $K_B(1+[C]/K_C)$.

PROBLEM 1.3

Here the scheme for receptor activation is as shown in Equation (1.38) in Section 1.4.6. There are three equilibria, and applying the law of mass action to each gives

$$[A]p_R = K_A p_{AR}$$

$$p_{AR^*} = E p_{AR}$$

$$[G]p_{AR^*} = K_{ARG} p_{AR^*G^*}$$

Also,

$$p_R + p_{AR} + p_{AR^*} + p_{AR^*G^*} = 1$$

Using the mass law equilibrium equations to substitute for p_R, p_{AR}, and p_{AR^*} in this expression, we obtain

$$p_{AR^*G^*} = \frac{E[G]_T[A]}{K_A K_{ARG} + \left\{ E[G]_T + K_{ARG}(1+E) \right\}[A]}$$

It has been assumed here that G is present in such excess that its total concentration $[G]_T$ does not fall appreciably when AR*G* is formed. [G] in the mass law equation can then be replaced by $[G]_T$.

If we now consider Furchgott's analysis of the effect of an irreversible antagonist on the response to an agonist, and make the same assumptions as in Section 1.6.4, we can write

$$\frac{E[R]_T[G]_T[A]}{K_A K_{ARG} + \left\{ E[G]_T + K_{ARG}(1+E) \right\}[A]} = \frac{qE[R]_T[G]_T[A]'}{K_A K_{ARG} + \left\{ E[G]_T + K_{ARG}(1+E) \right\}[A]'}$$

Here, just as before, [A] and [A]′ are the concentrations of the agonist A that produce the same response (assumed to correspond to the same concentrations of receptors in the active, AR*G*, form) before and after reducing the total concentration of receptors from $[R]_T$ to $q[R]_T$.

Cancelling E, $[G]_T$ and $[R]_T$ in the numerators, and inverting, we obtain

$$\frac{1}{[A]} = \frac{1}{q}\frac{1}{[A]'} + \left(\frac{E[G]_T + K_{ARG}(1+E)}{K_A K_{ARG}} \right)\left(\frac{1}{q} - 1 \right)$$

Hence a plot of 1/[A] against 1/[A]′ should again give a straight line of slope $1/q$, and the quantity estimated by (slope−1)/intercept would be

$$\frac{K_A K_{ARG}}{E[G]_T + K_{ARG}(1+E)}$$

This is just what would be estimated by a direct ligand binding experiment were this scheme for receptor occupation and activation to apply.

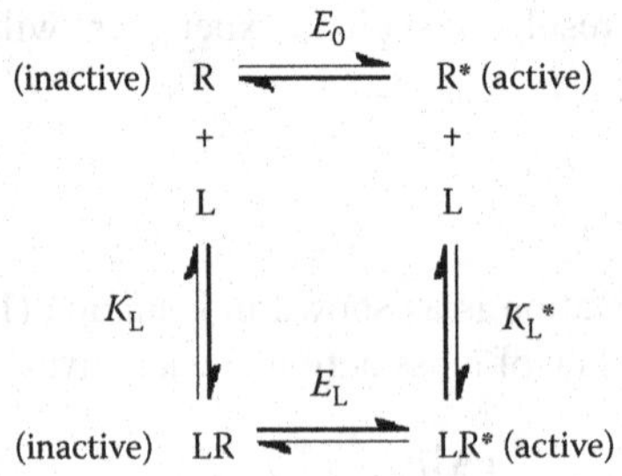

$$(\text{inactive}) \quad R \xrightleftharpoons{\quad E_0 \quad} R^* \ (\text{active})$$

$$+ \qquad\qquad +$$

$$L \qquad\qquad L$$

$$K_L \ \big\updownarrow \qquad\qquad \big\updownarrow \ K_L^*$$

$$(\text{inactive}) \quad LR \xrightleftharpoons{\quad E_L \quad} LR^* \ (\text{active})$$

FIGURE 1.31   Model for Problem 1.4.

PROBLEM 1.4

The model is shown in Figure 1.31, from which we see that there are three equilibria to consider (the fourth is determined by the position of the other three—see Appendix 1.6.2). Applying the law of mass action to three of the equilibria, we have

$$p_{R^*} = E_0 p_R$$

$$[L] p_R = K_L p_{LR}$$

$$[L] p_{R^*} = K_L^* p_{LR^*}$$

where the equilibrium constants E_0, K_L, and K_L^* are as defined in Section 1.4.7.

Also,

$$p_R + p_{R^*} + p_{LR} + p_{LR^*} = 1$$

By using the mass law equilibrium expressions to substitute for p_R, p_{R^*}, and p_{LR} in the last equation, we obtain

$$p_{LR^*} = \frac{E_0[L]}{E_0\left([L] + K_L^*\right) + K_L^*\left(1 + \dfrac{[L]}{K_L}\right)}.$$

From this, and using the third of the equilibrium expressions, we also have

$$p_{R^*} = \frac{E_0 K_L^*}{E_0\left([L] + K_L^*\right) + K_L^*\left(1 + \dfrac{[L]}{K_L}\right)}$$

We wish to know the total fraction of receptors in the active state,

$$p_{\text{active}} = p_{R^*} + p_{LR^*}$$

$$= \frac{E_0\left([L] + K_L^*\right)}{E_0\left([L] + K_L^*\right) + K_L^*\left(1 + \dfrac{[L]}{K_L}\right)}$$

$$= \frac{E_0}{E_0 + \left(\dfrac{1 + \dfrac{[L]}{K_L}}{1 + \dfrac{[L]}{K_L^*}}\right)}$$

This derivation has followed the same general procedure applied throughout this chapter. Another route is instructive:

$$p_{\text{active}} = p_{R^*} + p_{LR^*}$$

$$= \frac{[R^*]+[LR^*]}{[R^*]+[LR^*]+[R]+[LR]}$$

$$= \frac{1}{1+\left(\dfrac{[R]+[LR]}{[R^*]+[LR^*]}\right)}$$

Considering just the term in brackets, and making use of the three equilibrium equations, we have

$$\frac{[R]+[LR]}{[R^*]+[LR^*]} = \frac{[R]}{[R^*]}\left(\frac{1+\dfrac{[LR]}{[R]}}{1+\dfrac{[LR^*]}{[R^*]}}\right) = \frac{1}{E_0}\left(\frac{1+\dfrac{[L]}{K_L}}{1+\dfrac{[L]}{K_L^*}}\right)$$

Hence Equation (1.39) has been derived.

PROBLEM 1.5

Here the model is formally similar to the one discussed in Appendix 1.6.2, which describes the application of the law of mass action to a scheme (Figure 1.28) in which each receptor macromolecule carries a separate binding site for each of two ligands. However, in the mechanism for the action of a GPCR illustrated in Figure 1.14, only two (R*G and LR*G) of the eight possible conditions of the receptor are active. The diagram in Figure 1.32 reproduces Figure 1.14 with the addition of the twelve equilibrium constants.

Using the second approach introduced in the solution to the last problem, we can write the fraction of active receptors as

$$P_{\text{active}} = \frac{[R^*G]+[LR^*G]}{[R]+[R^*]+[LR]+[LR^*]+[RG]+[R^*G]+[LRG]+[LR^*G]}$$

$$= \frac{1}{1+\left(\dfrac{[R]+[R^*]+[LR]+[LR^*]+[RG]+[LRG]}{[R^*G]+[LR^*G]}\right)}$$

$$= \frac{1}{1+\dfrac{[R]}{[R^*]}\left(\dfrac{1+\dfrac{[R^*]}{[R]}+\dfrac{[LR]}{[R]}+\dfrac{[LR^*]}{[R]}+\dfrac{[RG]}{[R]}+\dfrac{[LRG]}{[R]}}{\dfrac{[R^*G]}{[R^*]}+\dfrac{[LR^*G]}{[R^*]}}\right)}$$

By using the relationships obtained from applying the law of mass action to the individual equilibria in the scheme (see Appendix 1.6.2), this can be rewritten as

$$p_{\text{active}} = \frac{E_0}{E_0+\left\{\dfrac{1+E_0+\dfrac{[L]}{K_L}+E_0\dfrac{[L]}{K_L^*}+\dfrac{[G]}{K_G}+\dfrac{[G]}{K_{GL}}\dfrac{[L]}{K_L}}{\dfrac{[G]}{K_G^*}+\dfrac{[G]}{K_{GL}^*}\dfrac{[L]}{K_L^*}}\right\}}$$

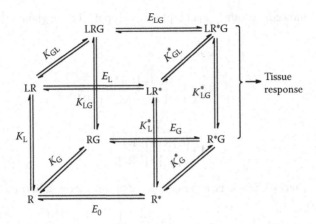

FIGURE 1.32   Model for Problem 1.5.

Rearrangement, and making use of the relationships between the equilibrium constants set out in Table 1.9 (see Appendix 1.6.2 for more detail), provides the expression we require:

$$p_{active} = \frac{E_G \dfrac{[G]}{K_G}\left(1 + \dfrac{[L]}{K_{LG}^*}\right)}{1 + E_0 + (1 + E_G)\dfrac{[G]}{K_G} + \left\{1 + E_L + (1 + E_{LG})\dfrac{[G]}{K_{GL}}\right\}\dfrac{[L]}{K_L}} \tag{1.60}$$

In the absence of the ligand L, Equation (1.60) reduces to

$$p_{active(min)} = \frac{E_G \dfrac{[G]}{K_G}}{1 + E_0 + (1 + E_G)\dfrac{[G]}{K_G}}$$

This predicts the constitutive activity of the GPCR. Note the dependence on the effective concentration of the G-protein.

If the concentration of L is made very large, the proportion of the receptors in the active state rises to

$$p_{active(max)} = \frac{E_{LG} \dfrac{[G]}{K_{GL}}}{1 + E_L + (1 + E_{LG})\dfrac{[G]}{K_{GL}}}$$

Assuming, finally, that we are fortunate enough to be dealing with a simple response that is directly proportional to the fraction of receptors in the active condition, we can go on to predict the EC$_{50}$. This is the concentration of L that causes the response to rise from its value, y_{min}, in the absence of L to y_{min} plus 50% of the maximum increase ($y_{max} - y_{min}$) that L can induce. More formally, and assuming direct proportionality between y and p_{active}, we can write

$$p_{active(EC_{50})} = p_{active(min)} + \frac{1}{2}\left(p_{active(max)} - p_{active(min)}\right)$$

$$= \frac{1}{2}\left(p_{active(max)} + p_{active(min)}\right)$$

Using Equation (1.60) and the expressions for $p_{\text{active(min)}}$ and $p_{\text{active(max)}}$ just derived, we find that the value of EC_{50} is given by

$$\left\{ \frac{1 + E_0 + (1 + E_G)\dfrac{[G]}{K_G}}{1 + E_L + (1 + E_{LG})\dfrac{[G]}{K_{GL}}} \right\} K_L$$

In Appendix 1.6.2 we obtained an expression for the macroscopic equilibrium dissociation constant, K_{eff}, for the binding of a ligand on the same scheme as in Figure 1.14. Allowing for the differences in terms, K_{eff} and EC_{50} are seen to be identical.

FURTHER READING

GENERAL

Terms and Symbols in Receptor Pharmacology

Neubig, R.R., Spedding, M., Kenakin, T.P. and Christopoulos, A., International Union of Pharmacology Committee on Receptor Nomenclature and Drug Classification. XXXVIII. Update on Terms and Symbols in Quantitative Pharmacology. *Pharmacol. Rev.*, 55, 597–606, 2003.

Three Useful Books

Kenakin, T.P. *A Pharmacology Primer: Theory, Applications and Methods.* 3rd ed. Elsevier Academic Press, Amsterdam, 2009.

Kenakin, T., and Angus, J.A. The Pharmacology of Functional, Biochemical and Recombinant Receptor Systems. In *Handbook of Experimental Pharmacology*, Vol. 148, 2000.

Limbird, L.E. *Cell Surface Receptors: A Short Course on Theory and Methods.* 3rd ed. Springer, New York, 2005.

EARLY WORK

General

Colquhoun, D. The quantitative analysis of drug-receptor interactions: A short history. *Trends Pharmacol. Sci.* 27, 149–157, 2006.

Prüll, C.-R., Maehle, A.-H., and Halliwell, R.F. *A Short History of the Drug Receptor Concept.* Palgrave Macmillan, Basingstoke, 2009.

The Hill–Langmuir Equation and the Application of the Law of Mass Action to the Kinetics of Drug-Receptor Interaction

Hill, A.V. The mode of action of nicotine and curari, determined by the form of the contraction curve and the method of temperature coefficients. *J. Physiol.* 39, 361–373, 1909.

The Hill Equation

Hill, A.V. The possible effects of the aggregation of the molecules of haemoglobin on its dissociation curve. *J. Physiol.* 40, iv–vii, 1910.

Clark's Modeling of the Concentration-Response Relationship

Clark, A.J. The reaction between acetylcholine and muscle cells. *J. Physiol.* 61, 530–547, 1926.

The Gaddum Equation

Gaddum, J.H. The quantitative effect of antagonistic drugs. *J. Physiol.* 89, 7–99P, 1937.

Gaddum, J.H. The antagonism of drugs. *Trans. Faraday Soc.* 39, 323–332, 1943.

The pA Scale

Schild, H.O. pA, a new scale for the measurement of drug antagonism. *Br. J. Pharmacol.* 2, 189–206, 1947.

The Schild Equation

Schild, H.O. pA_x and competitive drug antagonism. *Br. J. Pharmacol.* 4, 277–280, 1949.
Schild, H.O. Drug antagonism and pA_x. *Pharmacol. Rev.* 9, 242–246, 1957.

EFFICACY

Colquhoun, D. Binding, gating, affinity and efficacy. The interpretation of structure-activity relationships and of the effects of mutating receptors. *Br. J. Pharmacol.* 125, 924–947, 1998.
Samama, P., Cotecchia, S., Costa, T., and Lefkowitz, R.J. A mutation-induced activated state of the β_2-adrenergic receptor: Extending the ternary complex model. *J. Biol. Chem.* 268, 4625–4636, 1993.
Stephenson, R.P. A modification of receptor theory. *Br. J. Pharmacol.* 11, 379–393, 1956.
Vilardaga, J.-P., Bünemann, M., Feinstein, T.N., Lambert, N., Nikolaev, V.O., Engelhardt, S., Lohse, M.J., and Hoffmann, C. GPCR and G-proteins: Drug efficacy and activation in live cells. *Mol. Endocrinol.* 23, 590–599, 2009.

ANTAGONISM

General

Wyllie, D., and Chen, P.M. Taking the time to study competitive antagonism. *Br. J. Pharmacol.* 150, 541–551, 2007.

Examples of the Practical Application of Schild's Approach to the Study of Antagonism

Arunlakshana, O. and Schild, H.O. Some quantitative uses of drug antagonists. *Br. J. Pharmacol.* 14, 48–58, 1959.
Black, J.W., Duncan, W.A.M., Durant, C.J., Ganellin, C.R., and Parsons, E.M. Definition and antagonism of histamine H_2-receptors. *Nature* 236, 385–390, 1972.

Additional Example of Analysis of Deviations from the Schild Equation

Black, J.W., Leff, P., and Shankley, N.P. Further analysis of anomalous pK_B values for histamine H_2-receptor antagonists on the mouse isolated stomach assay. *Br. J. Pharmacol.* 86, 581–587, 1985.

Applications of Irreversible Antagonists (Receptor Protection Experiments, Attempted Determination of K_A for Agonists)

Bodenstein, J., Venter, D.P., and Brink, C.B. Phenoxybenzamine and benextramine, but not 4-diphenylacetoxy-N-[2-chloroethyl]piperidine hydrochloride, display irreversible noncompetitive antagonism at G protein-coupled receptors. *J Pharmacol. Exp. Ther.* 314, 891–905 (2005).
Eglen, R.M., and Harris, G.C. Selective inactivation of muscarinic M_2 and M_3 receptors in guinea-pig ileum and atria *in vitro*. *Br. J. Pharmacol.* 109, 946–952, 1993.
Furchgott, R.F. The use of β-haloalkylamines in the differentiation of receptors and in the determination of dissociation constants of receptor-agonist complexes. *Adv. Drug Res.* 3, 21–55, 1966.
Morey, T.E., Belardinelli, L., and Dennis, D.M. Validation of Furchgott's method to determine agonist-dependent A_1-adenosine receptor reserve in guinea-pig atrium. *Br. J. Pharmacol.* 123, 1425–1433, 1998.

Section II

Molecular Structure of Receptors

2 Structure and Function of 7-TM G-Protein Coupled Receptors

Alasdair J. Gibb

CONTENTS

2.1 INTRODUCTION

The G-protein coupled receptors (GPCRs) generate a response by linking drug binding at the extracellular part of the receptor protein to activation of particular intracellular guanosine triphosphate (GTP) binding proteins (Brown, Chapter 7). Many GPCRs are hormone receptors and respond to changes in hormone concentration circulating in the blood. Many other GPCRs respond to the release of neurotransmitters at synapses in the brain or in the periphery. GPCRs may be located at a synapse; pre-, post- or perisynaptically; and mediate slow synaptic transmission (on a time scale of 100 ms to seconds) whose characteristics will depend on the particular G-protein that couples to the receptor.

GPCRs represent the largest and most diverse class of membrane receptors: a superfamily of structurally related receptor proteins predicted to have seven transmembrane (7-TM) domains that range from rhodopsin to the odorant receptors. Some representative examples of the diversity of GPCRs are listed in Table 2.1. The human genome contains more than 800 7-TM protein sequences, some of which are still *orphan receptors* without an identified physiological ligand.

The importance of the GPCRs to healthcare is enormous: It is estimated that about 40% of prescription medicines in Europe and the United States are targeted at GPCRs.

TABLE 2.1

Common Examples of G-Protein Coupled Receptors

Amino acid receptors: metabtropic glutamate and GABA$_B$ receptors

Monoamine receptors: adrenoceptors, muscarinic receptors, 5HT receptors, etc.

Lipid receptors: prostaglandin, thromboxane, and PAF receptors

Purine receptors: adenosine and ATP receptors

Neuropeptide receptors: neuropeptide Y, opiate, cholecystokinin VIP receptors, etc.

Peptide hormone receptors: angiotensin, bradykinin, glucagon, parathyroid receptors, etc.

Chemokine receptors: interleukin receptors, CXCR receptors

Glycoprotein receptors: TSH, LH/FSH, choriongonadotropin receptors, etc.

Protease receptors: thrombin receptor

Wnt receptors: frizzled and smoothened receptors

2.1.1   G-Proteins

The G-proteins act as transducers between the receptor and the effector system and are presented in detail in Chapter 7. These are heterotrimeric proteins composed of α and βγ subunits. Both α and βγ subunits are involved in mediating the response to receptor activation. The α subunit determines which class the G-protein belongs to. Four general classes of G-protein are identified based on their sensitivity (or lack of) to cholera and pertussis toxins:

- G$_s$—Activates adenylyl cyclase (irreversibly activated by cholera toxin)
- G$_{i/0}$-G$_i$—Inhibits adenylyl cyclase (irreversibly inactivated by pertussis toxin); G$_o$ modulates Ca^{2+} and K$^+$ channels (irreversibly inactivated by pertussis toxin)
- G$_q$—Activates phospholipase-C (no modifying toxin)
- G$_{12/13}$—Activates the small GTPase Rho and phospholipase Cε (no modifying toxin)

Upon receptor activation following agonist binding, the G-protein splits into α and βγ subunits. The α subunits then bind to enzymes or βγ subunits to ion channels or other effectors, altering the effector activity and giving rise to the response. Typical examples of effector mechanism are as follows:

- G$_s$—Raising cAMP[*] and hence increasing PKA[†] activity
- G$_i$—Decreasing cAMP and hence reducing PKA activity; activates inward rectifier potassium channels (GIRK[‡] channels)
- G$_o$—Inhibition of voltage-dependent Ca^{2+} channels (N- and P/Q-type) and reduced neurotransmitter release
- G$_q$—IP$_3$[§] and DAG[¶] from membrane PIP$_2$[**] resulting in raised intracellular (Ca^{2+}) and PKC[††] activation. Decrease in membrane PIP$_2$ results in reduced activity of PIP$_2$ sensitive channels such as the KCNQ[‡‡] potassium channels (M-channels)
- G$_{12/13}$—Activation of Rho and stress fiber formation

Within each receptor family diversity of signaling is enhanced by selective coupling to different G-proteins (Table 2.2). For example, the five subtypes of the muscarinic receptor are separated neatly

---

[*] cAMP: Cyclic adenosine5′ monophosphate

[†] 2PKA: Protein kinase A

[‡] GIRK: G-protein activated inwardly activating potassium channel

[§] IP3: Inositol-3,4,5-trisphosphate

[¶] DAG: Diacylglycerol

[**] PIP2: Phosphatidylinositol-4,5-bisphosphate

[††] PKC: Protein kinase C

[‡‡] KCNQ: Potassium channels of the Kv7.2/7.3 subtype

TABLE 2.2
Examples of Receptor G-Protein Coupling

Receptor	G-Protein	Receptor	G-Protein
ACh-Muscarinic		Dopamine	
m1, m3, m5	G_q, $G_{12/13}$	D_1 D_5	G_s
m2, m4	G_o, G_i	D_2, D_3, D_4	G_o, G_i
Histamine		Opiate	
H_1, H_3	G_q	μ, δ, κ	G_o, G_i
H_2	G_s		
		$GABA_B$	G_o, G_i
Adrenoceptors		Glutamate-Metabotropic	
α_1	G_q, $G_{12/13}$	mGluR1, 5	G_q
α_2	G_o, G_i	mGluR2, 3	G_i
β_1, β_2, β_3, β_4	G_s	mGluR4, 6, 7,8	G_o, G_i

into even numbers (m_2 and m_4) coupling to G_i and G_o, and odd numbers (m_1, m_3, and m_5) coupling to G_q. Selectivity of G-protein coupling is determined primarily by the third intracellular loop (between transmembrane domains TM5 and TM6—Figure 2.1). $G_{12/13}$ signaling allows GPCR activation to link to cell shape changes and cell migration in the vasculature. Interestingly, most hormones can act on receptor subtypes that couple to two or three of the four G-protein classes, but rarely all four.

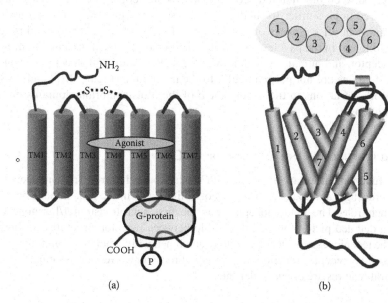

FIGURE 2.1 The molecular structure of rhodopsin-like 7-TM domain receptors. These receptors are characterized by the presence of seven membrane-spanning domains (TM1–TM7) with a short extracellular N-terminus and intracellular C-terminus shown in a two-dimensional schematic in (a). Agonist binding is predicted to be within the transmembrane domains. The extracellular structure is stabilized by a disulphide bond joining the first and second extracellular loops. The third intracellular loop is the main site of G-protein interaction, while both the third intracellular loop and carboxy tail are targets for phosphorylation by kinases responsible for initiating receptor desensitization and internalization. (b) Analysis of crystal structures has shown that the packing arrangement of the transmembrane domains is more complicated than that implied in (a) with transmembrane domains tilted to form the ligand binding pocket. (**See color insert following page 116.**)

2.1.2 G-Protein Independent Signaling

In addition to classical signaling via heterotrimeric G-proteins, several GPCRs can signal in a G-protein independent way via the arrestin adaptor proteins (see Section 2.5) to activate glycogen synthase kinase 3 (GSK-3), extracellular signal-regulated kinases (ERKs), or mitogen-activated protein (MAP) kinase. Transactivation of tyrosine kinases in response to cytokine signaling among immune cells is of particular note here. Some GPCRs can also transactivate growth factor receptors such as EGFR and so influence tyrosine kinase signaling (Kramer, Chapters 4 and 8).

2.2 GPCR TRANSMEMBRANE TOPOLOGY AND TERTIARY STRUCTURE

2.2.1 Electron Microscopy and X-Ray Crystallography

Amino acid sequence determination provides a definitive receptor classification, but it does not provide information on the three-dimensional structure of the protein necessary to understand drug binding and receptor activation. X-ray crystallography was for many years unsuccessful for any membrane receptor, but cryoelectron microscopy of two-dimensional membrane crystals successfully produced electron density maps of the nicotinic acetylcholine receptor from *Torpedo* electroplaque (Ejberg, Chapter 3) and of both bacteriorhodopsin and bovine rhodopsin. Bacteriorhodopsin is not a GPCR but a proton pump, while bovine rhodopsin is a true GPCR. Both proteins were shown to have seven alpha helices crossing the cell membrane giving rise to the fingerprint of the 7-TM domain receptors, illustrated in Figure 2.1a. Molecular modeling suggested a particular packing arrangement for the alpha helices that were stabilized by a disulphide bridge between the first and second extracellular loops. The structure of most other GPCRs was inferred to be similar to rhodopsin because of the presence of seven hydrophobic amino acid domains in all members of this receptor family. These early breakthroughs with rhodopsin were followed in the past few years with crystal structures of human β2-adrenoceptor, avian β1-adrenoceptor, and human adenosine A2 receptors. The crystal structures show that the transmembrane domains are not perpendicular to the membrane (Figure 2.1b) and showed also that there are subtle variations in the arrangement of the transmembrane domains between the receptors and rhodopsin.

2.2.2 Structure–Function Information for GPCRs

Most structure–function information for the GPCRs has been inferred from molecular genetic experiments where single amino acids or groups of amino acids in the protein have been changed to investigate their role. The β-adrenoceptor was the first neurotransmitter/hormone GPCR to be cloned, and a detailed picture of the relationship between receptor structure and function has emerged using the techniques of molecular biology combined with radioligand binding and classical pharmacology to study receptor function in a variety of receptor expression systems.

What structural features are of particular interest?

- Agonist and antagonist binding site
- Receptor activation—G-protein coupling
- Receptor dimerization
- Receptor modulation/desensitization

2.2.2.1 Ligand Binding Domain

In the monoamine receptors the ligand binding domain is located within the transmembrane helices. A pocket is formed between TM3, TM5, and TM6 where the agonist binds. A conserved aspartate residue in TM3 (Asp-113 in the β-adrenoceptor) and a conserved phenylalanine in TM6 (Phe-290) and two serine residues in TM5 (Ser-204 and 207) are known to be crucial for agonist binding. Antagonists have been shown to have extra interaction points on TM4 and TM7 but are thought to largely share the same binding sites as the agonist, and so can act by simple competition.

2.2.2.2 G-Protein Coupling

All rhodopsin-like GPCRs have a conserved arginine residue at the intracellular end of TM3, and this residue is thought to be crucial for G-protein activation. The third intracellular loop determines the class of G-protein activated by the receptor, with the second intracellular loop and C-terminus also influencing G-protein binding in some cases. Using chimeric receptors it has been shown that swapping the third intracellular loop between receptors (e.g., between α and β adrenoceptors) also swaps their G-protein selectivity. It has been shown in heterologous expression systems that when a GPCR is expressed at very high levels, the selectivity of G-protein coupling can be overruled, and, for example, a receptor that normally couples to G_o can be made to activate G_i. Surprisingly, some agonists (so-called protean agonists, after Proteus, the Greek god who could change shape and appearance at will) while acting at a single receptor may be an agonist for activating one class of G-protein (e.g., G_s) and yet be an inverse agonist for a different class of G-protein (e.g., G_i). Thus, the effect of the ligand depends on the identity of the interacting G-protein, something that might have been expected from the reciprocal nature of all molecular interactions but was surprising nonetheless. The G-protein binding domain and the carboxy terminal domain also contain a variable number of serine and threonine residues that are the target of specific GPCR protein kinases (GRKs) (e.g., β-adrenoceptor kinase, or βARK), as well as in some cases PKA and PKC, involved in receptor desensitization (Figure 2.3).

2.3 CLASSIFICATION OF GPCRS

Much of classical pharmacology developed this century before any knowledge of receptor structure was available. The concept of the receptor was developed to explain, in quantitative terms, the actions of drugs. Receptors came to be classified according to the actions of drugs. For example, the muscarinic receptor was defined as a receptor at which atropine had a dissociation equilibrium constant of about 1 nM.

The definitive receptor classification now depends on the amino acid sequence of the receptor protein. Molecular genetic techniques and the Human Genome Project have now provided the gene sequence for all receptors, and hence the amino acid sequence of the receptor proteins has been deduced.

Figure 2.2 shows diagrammatic illustrations of the proposed topology of the GPCR families. Three main families are identified based on the proposed location of the agonist binding domain:

1. Group A: Rhodopsin-like 7-TM receptors
   • Ligand binding within the transmembrane domains
   • Monoamine, nucleotide, and lipid receptors
2. Group B: Glucagon, VIP, and calcitonin family
   • Ligand binding outside the transmembrane domains on cell surface
3. Group C: Metabotropic glutamate receptors, $GABA_B$ receptors, and chemosensor (Ca^{2+}) receptors
   • Ligand binding on large extracellular N-terminus

2.3.1 GROUP A: RHODOPSIN-LIKE 7-TM RECEPTORS

By far the most studied family of the GPCRs are the rhodopsin-like receptors. These are also the largest group of receptors in number as they include receptors not only for the monoamines, nucleotides,

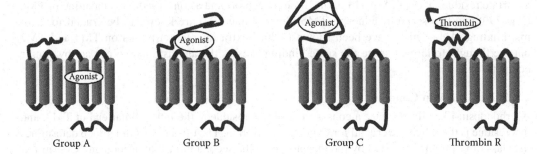

FIGURE 2.2 Agonist binding domains. Ligand binding to GPCRs varies between the different classes of receptors. Group A: Small ligands such as monoamines, nucleotides, and lipids bind within the transmembrane domains, but Group B receptors, peptide and glycoprotein hormones, bind outside the transmembrane region. Group C receptors: Metabotropic glutamate, glycine receptor γ-aminobutyric acid receptor (GABA$_B$) receptors and Ca2+ sensors have agonist binding on the large N-terminal domain while the thrombin receptor is activated by cleavage of the N-terminal domain by thrombin.

neuropeptides, and peptide hormones, but they also include the odorant receptors, which number several hundreds of related receptors. These receptors have short N-termini, a conserved disulphide bridge between the TM2–TM3 and TM4–TM5 extracellular domains, and variable length C-termini. In some cases the C-terminus is myristolyated, which, by tying the C-terminus to the cell membrane, generates a fourth intracellular loop. While the agonist binding domain is thought to be within the transmembrane domains for the monoamine and nucleotide receptors, neuropeptides are thought to bind close to the membrane surface on the extracellular domains of the receptor. It is still not clear whether nonpeptide antagonists bind at an overlapping or at a different site on the receptor.

2.3.2 Group B: Glucagon, VIP, and Calcitonin Family

These receptors are unlike the well-characterized rhodopsin-like family in that they have a large extracellular N-terminus and hormone binding seems to be dominated by this domain rather than the transmembrane domains. Receptors in this class include growth hormone releasing hormone (GHRH), adrenocorticotrophic hormone releasing factor, and the neuropeptide vasoactive intestinal polypeptide (VIP). All receptors in this family couple to G$_s$ to stimulate adenylyl cyclase and hence raise cAMP levels.

2.3.3 Group C: Metabotropic Glutamate, GABA$_B$, and Chemosensor (Ca^{2+}) Receptors

The metabotropic glutamate receptors (mGluR) and GABA$_B$ receptors are a distinct family of GPCRs that are homologous only to the Ca^{2+} sensors of the parathyroid and kidney. These receptors have an extremely large extracellular N-terminal domain of 500–600 amino acids (cf. 30–40 amino acids for the monoamine receptors). The binding of glutamate is thought to be within a clamshell region formed by two subdomains of the N-terminal region in an analogous manner to the binding of glutamate to the extracellular domain of the kainate, AMPA, and NMDA receptor NR2 subunits (Ejberg, Chapter 2).

2.3.4 Thrombin Receptors

The thrombin receptor is unusual in that the receptor is activated by the enzymatic action of thrombin, which cleaves the N-terminus of the receptor, leaving the receptor constitutively active.

2.4 RECEPTOR DIMERIZATION—QUATERNARY STRUCTURE

The GABA$_B$ receptors were the first GPCRs to be observed to form functional heterodimers where two GPCR monomers (GBR1 and GBR2) come together as a dimer to enhance their combined response. GBR1 and GBR2 do not function when expressed individually, but when expressed together they can efficiently activate G-protein activated inwardly-rectifying potassium channel (GIRK) potassium currents. The sweet and umami taste receptors also function as heterodimers; and similarly, the dopamine and somatostatin receptors, neurokinin NK1, and mu-opioid receptors may function as heterodimers. It is likely that this phenomenon occurs with a number of other GPCR pairs. It is more difficult to show that GPCRs may form functional homodimers, and the existence of these remains uncertain. The significance of dimerization in terms of the pharmacology of the receptors is unclear (e.g., there may be cooperativity between the two binding sites of a dimer), as well as whether dimerization affects mechanisms such as partial agonism, inverse agonism, or constitutive activity. Dimerization may affect the trafficking and delivery of receptors to the cell surface or influence desensitization and receptor internalization processes. A good example of this is that NK1 receptors regulate morphine-induced endocytosis and desensitization of mu-opioid receptors in CNS neurons.

2.5 RECEPTOR DESENSITIZATION

When the receptor is activated, there are immediately physiological mechanisms that come into play to limit overstimulation of the receptor signalling pathway. These mechanisms serve to regulate the density of functional receptors on the cell surface. Controlling the density of surface receptors is the main mechanism determining the sensitivity of the cell to a particular hormone or neurotransmitter. Serine and threonine residues on the third intracellular loop and on the carboxy tail are targets for phosphorylation by second messenger-dependent protein kinases and specific GRKs that phosphorylate agonist-occupied receptors. Receptor phosphorylation leads to receptor desensitization by inhibiting G-protein coupling to the receptor and promoting receptor internalization (removing receptors away from their plasma membrane located effectors). GRK-mediated phosphorylation and desensitization is illustrated in Figure 2.3. Phosphorylation of the agonist-occupied receptor leads to recruitment of the adaptor protein *arrestin* and G-protein uncoupling. Arrestin binding subsequently

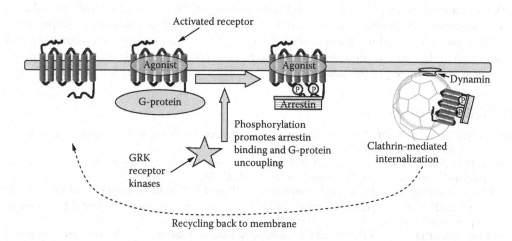

FIGURE 2.3 GRK-mediated desensitization and trafficking of GPCRs. Ligand binding to GPCRs not only promotes G-protein activation but makes the receptor a substrate for phosphorylation by GRKs. GRK phosphorylation promotes arrestin binding, which causes G-protein uncoupling and promotes receptor internalization via clathrin-mediated endocytosis.

targets the receptor for internalization via dynamin-dependent clathrin-mediated endocytosis, and the number of surface receptors decrease (Figure 2.3).

2.6 CONSTITUTIVELY ACTIVE RECEPTORS

One current model of G-protein receptor activation is the *allosteric ternary complex* model (see the "Further Reading" section). The agonist, receptor, and G-protein must combine to form a *ternary* complex in order to generate a response. Thermodynamically, this freely reversible mechanism means receptors may occasionally adopt the active conformation in the absence of ligand and may then cause G-protein activation. Such constitutive activity can be demonstrated by the effect of *antagonists*, which inhibit the unstimulated activity of the receptor and so are known as *inverse agonists* (Jenkinson, Chapter 1). Constitutive activity has been produced by specific point mutations of the β-adrenoceptor where, for example, conversion of Ala-293 to Glu-293 results in a 10-fold increase in constitutive activity. For many GPCRs, this constitutive activity has only been demonstrated convincingly in heterologous receptor expression systems where, with a very high level of receptor expression, a low level of basal activity becomes apparent. However, a number of rare mutations producing constitutively active receptors have been found recently in several genetic diseases.

- *TSH receptor*—Hyperthyroidism
- *LH receptor*—Precocious puberty
- *Rhodopsin*—Retinitis pigmentosa

Clearly the ability to manipulate the degree of constitutive receptor activity using drugs could provide a therapeutic strategy in these and perhaps other diseases.

2.7 FUTURE DIRECTIONS

The preceding 30 years have been a marvelous period of combined academic and pharmaceutical research into the structure and function of GPCRs. Gene sequence cloning and receptor expression have allowed receptor function and pharmacology to be studied at a level of detail previously unimaginable. When combined with high-resolution structural information, this has placed the GPCRs ever closer to providing a structural understanding of the actions of agonists, partial agonists, antagonists, and inverse agonists. The ability of inverse agonists to stabilize the receptor inactive state has been crucial in obtaining crystals of receptor protein, but high-resolution structural information of the active conformation has yet to be achieved except for rhodopsin. The next few years may see attainment of this goal and a structural understanding of drug action at GPCRs.

FURTHER READING

Bowery NG, Enna SJ (2000). Gamma-aminobutyric acid (B) receptors: First of the functional metabotropic heterodimers. *J Pharmacol Exp Ther* 292:2–7.

Carrillo JJ, Pediani J, Milligan G (2003). Dimers of class A G-protein-coupled receptors function via agonist-mediated transactivation. *J Biol Chem* 278(43):42578–42587.

Cherezov V, Rosenbaum DM, Hanson MA, Rasmussen SG, Thian FS, Kobilka TS, Choi HJ, Kuhn P, Weis WI, Kobilka BK, Stevens RC (2007). High-resolution crystal structure of an engineered human β_2-adrenergic G-protein coupled receptor. *Science* 318:1258–1265.

Foord SM, Bonner TI, Neubig RR et al. (2005). International Union of Pharmacology. XLVI. G-protein coupled receptor list. *Pharmacological Reviews* 57(2):279–288.

Lane JR, Powney B, Wise A, Rees S, Milligan G (2007). Protean agonism at the dopamine D2 receptor: (S)-3-(3-hydroxyphenyl)-*N*-propylpiperidine is an agonist for activation of G_{o1} but an antagonist/inverse agonist for G_{i1},G_{i2}, and G_{i3}. *Mol Pharmacol* 71(5):1349–1359.

Lefkowitz RJ, Cotecchia S, Samama P, Costa T (1993). Constitutive activity of receptors coupled to guanine nucleotide regulatory proteins. *TIPS* 14:303–307.

Lefkowitz RJ (2004). Historical review: A brief history and personal retrospective of seven-transmembrane receptors. *Trends in Pharmacological Sciences* 25:413–422.

Milligan G, Bond RA (1997). Inverse agonism and the regulation of receptor number. *TIPS* 18:468–474.

Milligan G (2004). G-protein coupled receptor dimerization: Function and ligand pharmacology. *Mol Pharmacol* 66(1):1–7.

Milligan G (2008). A day in the life of a G-protein coupled receptor: The contribution to function of G-protein coupled receptor dimerization. *Br J Pharmacol* 153 Suppl 1:S216–S229.

Milligan G (2009). G-protein coupled receptor hetero-dimerization: Contribution to pharmacology and function. *Br J Pharmacol* [Epub ahead of print].

Palczewski K, Kumasaka T, Hori T, Behnke CA, Motoshima H, Fox BA, Le Trong I, Teller DC, Okada T, Stenkamp RE, Yamamoto M, Miyano M (2000). Crystal structure of rhodopsin: A G-protein coupled receptor. *Science* 289:739–745.

Rocheville M, Lange DC, Kumar U, Patel SC, Patel RC, Patel YC (2000). Receptors for dopamine and somatostatin: Formation of hetero-oligomers with enhanced functional activity. *Science* 288(5463):154–157.

Rosenbaum DM, Rasmussen SG, Kobilka BK (2009). The structure and function of G-protein coupled receptors. *Nature* 459:356–363.

Schertler GF, Villa C, Henderson R (1993). Projection structure of rhodopsin. *Nature* 362:770–772.

Schwartz TW, Rosenkilde MM (1996). Is there a "lock" for all agonist "keys" in 7TM receptors? *TIPS* 17:213–216.

Seifert R, Wenzel-Seifert K (2002). Constitutive activity of G-protein coupled receptors: Cause of disease and common property of wild-type receptors. *Naunyn Schmiedebergs Arch Pharmacol* 366(5):381–416.

3 The Structure of Ligand-Gated Ion Channels

Jan Egebjerg

CONTENTS

3.1 INTRODUCTION

Ligand-gated ion channels are integral glycoproteins that transverse the cell membrane. All molecularly characterized ligand-gated ion channel receptors are multi-subunit complexes. Ligand-gated ion channels generally exist in one of three functional states: resting (or closed), open, and desensitized. Each functional state may reflect many discrete conformational states with different pharmacological properties. The receptors in the resting state will in the presence of agonist undergo a fast transition to the open state, called gating, and most agonists will also induce a transition to the desensitized state. Because the desensitized state often exhibits higher agonist affinities than the open state, most of the receptors will be in the desensitized state after prolonged agonist exposure.

Receptors have three important properties: (1) they are activated in response to specific ligands, (2) they conduct ions through the otherwise impermeable cell membrane, and (3) they select among different ions.

Molecular cloning combined with a variety of different techniques has revealed the existence of at least three structurally different families of ligand-gated channels. These families can be classified as the four transmembrane (4-TM) receptors, the excitatory amino acid receptors (3-TM), and the ATP receptors (2-TM). These receptors constitute the major classes of ligand-gated ion channel receptors in the plasma membrane. Other receptors such as the capsaicin-activated vanilloid receptor (6-TM), for which no endogenous ligands have been identified; cyclic nucleotide-gated channels; the intracellular Ca^{2+}-activated ryanodine receptor; and the IP_3- activated receptor are also ligand-gated channels but will not be discussed in this chapter.

3.2 THE 4-TM RECEPTORS

The 4-TM family of receptors, also called the *Cys-loop* receptors after a 13 amino acid loop limited by two conserved cysteines, consists of the nicotinic acetylcholine receptors (nAChR), serotonin receptors ($5HT_3$), and glycine receptors and γ-aminobutyric acid receptors ($GABA_A$ and $GABA_C$).

nAChRs are the primary excitatory receptors in skeletal muscle and the peripheral nervous system of vertebrates. $5HT_3$ receptors are also cation selective.

Glycine and GABA are the major inhibitory neurotransmitters. GABA predominates in the cortex and cerebellum, whereas glycine and GABA are both abundant in the spinal cord and brain stem. Both GABA and glycine receptor channels conduct chloride selective currents.

These neurotransmitters, except glycine, also activate G-protein coupled receptors.

3.2.1 MOLECULAR CLONING

The 4-TM receptors are pentameric complexes composed of subunits of 420 to 550 amino acids. The subunits exhibit sequence identities from 25 to 75% with a similar orientation of hydrophobic and hydrophilic domains (Figure 3.1). The hydrophilic 210–230 amino acid N-terminal domain is followed by three closely spaced hydrophobic transmembrane domains, then a variable length intracellular loop, and finally a fourth transmembrane region shortly before the C-terminus (Figure 3.1).

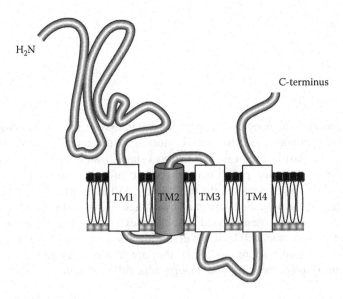

FIGURE 3.1 Schematic representation of the transmembrane topology of the 4-TM receptor family. TM2 forms the pore. Both the N-terminus (indicated by H_2N) and the C-terminus are located extracellularly. The cytoplasmic loop between TM3 and TM4 is variable in size and contains putative phosphorylation sites.

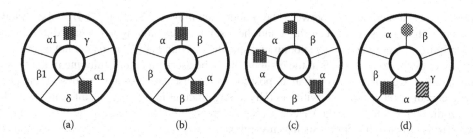

(a)   (b)   (c)   (d)

FIGURE 3.2   Schematic representation of the subunit organization in the most abundant heteromeric receptor complex: (a) adult muscle nAChR, (b) neuronal nAChR, (c) glycine receptors, and (d) GABA$_A$ receptors. The squares indicate the location of the agonist binding site at the interface between the subunits in nAChR and GABA$_A$ receptors. The square indicates the location of the benzodiazepine binding site. The depicted GABA$_A$ receptor model is the general model with at least one GABA and one benzodiazepine binding site. The number of different binding sites on the GABA$_A$ receptor depends on the final stoichiometry of the pentameric complex. Embryonic muscle nAChR has the stoichiometry $(\alpha 1)2\beta\gamma\varepsilon$.

The 4-TM regions form α-helices with TM2 lining the pore and the other three helices forming an outer layer to the lipid layer.

Molecular cloning has resulted in the identification of the muscle nAChR subunits α_1, β_1, γ, δ, and ε and the structurally related neuronal α_2–α_{10} and β_2–β_4. The neuronal nAChR subunits α_2–α_5 can assemble with β_2–β_4 and generate functional heteromeric receptors, while the α_7–α_9 subunits can generate functional homomeric receptors and the α_{10} subunit only forms functional channels in combination with α_9 subunits. The neuronal nAChRs assemble according to the general stoichiometry $2\alpha : 3\beta$ with a β subunit between the α subunits (Figure 3.2). Obviously, the properties of the receptor depend on the subunit composition, and the assembly process seems to be controlled in cells that express more than two different subunits. At least in muscle cells where four different subunits are expressed at the same time, the subunits are assembled in an ordered sequence to achieve the correct stochiometry and neighborhood relationship.

The 5-HT$_{3A}$ subunit can, in contrast to the other 5-HT$_3$ subunits, form functional homomeric receptors. The heteromeric 5-HT$_{3A-B}$ receptor differs from the homomeric 5-HT$_{3A}$ receptor in several aspects, but most striking is an increase from approximately 0.4 pS single channel conductance in the homomeric receptor to 16 pS in the heteromeric receptor. The difference has been attributed to a small arginine rich sequence in the intracellular domain of 5-HT$_{3A}$ between TM3 and TM4.

Five mammalian glycine receptor subunits have been identified: four α-subunits and one β-subunit. When expressed in heterologous systems homomeric α receptors, but not homomeric β, generate functional channels inhibited by strychnine and picrotoxinin. The β subunit is required for postsynaptic clustering of glycine receptors, due to interaction with the postsynaptic scaffolding protein *gephyrin*. The receptors in adult spinal cord neurons are heteromers, most likely, with the stoichiometry $2\alpha : 3\beta$, while the embryonic glycine receptors are more likely homomeric α receptors.

The diversity of the GABA$_A$ subunits (Figure 3.2d) is reflected in a very complex pharmacology. The GABA receptors can in a subtype selective manner be modulated by a number of agents that either enhance the agonist-induced current (benzodiazepines, barbiturates) or reduce the current (bicuculline, β-carbolines, picrotoxin). When expressed in heterologous systems a combination of α and β subunits yields functional receptors, but the pharmacological and physiological properties are modulated by the presence of other subunits in the receptor complex. As examples, the $(\alpha_1)_2(\beta_2)_2\gamma_2$ receptor is the most abundant GABA receptor in the brain, and due to the γ subunit mainly localized at synapses, mediates phasic inhibition after fast release of high concentrations of GABA from presynaptic terminals. In contrast, the δ containing receptors are mainly located extrasynaptically, mediating a tonic inhibition induced by the low concentrations of ambient GABA. The $\rho 1$–$\rho 3$ subunits coassemble with each other to form the GABA$_C$ receptors.

GABA binds at the interface between the α and β subunits (see Section 3.2.4), and the binding site for benzodiazepines is between the α and the γ subunits, explaining why benzodiazepine sensitivity requires the presence of a γ subunit and specific α subunits (α_{1-3} or α_5) but not α_4 or α_6. The selectivity of the benzodiazepines at the α subunits can be ascribed to a methionine in the sensitive subunits, but an arginine at the equivalent position in the insensitive subunits. Substituting part of the gene encoding the α1 subunit with the (His to Arg) mutant in the mice resulted in mice where the benzodiazepine effects on the α1 containing receptors are eliminated. In the mutant mice the known effects of benzodiazepines such as myorelaxation, motor impairments, anxiolysis, and ethanol potentiation remained, while other benzodiazepine effects such as sedation and amnesia were not induced, indicating the α1 containing receptors contribute to these behaviors. Similar studies were performed for the other benzodiazepine-sensitive subunits providing insight into the contribution of the different $GABA_A$ α-subunits to the wide spectrum of actions elicited by the clinically used benzodiazepines.

3.2.2 THE THREE-DIMENSIONAL STRUCTURE

The nAChRs of skeletal muscles and fish electric organs are the best characterized 4-TM ligand-gated ion channels. The receptor is a 290 kD complex, composed of four distinct subunits assembled into a heterologous $(\alpha_1)_2\beta_1\gamma\delta$ pentameric complex. In skeletal muscles, the embryonic γ-subunit is replaced by the ε-subunit in adult tissue. The receptor complex in the resting state, in electron micrographs from the synaptic site viewed perpendicular to the plane of the membrane, appears as a ring-like particle with an outer diameter of 80 Å and an inner tube of 20–25 Å. Viewed from the side (Figure 3.3), the receptor looks like a 125 Å-long cylinder protruding 60 Å into the synaptic cleft and 20 Å into the cytoplasm, with square-like density located beneath the cytoplasmatic vestibule. The cation conducting pathway consist of three parts: In the synaptic portion, it forms a water-filled tube 20 Å in diameter and 60 Å long. In the next part, across the membrane, it forms a more constricted region about 30 Å long (the pore). Near the middle of the membrane the pathway becomes constricted in a region where the pathway is blocked when the channel is closed (the gate). In the cytoplasmic part of the pathway, it forms a cylinder 20 Å in diameter and 20 Å long with four exit points corresponding to 10 Å-diameter openings between the intracellular domains of the individual subunits. A close inspection of the electron micrographs revealed that each subunit has an α-helical-like segment lining the pore. This segment consists of two α-helices separated by a kink around the midpoint pointing into the pore (in the resting state), giving the pore an hourglass shape with the kink located at the most constricted point. When the receptor is activated by acetylcholine, each of the helical TM2 segments rotates, opening the gate. In the open state the pore narrows from the outside to the cytoplasmic side where the diameter is roughly 11 Å. Thus the flexure between the TM2 α-helices provides an effective way of altering the shape and size of the pore (Figure 3.4).

3.2.3 THE RECEPTOR PORE

The ability of a receptor channel to permeate ions, which is measured as the conductance (the reciprocal of resistance) of the channel, depends on TM2. The key experiment was based on the observation that receptors made of *Torpedo* α, β, γ, and δ subunits had a different conductance than receptors made of *Torpedo* α, β, γ, and calf δ subunits. Using chimeric δ subunits, where *Torpedo* sequences were replaced by the corresponding calf sequence, showed that the entire difference in conductance could be attributed to the TM2 region.

The structure of the TM2 regions is not a perfect α-helix. However, assuming a symmetric pentameric distribution of α-helices gives a useful structural model to describe the molecular environment an ion has to pass when permeating the receptor channel. Amino acids assigned to the same position in the sequence alignments would then, due to the symmetric distribution around the pore, form a ring in the three-dimensional model (Figure 3.5).

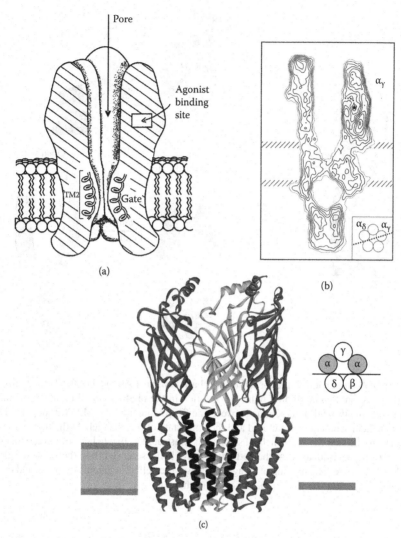

FIGURE 3.3 (a) Model of the 4-TM receptors. The model shows the ligand binding site, the membrane bilayer, and the position of the channel gate. (b) Electron density map of the nAChR in profile at 4.6 Å resolution. The electron density is shown through a cross-section of an α-subunit and the interface between the other α-subunit and the δ subunit. The asterisk indicates the proposed ACh binding site. (c) A 4 Å model of the receptor. Only the two α and the γ subunits are shown. The TM2 is shown dark.

Important clues to how the pore is structurally organized were obtained by examining the distribution of the charged and uncharged residues in the *Torpedo* nAChR subunits. As expected for hydrophobic segments, TM2 contains no charged residues, but a number of charged and polar residues are located at both ends of TM2 (Figure 3.5). According to the 4-TM model, the charged residues in the TM1–TM2 loop will be located at the entrance to the pore from the cytoplasmic side while the charged residues in the TM2–TM3 loop are located at the pore entrance from the extracellular side. Since nAChRs conduct cations, the negatively charged rings were expected to line the channel and also attract permeant cations to the pore. Indeed, when the number of charged amino acids in the intermediate ring (Figure 3.5) was reduced from the four negative charges in the native *Torpedo* receptor, there was a clear reduction in the conductance of the channel. Mutations that altered the charge of the inner and the outer ring also changed the conductance but to a much lesser extent. This suggests that the residues are exposed to the lumen of the pore, although additional

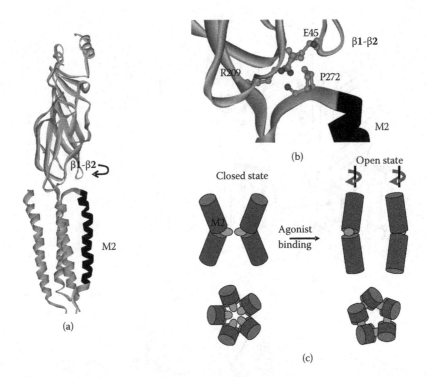

FIGURE 3.4 (a,b) A model of a single α-subunit. It is based on the 4 Å model of the Torpedo nAChR where it has been proposed that ligand binding induces a rotation in the binding domain that is transmitted to the transmembrane regions through interactions between the β1–β2 loop and the M2–M3 loop. (c) The orientation of the TM2 helical segment in the closed and the open state of the channel. At the top: A view of two of the five helices from the side where the helical segment is illustrated as two helices (rods) separated by a kink where the leucine (ellipse) is located. At the bottom: The five helices viewed from the synaptic side where the leucines will block the pore. The binding of an agonist causes the helical segments to rotate, and the narrowest region is then in the open state at the cytoplasmic part of the pore.

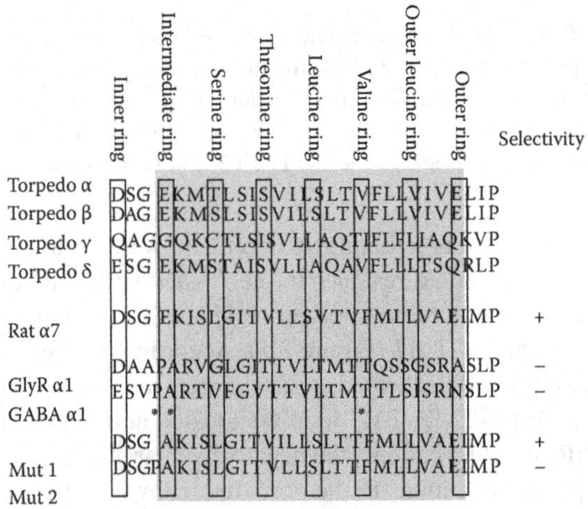

FIGURE 3.5 Alignment of the TM2 amino acid sequences. The nomenclature of the rings is based on the α7 sequence. Selectivity indicates the charge of the permeant ions. Mut1 and Mut2 are site-directed mutants (indicated by asterisk) of the α7 subunit (see text).

experiments indicate that the inner and outer rings are more involved in regulating the access of the cations to the channel than being in direct contact with the permeating ions. The optimal effect of the negatively charged rings on the current is a subtle balance between attracting monovalent ions and boosting the current versus attracting divalent ions that bind to the residues in the charged rings with high affinity, thereby reducing the current. These counteracting effects might explain why some functional nAChR subunits encode positively charged amino acids at some of the ring positions.

In the GABA and glycine receptors, where the permeant ion is negatively charged, the inner ring remains negatively charged and the outer is either negative or neutral. The question is then: What determines the ion selectivity of the channel? An alignment of the TM2 region between the nAChR subunit $\alpha 7$, and the glycine and GABA subunits revealed amino acid differences at five of the positions that line the pore, and in addition an extra amino acid was present at the N-terminal end of the TM2 segment in the anion-selective channels (Figure 3.5). Mutagenesis studies showed that substitutions of the amino acids lining the pore did not influence the cation selectivity of nAChR$\alpha 7$ (Mut1, Figure 3.5). But insertion of a proline into Mut1 at the N-terminus end of TM2, similar to the GABA receptors, changed the channel to be anion selective. Thus the pore can be permeable to both cations and anions, and the ion selectivity seems not to depend on the amino acid sequence within the pore, but on changes in the position of the TM2 relative to the surrounding amino acids. It is important that conclusions based on mutagenesis studies are confirmed by other experiments, since mutations involving residues in key positions for structure or for function may cause their effect not only as a result of changes at the site of substitution, but also as a result of nonlocalized structural perturbations created to accommodate the mutation. In fact, most of the residues facing the lumen of the pore were also identified in labeling experiments using noncompetitive antagonists known to bind in the pore. When the noncompetitive antagonist [3H]chlorpromazine was photolabeled to the receptor, the cross-linked amino acids were located in the serine, threonine, and leucine rings (Figure 3.5). Evidence for structural changes in the pore were obtained by the antagonist trifluoromethyl-iodophenyldiazirine, which in the absence of agonist cross-linked to amino acids equivalent to the valine and the leucine ring. In the presence of agonist the labeling pattern extended down to the threonine and serine rings indicating that the central valine, leucine, and threonine rings may correspond to the constricted region observed in the electron micrographs. The leucine is suggested to be the gate-forming residue pointing into the pore from the kink in TM2. This is supported by mutagenesis studies, which demonstrated that a substitution of the leucine with a smaller amino acid affects the ability of the channel to close when the receptor enters the desensitized conformation. The accessibility of the residues in the pore has also been examined by systematic SCAM (substituted cysteine accessibility modification) studies, where each amino acid (one at a time) in the pore is replaced by a cysteine, and the accessibility is assessed by the cysteine's ability to form a disulfide bridge with compounds of different charge and size. However, results from the SCAM methods suggest that the gate might be located deeper in the pore, closer to the intracellular interface.

3.2.4 The Ligand Binding Site

For studies of the binding site properties it is important to keep in mind that receptors exist in a number of conformations, which may exhibit different binding properties. As mentioned, the affinity of the ligand for the open state is usually much lower (10- to 1000-fold) than the affinity for the desensitized state. Thus in biochemical experiments where the receptor is exposed to a ligand for prolonged time periods, agonists–receptor interactions will reflect the receptor conformations of the desensitized state while antagonist interaction may reflect conformations of either the resting state or the desensitized states. In contrast, electrophysiological evaluations of the agonist interactions reflect the low-affinity binding state of the resting or open state except for certain mutants. As an example, studies of a mutant nAChR$\alpha 7$ subunit where the leucine ring (at the gate) is substituted for a smaller amino acid, the potency for ACh measured in electrophysiological recordings increases 150-fold. In addition, the apparent desensitization is almost eliminated. The simple interpretation would be that the leucine directly enhances the binding of ACh. However, the single channel conductance activated at low ACh concentrations is different from the conductance states activated at higher concentrations, supporting an alternative explanation that the leucine mutation at the gate means the channel cannot close in one of the desensitized conformations, which bind ACh with high affinity.

Insights into the three-dimensional structure of the agonist binding site of the 4-TM receptors have been obtained from comparisons with the crystal structure of a soluble acetylcholine-binding protein (AChBP) found in the snail *Lymnaea stagnalis* or *Aplysia*. The AChBP exhibits the highest sequence identity with the N-terminal domain of the nAChR α7 subunit (24%). Obviously, comparisons between proteins with low sequence identity should be treated with caution, but the residues that are conserved between the members of the 4-TM superfamily are nearly all conserved in the AChBP, and a number of competitive agonists and antagonists also bind the AChBP, suggesting that the structures might be similar.

AChBPs crystallize as a pentameric complex, with dimensions similar to the extracellular part of the nAChR. The subunits form a ring, thereby generating a central hydrophilic pore similar to the extracellular vestibule observed in the EM studies. The central part of each subunit is formed by 10 β-sheets, forming a β-sandwich. The five ligand binding sites in the pentameric complex are situated between subunits and formed by a principal side formed by three loop regions (loop A–C), between the β-strands from one subunit, and residues located in two β-strands and a loop from the adjacent subunit. In the nAChR, GlyR, and GABA the principal side is located at the α-subunits and the adjacent subunits are the β-subunits for the neuronal nAChR, glycine and GABA receptors and the γ and ε (or δ) subunits for the muscle nAChRs. The binding site is mainly formed by aromatic residues stabilizing the cation of the ligands by π-interactions in addition to a few ligand-specific hydrogen bonds to the peptide backbone. All the residues involved in ligand binding have also been identified in mutagenesis or cross-linking experiments on the nAChR. Apart from one residue, all the potential ligand-interacting residues are conserved among the nAChR. As expected these residues vary between pharmacologically different classes within the 4-TM superfamily. The inter-subunit localization of the ligand binding site provides an explanation for the pharmacological diversity observed in receptors formed from different subunits. Interestingly, the conserved residues, which mostly are hydrophobic, are involved in maintaining the overall structure of the subunits, further supporting the similar three-dimensional structure of the members of the 4-TM superfamily.

The ACh binding cavity is located approximately 30 Å above the membrane, raising the question: How can agonist-induced changes induce pore opening? Comparisons of the x-ray structures of the *Aplysia* AChBP (Figure 3.6) in the apo-form and in complex with antagonists and agonists revealed, apart from a large agonist-induced change in loop C, only small changes in the binding pocket. Loop C is formed between the β-sheets 9 and 10 and acts as an "induced-fit sensor" adopting a configuration dependent on the bound ligand. The antagonist α-conotoxin ImI induces a 4.3 Å opening of the tip of loop C compared to the apo form, while the agonist epibatidine induces a 7.3 Å closure (Figure 3.6b,c), completely burying the agonist in the binding cavity. To investigate if the transitions in the AChBP were relevant and sufficient to activate the channel, a chimeric receptor between the AChBP and the transmembrane region of the 5HT₃ receptor was studied. Despite excellent expression and binding, ACh failed to activate the channel, unless the three loops between β1–β2, β6–β7 (the conserved Cys loop) and β8–β9, in the binding AChBP were substituted with the equivalent residues from the 5HT₃ receptor, in which case ACh could activate the receptor. Interestingly, the binding affinity for ACh dropped 20-fold in the chimera that couples functionally to the channel compared to the AChBP-5HT₃ chimera. Using the structural changes observed in the isolated AChBP directly as a mechanism for activation of the functional chimeras should be done with caution, since fusion of the pore region might induce different conformations of the binding domain. However, the detailed structural information combined with the model of the *Torpedo* receptor at 4 Å resolution has generated an intriguing model for receptor activation, which partly has been confirmed by mutagenesis studies. The model predicts that the agonist-induced changes in

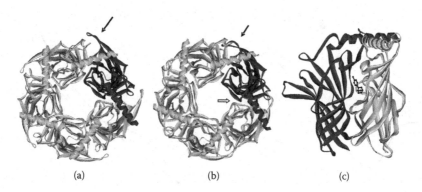

(a)　　　　　　　　　　　(b)　　　　　　　　　　　(c)

FIGURE 3.6 Crystal structure of the *Aplysia* AChBP. (a,b) The complex, as viewed into the extracellular vestibule formed by the subunits in the apo form (a) or with epibatidine (b). The complex consists of five identical subunits. One of the subunits is highlighted (as shown in the insert), and the open arrow indicates the agonist binding site, the black arrow indicates loop C. (c) View of the epibatidine binding site viewed from the pore side (along the open arrow in b).

loop C are transmitted through the β10 sheet to Arg209, which is proximal to Glu45 in the β1–β2 loop (Figure 3.4b). Both Arg 209 and Glu45 are universally conserved in the 4-TM receptor family, and mutations of these residues abolished receptor function; but double mutations where the charge is reversed restored activity, strongly supporting interaction between the residues. Mutagenesis studies in several of the 4-TM receptors suggest an interaction between the β1–β2 loop and the M2–M3 linker at the top of the channel forming M2 helix, thereby establishing a link between the binding domain and the transmembrane region apart from the direct connection to TM1.

3.3　THE EXCITATORY AMINO ACIDS RECEPTORS—3-TM RECEPTORS

L-glutamate acts as an excitatory neurotransmitter at many synapses in the mammalian central nervous system. Electrophysiological measurements and the use of different selective agonists and antagonists indicate that different glutamate receptors coexist on many neurons.

The exogenous agonist N-methyl-D-aspartate (NMDA) activates receptors, which are characterized by slow kinetics and a high Ca^{2+} permeability. These receptors require (in addition to glutamate or NMDA) glycine as a co-agonist. The currents conducted by NMDA receptors are blocked by extracellular Mg^{2+} in a voltage-dependent manner. At resting membrane potential ($\approx$ –70 mV) activation of the channel will only result in a small current because entry of Mg^{2+} ions into the channel will block the current. The affinity for the Mg^{2+} ions decreases at less negative membrane potentials as the electrical driving force for Mg^{2+} is reduced and the block becomes ineffective (Figure 3.7a).

Another class of ionotropic glutamate receptors, called AMPA receptors, exhibit fast kinetics, and in most neurons, a low Ca^{2+} permeability when activated by glutamate. The selective agonist α-amino-3-hydroxy-5-methyl-4-isoxazole propionate (AMPA) activates a fast desensitizing current, as does glutamate. Kainate activates a nondesensitizing current when applied to AMPA receptors, but it binds with high affinity to the third glutamate receptor subtype, the kainate receptors. Kainate activates a fast desensitizing current on the kainate receptors (Figure 3.8).

In addition to the three groups of ionotropic receptors, glutamate also activates GPCRs called metabotropic glutamate receptors (see Chapter 2).

AMPA receptors mediate the majority of fast excitatory neurotransmission in the mammalian brain. The rapid kinetics and the low Ca permeability make these receptors ideal for fast neurotransmission without sufficient changes in the intracellular calcium concentration to activate Ca^{2+} dependent processes. NMDA receptors are colocalized with AMPA receptors at most glutamategic

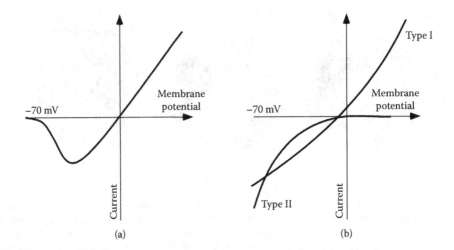

FIGURE 3.7 Current–voltage relationships for the NMDA and the non-NMDA glutamate receptors. (a) Current–voltage relationship of the NMDA receptor recorded in the presence of Mg2+. The current through the channel becomes progressively smaller at negative membrane potentials due to the Mg2+ block. (b) Expression of the AMPA and kainate receptor subunits generates either linear (Type I) or an inwardly rectifying (Type II) current–voltage relationships depending on the subunit composition of the receptor. If the receptor contains subunits edited at the Q/R site (i.e., GluR2 for the AMPA receptors, GluR5R or GluR6R for the kainate receptors) the current–voltage relationship is linear. Receptors made of unedited subunits alone or in combinations with each other exhibit an inwardly rectifying current–voltage relationship.

synapses, but the slow kinetics of the NMDA receptor minimize the receptor activation after a single presynaptic glutamate release where the neuron quickly repolarizes, resulting in Mg^{2+} block of the NMDA receptor. However, the NMDA receptor will be fully activated after extensive stimulation of the synapse when repetitive activation of the AMPA receptors evokes sufficient depolarization of the postsynaptic membrane to relieve the NMDA receptors of the Mg2+ block. This creates a use-dependent Ca2+ influx that triggers processes leading to synaptic plasticity, such as long-term potentiation and depression, which are interpreted as the underlying mechanism for many different neuronal processes including learning and memory.

3.3.1 MOLECULAR CLONING

Eighteen genes encoding glutamate receptor subunits have been identified in the human genome. Based on sequence identities these subunits are grouped into seven different classes. All the subunits have similar profiles in hydrophobicity plots and presumably the same topology with a 400–500 amino acid extracellular N-terminal part followed by a 400 amino acid region encoding the transmembrane domains. The C-terminus is intracellular and varies in size from 50 to 750 amino acids. The glutamate receptor subunits exhibit, in contrast to the 4-TM receptors, the highest sequence variability at the N-terminal region while the transmembrane domain is highly conserved.

The stoichiometry of the receptor was a controversial issue although most of the recent data strongly support a tetrameric structure formed of two pairs.

3.3.1.1 AMPA Receptors

The GluR1–GluR4 subunits (also named GluRA–GluRD) coassemble with one another but not with subunits from the other classes. The functional profile of these cloned receptors demonstrated a desensitizing response to AMPA, or glutamate, but a nondesensitizing response to kainate (EC50 > 30 µM), features similar to studies of AMPA receptors from the brain. The affinity for AMPA in binding experiments also resembles the affinities observed in brain tissue.

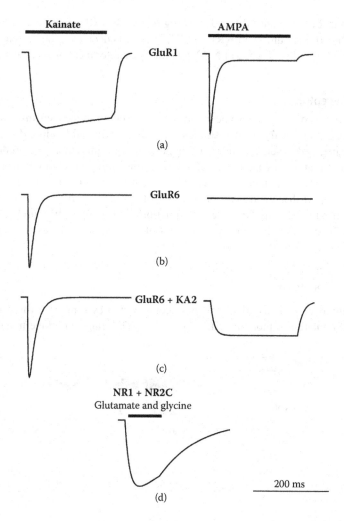

FIGURE 3.8 AMPA and kainate activate different current responses in the different classes of AMPA and kainate receptors: (a) the AMPA receptor GluR1, (b,c) kainate receptors, (d) glutamate + glycine activation of the NMDA receptor. The current response is characterized by a slow onset and offset compared to the AMPA and kainate receptors.

3.3.1.2 Kainate Receptors

The kainate receptors are composed of subunits from the GluR5–GluR7 class and the KA1–KA2 class of subunits. Homomeric receptors of the former class generate functional receptors and bind kainate with an affinity of 50 to 100 nM. KA1 or KA2 does not generate functional channels, but the receptors bind kainate with an affinity of 5 to 10 nM. Homomeric GluR6 and KA2 receptors are neither activated by AMPA nor bind AMPA. Interestingly, when they are coexpressed, they form heteromeric receptors that respond to AMPA (Figure 3.8).

3.3.1.3 NMDA Receptors

Functional NMDA receptor complexes contain at least one NR1 and one NR2 subunit. The heteromeric composition requires, at nearly all NMDA receptors, two agonists for activation: glycine binding to the NR1 subunit and glutamate binding to the NR2 subunit. The NR2 subunits have the same basic structure as the other glutamate subunits, except for a large 400–630 amino acid C-terminal domain. Many of the receptor features such as Mg^{2+} block, glycine sensitivity, deactivation kinetics, and the single-channel conductance differ depending on which NR2 subunit coassembles with NR1. Coexpression of the NR3 subunit with NR1 and NR2 subunits decreases the current amplitude, and coexpression with NR1, in the absence of NR2 subunits, generates a cation channel activated by glycine alone.

3.3.1.4 Delta Receptors

Two additional subunits δ1 and δ2 have been identified. Based on sequence similarities they belong to the glutamate receptor family. Recent studies show that the ligand binding domain can cocrystallize with D-serine, and several amino acid ligands (but not glutamate) can reduce the current through the Lurcher mutant, a constitutive δ2 receptor, indicating an interaction with the binding domain. Neither of the ligands induce a detectable current in the normal δ2 receptors. At least two lines of evidence support the functional importance of the channels: first, genetic knock-out of the δ2 results in impaired cerebellar Purkinje cell function; and second, the Lurcher mutant mouse, which shows significant cerebellar atropy, is a result of a mutation in the extracellular part of M3 that renders the receptor constitutive active.

3.3.2 Receptor Topology

Results from a number of biochemical and mutagenesis studies support a three transmembrane topology of the glutamate receptor subunits (Figure 3.9). The transmembrane nomenclature in the

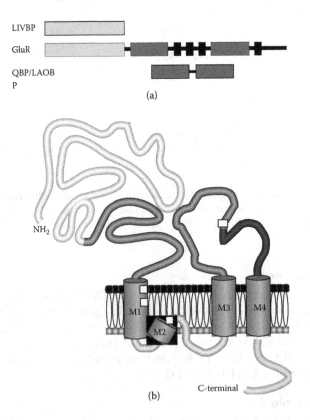

FIGURE 3.9 (a) Diagram showing the regions of glutamate receptors that exhibit sequence homology to bacterial plasma membrane binding proteins. (b) Schematic representation of the transmembrane topology of the excitatory amino acid receptors. The dark extracellular regions indicate the two lobes forming the agonist binding site. The darkest region represents the alternatively spliced element (flip/flop) in the AMPA class of receptors. The edited sites are indicated by squares.

literature is confused by the early proposed four transmembrane topology using TM1–TM4. Most literature will use membrane regions M1–M4 for the same segments, but only M1, M3, and M4 are transmembrane spanning, while M2 forms a reentrant loop.

The M2 is proposed to be structurally similar to the P-loop found in the voltage gated channels. However, the loop enters the membrane from the cytoplasmic side in the glutamate receptors, while it is located at the extracellular side of the voltage gated channels.

3.3.3 THE EXTRACELLULAR PART OF THE RECEPTOR: THE AGONIST BINDING SITE

Sequence comparisons between the glutamate receptors and other proteins revealed that the N-terminal part of the receptor exhibited a low level of sequence similarity to a bacterial periplasmic Leucine-Isoleucine-Valine binding protein (LIV-BP), while the region N-terminal of M1 (130 amino acids) and the region between M3 and M4 showed sequence similarity to another bacterial amino acid binding protein, Lysine-arginine-ornithine binding protein (Figure 3.9). These sequence similarities and the resemblance of the M1–M3 segment with the pore region of the voltage-gated channels suggest that the glutamate receptor might have evolved as a chimera of two evolutionary ancient modules. Identification of a bacterial potassium selective glutamate receptor, GluR0, containing only the binding domain intersected by the pore region, strongly supports the evolutionary model.

The sequence similarity to the soluble periplasmic binding protein and a number of chimeric receptors formed between the AMPA and kainate receptors suggested that a soluble form of the binding domain could be engineered by replacing the M1–M3 segment with a hydrophilic linker and truncating the N-terminal part and M4 and the C-terminal tail. When examined initially for the GluR2 subunit, the soluble binding domain exhibits the same pharmacological characteristics as the whole receptor, and it was possible to cocrystallize the GluR2 binding domain with different ligands. Since then, crystal structures of the binding domain from all the subunit classes have been obtained.

The structures are remarkably similar to the bacterial periplasmic binding proteins. The overall structure of the binding domain is two domains, called domain 1 (D1) and domain 2 (D2), and a hinge, where the agonist binds between the domains. Most of the segment N-terminal to M1 form part of D1, while the C-terminal part crosses the hinge between the two domains and the C-terminus protrudes from D2 into M1 (in the whole receptor). The N-terminal part of the segment between M3 and M4 forms D2, and the C-terminal part crosses the hinge and forms part of lobe D1. The binding domains crystallize as dimers back-to-back with the inter-subunit interactions formed between D1 from each subunit. In the unbound condition (apo-form) the domains are separated and the protrusions extending into the pore region (in the whole receptor) are separated by 32 Å.

Binding of an agonist stabilizes a closed conformation of the binding domain where D2 is brought closer to D1 and, consequently, the separation between the protrusion extending from D2 into the membrane domains is increased. The closure is described by the angle between D1 and D2, where the degree depends on the agonist. Partial agonists such as kainate induce a closure of 8 degrees while full agonists like glutamate and AMPA induce a tighter closure resulting from a 20-degree closure. Interestingly, antagonists, like DNQX or ATPO, also induce a closure of the domains but only by 3 degrees, apparently insufficient to open the pore. The interactions, which stabilize the closed binding domain, can be divided into three different contributions. First, the glutamate-like moiety found in all the agonists forms a bridge between the domains (Figure 3.10b); and second, the unique structures of the agonists, such as the pyrrolidine ring and isopropenyl in kainate (Figure 3.10c), contribute to the selective binding either by direct interactions with the binding domain, binding through water molecules, or by confining the conformation of the glutamate moiety. Finally, the proximity of the domains in the closed form promotes direct interactions between D1 and D2.

Competitive antagonists and agonists selecting between the NMDA receptors and the AMPA/kainate receptors have been identified, where APV and NBQX or CNQX are the most commonly used selective NMDA and AMPA/kainate receptor antagonists, respectively. However, the high degree of conservation in the binding pocket has made identification of subtype selective competitive

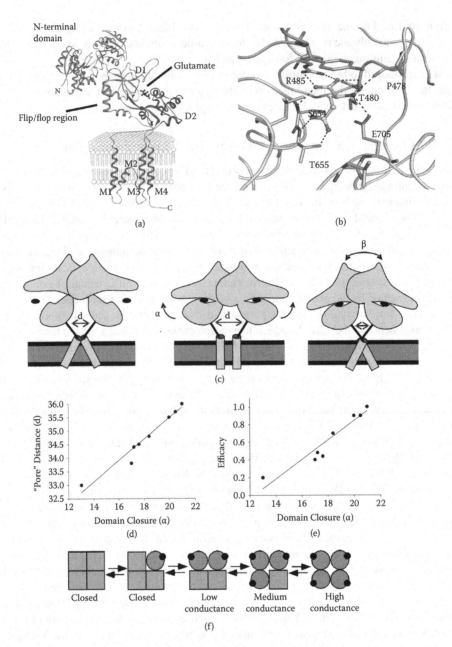

FIGURE 3.10 (a) A model of a glutamate receptor subunit. (b) Binding of glutamate at the GluR2 binding pocket. Glutamate interacts directly with residues in both domain 1 (R485, P478, and T480) and domain 2 (S654, T655, and E750), thereby stabilizing the domain closure. (c) Schematic illustration of the proposed model for subunit activation. Two subunits are shown. Agonist binding stabilizes a closed conformation of the lobes in the binding domain, thereby inducing an opening of the pore. Agonist stabilizing a high degree of domain closure (α) will subsequently induce a twist (β) between the subunits resulting in a conformational change that reduces the distance between the domains projecting to the pore. (d) Relationship between the degree of domain closure (α) and distance for the regions projecting to the pore (d) for eight agonists. (e) The relationship between efficacy, measured as the relative (to the full agonist glutamate) maximal response in a nondesensitizing mutant of the receptor and the domain closure. (f) Activation of the receptor is proposed to require activation of at least two sub-units, and activation of more subunits opens the channels to a higher conductance level, that is, approximately 6 pS, 12 pS, or 17 pS, when 2, 3, or 4 subunits are activated, respectively. **(See color insert following page 116.)**

antagonists very difficult. As a result, nearly all the known selective compounds act through non-competitive mechanisms, such as the AMPA receptor selective GYKI-53655, cyclothiazide which potentiates AMPA receptors in a splice variant dependent manner, or the polyamines which block AMPA and kainate receptors depending on the presence of an edited subunit (see Section 3.3.4).

An important question is how changes in the agonist binding domain are transmitted to the pore region and how this can result in different efficacy. The three-dimensional structure of more than 30 agonist–GluR2 complexes has been resolved, and there is a striking correlation between the degree of domain closure and efficacy, that is, agonists inducing the largest degree of closure, as glutamates (20 degree) are the most efficacious. Examination of the structure also shows an almost linear correlation (Figure 3.10a) between the degree of closure, the separation between the protrusions into the pore region, and the agonist efficacy (Figure 3.10e). Single channel studies show that AMPA receptors exhibit three conductance states of approximately 6 pS, 11 pS, and 17 pS, and the more efficacious an agonist the more frequently the receptor will occupy the high-conductance state. The distribution between the different conductance states can be described as each subunit independently can obtain one of two states—a closed or an open state. Activation of the receptor will require at least two of the subunits in the receptor complex, simultaneously, to be in the open state, resulting in the 6 pS conductance state. The 11 and 17 pS conductance states are obtained when three or four of the subunits simultaneously are in the open state. The transition between the open and closed states is very fast, and the probability for an agonist-bound subunit to be in the open state is characterized by a coupling efficiency ε, which depends on the degree of domain closure. For full agonists like glutamate, ε is 0.63, while the partial agonist, iodowillardiine, which closes the binding domain to 11 degrees, exhibits an ε of 0.4. Consequently the distribution of the conductance states can be described as a binomial distribution with the likelihood ε for each of the subunits to be in the active state (Figure 3.10f).

The x-ray structures have also provided important information on the mechanisms for desensitization and positive allosteric modulation. Kainate, which induces a minor closure, activates a non-desensitizing current, while glutamate activates a larger but transient current before entering into a desensitized state (Figure 3.8). The tighter closure of the binding domain induced by glutamate also induces a tension at the D1–D1 interface between the two binding domains, resulting in a subsequent rotation of the binding domains relative to each other. This interdomain rotation reduces the distance between the protrusion to the pore region from 37 Å in the open form to 26 Å in the desensitized state, which is less than observed in the closed state. Mutations stabilizing the interdomain interface reduce the rate of desensitization, and positive modulators like cyclothiazide prevent the transition to the desensitized state by stabilizing the D1–D1 interdomain interface. Another type of positive modulator, aniracetam or CX614, which slows the receptor deactivation, also binds at the interface between the subunits but in addition interacts with residues in the hinge between D1 and D2, thereby stabilizing the closed conformation of the binding domain, and subsequently reducing the agonist off-rates (Figure 3.10c).

A group of noncompetitive antagonists, GYKI-53655 and CP-465,022, act by binding at the linkers between the binding domain and the transmembrane regions. They bind with high affinity to the receptor conformations obtained in the resting and the desensitized state, but only with low affinity at the activated receptors, thereby shifting the equilibrium to the inactive forms.

The size of the agonist-activated current is not solely dependent on the degree of domain closure, since a number of modulatory sites have, in particular for the NMDA receptor, been located in the N-terminal part of the receptor. Zinc ions inhibit NR2A containing receptors, while a number of compounds, such as ifenprodil, selectively inhibit NR2B containing receptors, and a splice variant in the N-terminal part of NR1 affects the pH and spermidine sensitivity of the receptor. The strong correlation between domain closure and efficacy observed for the AMPA receptors is not as clear for the NMDA receptors, since different partial agonists at the glycine site induce the same degree of domain closure in NR1.

The crystallographic data obtained from the other glutamate receptor subtypes show a very similar overall structure, but more than five-fold differences in the size of the ligand binding cavity.

The smallest binding cavity, in NR1, contains no water molecules, while the additional space in the AMPA and kainate receptors, when cocrystallized with glutamate, is occupied by water molecules. The water molecules are displaced to accommodate binding of large heterocyclic ligands. Even small changes in the configuration of the water molecules influence the selectivity of agonist interaction, complicating modeling and prediction of ligand receptor interactions.

3.3.4 Posttranscriptional Modifications

One important form of regulation is achieved by splice variants. For instance, a 38 amino acid segment preceding M4 is present in one of two alternatively spliced forms called "flip or flop" in GluR1–GluR4. The flip/flop insert is located at the D1–D1 interface between the binding domains, thereby affecting the receptor kinetics. The current amplitude is smaller at the flop receptors compared with the flip receptors. This might be a mechanism that could enable the neurons to switch from a low-gain flop version to a high-gain flip receptor simply by alternative splicing of the transcripts. Splice variation at the C-terminus strongly influences the trafficking properties of several of the receptor subunits.

Another form of regulation is editing of the RNA transcript. When GluR1, GluR3 or GluR4 is expressed individually or in combination, the current voltage relationship exhibits an inwardly rectifying relationship and the receptor channel is permeable to Ca2+. However, if the GluR2 subunit is part of the receptor, the current–voltage relationship is linear and the channel is impermeable to Ca2+ (Figure 3.7b). Site-directed mutagenesis demonstrated that the channel properties were determined by a single amino acid difference in the putative TM2. GluR2 encodes an arginine (R) at that position while the other AMPA receptor subunits encode a glutamine (Q). Hence the name Q/R site. Analysis of the genomic sequences revealed that GluR2, like the other AMPA receptor subunits, encodes a glutamine (codon GAC) but the mRNA encodes an arginine (GGC) at that position. The A to G transition is catalyzed by an enzyme that recognizes an RNA structural element in the GluR2 transcript and then specifically deaminates the adenosine to an inosine (which is equivalent to a G). The presence of an edited subunit in the receptor complex prevents interaction with channel blockers, like Joro spider toxin and philantotoxins.

GluR6 is in addition to the editing at the Q/R site in TM2, also edited at two sites in TM1, which also influences the Ca2+ permeability. This suggests that TM1 might contribute to the pore in the glutamate receptors. Another A to G editing, designated the R/G site, can occur immediately preceding the "flip/flop" segment in GluR2–GluR4. The "flip-flop" segment influences the rate of desensitization while the rate of recovery from the desensitized state depends on the R/G site where the edited form (G) recovers faster than the unedited R form.

3.3.5 The Pore Region

The pore region has been studied extensively using mutagenesis and the substituted cysteine accessibility method (SCAM) in combination with electrophysiological measurements. These studies have provided some insight into the architecture of the glutamate receptor pore, and the data are to a large extent compatible with the overall three-dimensional structure of the potassium channel KcsA. The pore forms a cone-like structure, where the tip formed by the C-terminal part of M3 is located at the extracellular surface and the M2 region is inserted from the cytoplasmic side. The three transmembrane regions are directly linked to the binding domain, and mutations in these domains affect gating. However, two regions seem to be involved in structure that prevent ion permeation; the C-terminal part of M3 where mutations make the receptor constitutively active, and a part of M3 located deeper in the pore, close to M2. The latter region only becomes accessible using SCAM when the receptor is activated.

The experimental data also support a similar overall structure of the M2 region and the P-element in KcsA, where the N-terminal part of M2 forms an α-helical structure located parallel with the wall of the cone formed by the transmembrane regions. However, there are also differences between the glutamate receptor pore and the KcsA channel. The α-helical structure in M2 is followed by a random coiled structure pointing toward the center of the pore. That region forms the selectivity filter for potassium in the KcsA channel; however, the lack of discrimination between potassium and sodium ions in the glutamate receptor channel argues for a different structure. The Q/R site (see above) is located at the tip of the reentrant loop. That position determines the permeability of divalent ions relative to monovalent ions. The equivalent position in the NMDA receptors is occupied by an asparagine, which is involved in discrimination between the impermeable Mg^{2+} and the permeable Ca^{2+} ions. Additional amino acids are also involved, but they are not located at equivalent positions on the NR1 and the NR2 subunits, suggesting an asymmetry in the pore at that position compared to a symmetric configuration in the KscA channel. Finally, the overall symmetry differs since the K channels show a fourfold symmetry, while the dimer of dimers configuration in the glutamate receptors suggest a twofold symmetry.

3.3.6 THE INTRACELLULAR SIDE OF THE RECEPTOR

Long-term potentiation and depression of glutamatergic synapses are involved in many models for brain function and development. A key factor in the plasticity is changes in the AMPA and kainate receptor activities induced after NMDA receptor dependent elevations of the intracellular Ca^{2+} concentration. There is strong evidence for two receptor-dependent mechanisms involved in the changes in the receptor activity. Glutamate receptors are, as are most ion channels, regulated by phosphorylation. Phosphorylation and dephosphorylation have been shown to alter both the probability for opening and the distribution of different conductance states. The second mechanism involves dynamic changes in the number of AMPA receptors at the synapse regulated by interaction of a large number of trafficking and anchoring proteins at the C-terminus. The trafficking of the AMPA receptors does not solely depend on modification of the receptors, but a number of auxiliary subunits also called transmembrane AMPA receptor regulatory proteins (TARPs) have been identified. In addition to guiding the trafficking of AMPA receptors, TARPs also change basic receptor kinetic properties such as desensitization and deactivation.

3.4 ATP RECEPTORS—2-TM RECEPTORS

Extracellular ATP has been demonstrated to activate a depolarizing current in different neuronal and nonneuronal cell types. These receptors are referred to as P2 receptors. The receptors can further be divided into the G-protein coupled P2Y receptors and the ligand-gated ion channels, P2X. Currently, seven P2X receptors ($P2X_1$–$P2X_7$) have been cloned. The receptors exhibit between 26% and 50% overall amino acid identities, with the highest level of conservation in the extracellular and transmembrane regions. $P2X_7$ (also called P2Z) is the most distant member of the family.

The receptors range in size from 379 to 595 amino acids. The receptors have two transmembrane regions with intracellular N- and C-termini (Figure 3.11). The crystal structure of the orthologue zebrafish $P2X_4$ receptor has been solved in the closed state (Figure 3.11), and it shows strong structural similarity to the acid-sensing ion channel (ASIC). The receptor is organized as a trimer, and each subunit has two transmembrane helices, where the second helix (TM2) appears to form the pore. The pathways for ions to access the pore is not clear from the closed state; however, two potential pathways appear, either through three holes connecting the surroundings and a negatively charged vestibule located just above the pore (arrow at Figure 3.11b), or alternatively through a pathway running through the length of the extracellular domain. The latter is not permeable in the crystallized form, but contains two cavities surrounded by negatively charged residues.

The ATP binding site cannot be determined from the structure, but conserved residues supported by mutagenesis as contributing to the ATP binding site are located around a cavity formed at the interface between two subunits.

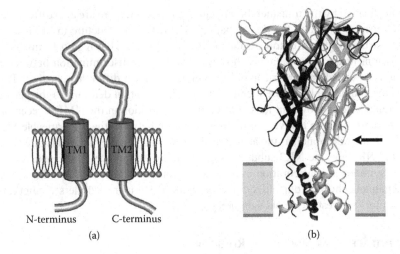

FIGURE 3.11 (a) Schematic representation of the transmembrane topology of a P2X ATP receptor subunit. (b) Three-dimensional structure of the Zebrafish P2X$_4$ receptor complex. The arrows show the holes connecting the vestibule and the surrounding medium. The circle indicates the putative ATP bindings site located between two subunits.

The number of selective compounds acting on the different P2X subtypes is very limited. P2X channels can be distinguished from the P2Y receptors by their much faster kinetics. Kinetic properties, such as desensitization can also be used in electrophysiological recordings to distinguish between the different subtypes; for example, P2X$_1$ and P2X$_3$ desensitize fast at saturating ATP concentrations, while P2X$_2$ and P2X$_4$ only desensitize very slowly. However, desensitization is not an optimal criterion for characterization of the receptors in general. First, different receptor-independent mechanisms (phosphorylation, binding proteins, etc.) might influence the desensitization. Secondly, desensitization is difficult to measure accurately in multicellular systems and with methods other than electrophysiology. Thirdly, different channel substates may have different desensitization properties.

P2X receptors are cation selective channels. It is generally assumed that ion selectivity is conserved for a given channel. However, studies on the P2X$_2$, P2X$_4$, and the P2X$_7$ receptors have revealed a shift in the ion selectivity after prolonged receptor activation. A short agonist application opens the channel pore to be permeable only for small cations, while longer activation (hundreds of milliseconds to seconds) induces a pore conformation permeable to large dyes (>630 Da). The larger pore conformation can be obtained by sustained application or by repetitive pulse. Interestingly, despite the change in pore size, the channel remains cation selective. Similar changes in conductance levels have been observed for a few other channels, but it remains to be shown how general the phenomenon is and whether it exhibits agonist specificity.

PROBLEMS

PROBLEM 3.1

Three agonists are developed for the AMPA receptor GluR2.

Agonist A has a coupling efficiency ε of 1.
Agonist B has a coupling efficiency ε of 0.7.
Agonist C has a coupling efficiency ε of 0.1.

- Calculate the maximal currents of B and C relative to A.
- Calculate the relative current at 50% occupancy for A–C.

PROBLEM 3.2

Assume the assembly of nicotine acetylcholine receptor subunits is completely permissive. How many different receptors can be assembled in a cell expressing $\alpha 3$, $\beta 2$, and $\beta 4$ if there must be two alpha and three beta subunits in each receptor? Group the receptors according to which are likely to have similar single-channel conductance and pharmacology.

SOLUTIONS TO PROBLEMS

PROBLEM 3.1

The distribution between the conductance states can be described (assuming all subunits bind the agonist) by a binomial distribution, that is,

$$(1-\varepsilon)^4, \ 4\varepsilon(1-\varepsilon)^3, \ 6\varepsilon^2(1-\varepsilon)^2, \ 4\varepsilon(1-\varepsilon)^3, \ \varepsilon^4,$$

where $(1-\varepsilon)^4$ is the likelihood that all subunits are in the inactive state, $4\varepsilon(1-\varepsilon)^3$ the likelihood that 1 is the active conformation and 3 is the inactive, and so forth.

The current associated with the different states is proportional to the conductance, that is, 0 for states where 0 or only 1 subunit is in the active conformation, when 2, 3, or 4 subunits are activated, the conductance is 6 pS, 11 pS, and 17 pS, respectively.

$$I_\varepsilon \propto 0 \cdot (1-\varepsilon)^4 + 0 \cdot 4\varepsilon(1-\varepsilon)^3 + 6pS \cdot 6\varepsilon^2(1-\varepsilon)^2 + 11pS \cdot 4\varepsilon^3(1-\varepsilon) + 17pS \cdot \varepsilon^4$$

$$\frac{I_{\varepsilon=0.7}}{I_{\varepsilon=1}} = \frac{6pS \cdot 6 \cdot 0.7^2(1-0.7)^2 + 12pS \cdot 4 \cdot 0.7^3(1-0.7) + 17pS \cdot 0.7^4}{17pS \cdot 1^4} = 0.60$$

$$\frac{I_{\varepsilon=0.1}}{I_{\varepsilon=1}} = \frac{6pS \cdot 6 \cdot 0.1^2(1-0.1)^2 + 12pS \cdot 4 \cdot 0.1^3(1-0.1) + 17pS \cdot 0.1^4}{17pS \cdot 1^4} = 0.60$$

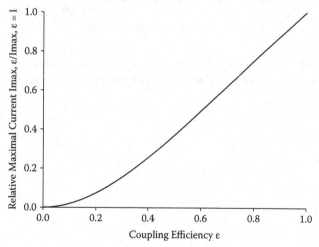

If each subunit is occupied by a fraction p, the distribution of receptors with 0–4 subunits occupied can also be described by a binomial distribution:

$$(1-p)^4, \ 4p(1-p)^3, \ 6p^2(1-p)^2, \ 4p(1-p)^3, \ p^4$$

For the receptors where all the subunits are occupied, the current can be described as in 1. If only three subunits are occupied by a ligand, then only the 0–3 conductance states can be present:

$$I_\varepsilon^{occ=4} \propto 0 \cdot (1-\varepsilon)^4 + 0 \cdot 4\varepsilon(1-\varepsilon)^3 + 6pS \cdot 6\varepsilon^2(1-\varepsilon)^2 + 11pS \cdot 4\varepsilon^3(1-\varepsilon) + 17pS \cdot \varepsilon^4$$

$$I_\varepsilon^{occ=3} \propto 0 \cdot (1-\varepsilon)^3 + 0 \cdot 3\varepsilon(1-\varepsilon)^2 + 6pS \cdot 3\varepsilon^2(1-\varepsilon) + 11pS \cdot \varepsilon^3$$

$$I_\varepsilon^{occ=2} \propto 0 \cdot (1-\varepsilon)^2 + 0 \cdot 2\varepsilon(1-\varepsilon) + 6pS \cdot \varepsilon^2$$

$$I_\varepsilon^{occ=1} \propto 0 \cdot (1-\varepsilon) + 0 \cdot \varepsilon$$

$$I_\varepsilon^{occ=0} \propto 0$$

$$\frac{I_{\varepsilon,p}}{I_{\varepsilon,p=1}} = \frac{(1-p)^4 \cdot I_\varepsilon^{occ=0} + 4p(1-p)^3 \cdot I_\varepsilon^{occ=1} + 6p^2(1-p)^2 \cdot I_\varepsilon^{occ=2} + 4p^3(1-p) \cdot I_\varepsilon^{occ=3} + p^4 \cdot I_\varepsilon^{occ=4}}{I_\varepsilon^{occ=4}}$$

For an occupancy $p = 0,5$; $I/I_{,p=1}$ is 0.26; 0.32 and 0.37 for ε 0.1, 0.7, and 1.0, respectively.

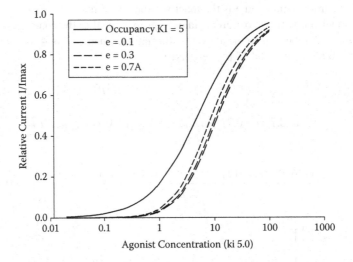

The graph illustrates the calculated normalized dose response relation for three agonists with coupling efficiencies of 0.1, 0.3, or 0.7, respectively, and the occupancy at the single subunit assuming a Ki of 5.0.

PROBLEM 3.2

Eight. In linear representation:
   (1) α_3-β_2-α_3-β_2-β_2
   (2) α_3-β_2-α_3-β_2-β_4
   (3) α_3-β_2-α_3-β_4-β_2
   (4) α_3-β_4-α_3-β_2-β_2
   (5) α_3-β_2-α_3-β_4-β_4
   (6) α_3-β_4-α_2-β_2-β_4
   (7) α_3-β_4-α_3-β_4-β_2
   (8) α_3-β_4-α_3-β_4-β_4
Combinations with similar stoichiometry would be likely to have similar conductance, i.e., four groups 1, 2-4, 5-7, and 8, while the subunit arrangement may be more important for the receptor

pharmacology since the agonist binding site is located between an α and a β subunit. If the binding site is assumed to be between the α subunit and the β subunit on the right (in this linear representation) there are 3 groups 1-2, $2x(\alpha_3-\beta_2)$; 3-6, $(\alpha_3-\beta_2)(\alpha_3-\beta_4)$; and 7-8, $2x(\alpha_3-\beta_4)$.

FURTHER READING

Barrera NP, Edwardson JM (2008). The subunit arrangement and assembly of ionotropic receptors. *Trends Neurosci.* 31, 569–576.

Celie PHN, Klaassen RV, van Rossum-Fikkert SE, van Elk R, van Nierop P, Smit AB, Sixma TK (2005). Crystal structure of acetylcholine-binding protein from *Bulinus truncatus* reveals the conserved structural scaffold and sites of variation in nicotinic acetylcholine receptors. *J Biol Chem.* 280, 26457–26466.

Dingledine R, Borges K, Bowie D, Traynelis SF (1999). The glutamate receptor ion channels. *Pharmacol Rev.* 51, 7–61.

Furukawa H, Singh SK, Mancusso R, Gouaux E (2005). Subunit arrangement and function in NMDA receptors. *Nature* 438, 185–192.

Gonzales EB, Kawate T, Gouaux E (2009). Pore architecture and ion sites in acid-sensing ion channels and P2X receptors. *Nature* 460, 599–604.

Hilf RJ, Dutzler R (2008). X-ray structure of a prokaryotic pentameric ligand-gated ion channel. *Nature* 452; 375–379.

Jin R, Banke TG, Mayer ML, Traynelis SF, Gouaux E (2003). Structural basis for partial agonist action at ionotropic glutamate receptors. *Nat Neurosci.* 6, 803–810.

Kawate T, Michel JC, Birdsong WT, Gouaux E. (2009). Crystal structure of the ATP-gated P2X(4) ion channel in the closed state. *Nature* 460, 592–598.

Kessels HW, Malinow R (2009). Synaptic AMPA receptor plasticity and behavior. *Neuron.* 61, 340–350.

Kuner T, Beck C, Sakmann B, Seeburg PH (2001). Channel-lining residues of the AMPA receptor M2 segment: Structural environment of the Q/R site and identification of the selectivity filter. *J Neurosci.* 21, 4162–4172.

Mayer ML (2006). Glutamate receptors at atomic resolution. *Nature* 440, 456–462.

Rudolph U, Crestani F, Möhler H (2001). $GABA_A$ receptor subtypes: Dissecting their pharmacological functions. *Trends Pharmacol Sci.* 22, 188–194.

Surprenant A, North RA (2009). Signaling at purinergic P2X receptors. *Annu Rev Physiol.* 71, 333–359.

Taly A, Corringer PJ, Guedin D, Lestage P, Changeux JP (2009). Nicotinic receptors: Allosteric transitions and therapeutic targets in the nervous system. *Nat Rev Drug Discov.* 8, 733–750.

4 Molecular Structure of Receptor Tyrosine Kinases

IJsbrand Kramer and Michel Laguerre

CONTENTS

4.1 INTRODUCTION

In this chapter we will describe structural features of a family of glycosylated cell surface receptors that cross the membrane through a single helix and carry a tyrosine protein kinase domain in their intracellular segment. Tyrosine kinases transfer gamma-phosphate of adenosine triphosphate (ATP) to tyrosine residues but not serine or threonine. The majority of ligands for these receptors are classified as growth factors, of which epidermal growth factor (EGF), fibroblast growth factor (FGF), insulin-like growth factor (IGF), platelet-derived growth factor (PDGF), vascular-endothelial growth factor (VEGF), and insulin are the most cited examples. The domain architecture of the members of this family of receptors is illustrated in Figure 4.1. As their name indicates, they play a role in the regulation of cell proliferation (growth), and that is a research area in which they are best studied, but they certainly play other roles. Insulin regulates glucose uptake and storage into glycogen but also imposes survival signals upon cells. Other growth factors, too, provide survival signals but are also implicated in cell motility, differentiation, and cell matrix reconstruction. In the case of aberrant functioning, certain growth factor receptors not only cause an excess of cells, or tumor

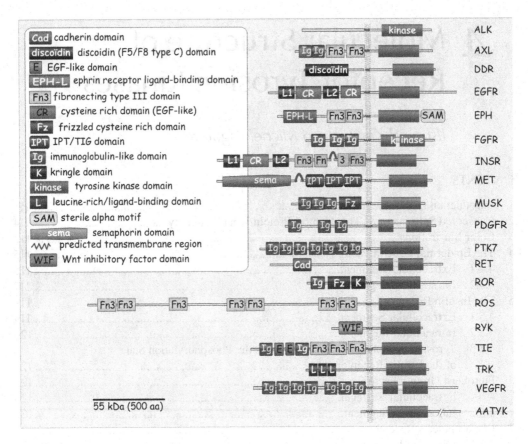

FIGURE 4.1 Classification of tyrosine protein kinase–containing receptors.

formation, but they also contribute toward malignant cell transformation, leading to subsequent dissemination of cells in other tissues (metastases).

All these receptors possess a single membrane-spanning segment, and all of them incorporate a kinase catalytic domain, in some cases interrupted by an *insert*. The extracellular domains vary as indicated but many contain an immunoglobulin motif that acts as a ligand binding site. Some of these receptors exist in various isoforms.

Tyrosine kinase receptors also share a characteristic mode of activation that seems to be best described as bringing two kinase domains of homologous receptors in close proximity so that they can render each other catalytically competent. In the majority of cases rendering competent involves phosphorylation of residues in the so-called activation segment; one kinase phosphorylates the other, a process also referred to as phosphorylation in *trans*. The requirement for dimerization is most likely put into place to reduce unsolicited receptor signaling (reduce background noise). The mechanism by which the tyrosine kinase domains are brought together and how they activate each other varies from receptor to receptor. In many cases the ligand acts as glue, combining two receptors. This may involve one ligand with two binding sites (insulin), two ligands with one binding site but linked together by disulphide bonds (PDGF), or two ligands plus heparin (FGF). The ligand may also act indirectly by changing receptor conformation, thereby exposing dimerization motifs (EGF) (Figure 4.2). Once activated, the kinase domains continue to phosphorylate each other on particular tyrosine residues that subsequently act as docking sites for adaptor/effector proteins. These attached proteins transmit the signal into the cell. In certain cases the substrate is a docking protein, with numerous tyrosine residues, which, in turn, attract numerous adaptors/effectors,

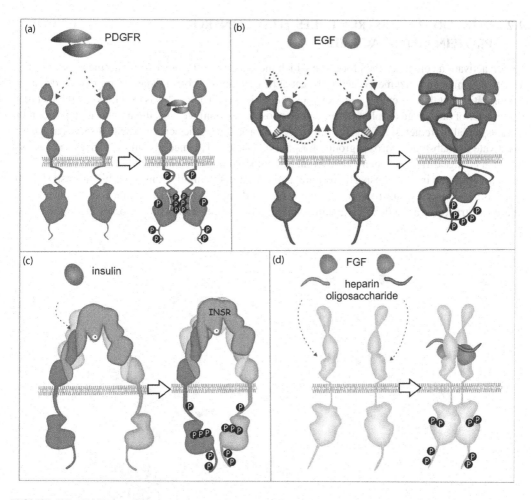

FIGURE 4.2 Different dimerization strategies receptors employ. (a) PDGF forms a ligand dimer of which each growth factor engages one receptor. (b) EGF has one binding site, and its binding reveals a receptor dimerization motif. (c) Insulin has two binding sites, and its action somehow must change the conformation of an existing receptor dimer. (d) FGF has two binding sites, but two ligands are needed to bring two receptors together. Stable dimers only form when two heparin sulfphate oligosaccharides combine with receptor-ligand complexes.

giving rise to an elaborate signaling complex. The assembly of signaling complexes and how they signal into the cell are discussed in Chapter 8 ("Signal Transduction through Protein Tyrosine Kinases," Kramer and Genot). Finally, although the majority of studies show that the activation process involves *trans*-phosphorylation events, true autophosphorylation, or phosphorylation in *cis*, is not entirely excluded. In particular, tyrosine residues located in the long and flexible C-terminal region of certain receptor tyrosine kinases appear not to be sterically hindered in reaching their *own* catalytic cleft.

Here we aim to illustrate the structure–function relationship of receptor tyrosine kinases through the description of the receptors for epidermal growth factor (EGF), insulin, and fibroblast growth factor (FGF). For pedagogical reasons we have included the structure–function relationship of the erythropoietin (Epo) receptor, which lacks an intrinsic tyrosine kinase domain but has an appended tyrosine kinase. We show that although being classified in a different family, this cytokine receptor has adapted a similar strategy to control signaling into the cell. We will also briefly discuss inhibitors of these receptors, which have been developed for the purpose of controlling their oncogenic potential.

4.2 CONSERVED SUBSTRUCTURES THAT CONTROL PROTEIN KINASE ACTIVITY

Kinase activation comprises the process in which the kinases shift from a dormant (incompetent) into an active (competent) enzyme. Structurally, catalytic domains of protein kinases vary in their dormant conformation but they resemble each other a lot once they are active. This is explained by the fact that the transfer of phosphate (or phosphoryl, hence phosphorylation) requires the precise juxtaposition of three essential ingredients: ATP, substrate, and an invariant aspartic acid residue that serves as a base to activate the substrate hydroxyl group phosphoryl acceptor. The mechanism that drives the conformational change differs between the different protein kinases (even within subfamilies).

Apart from the invariant aspartic residue, embedded in the highly conserved his-arg-asp (HRD) motif, other conserved substructures of the catalytic domain play an important role (Figure 4.3a). These substructures are a flexible, glycine-rich loop (between strands β1 and β2 of the N-lobe) that

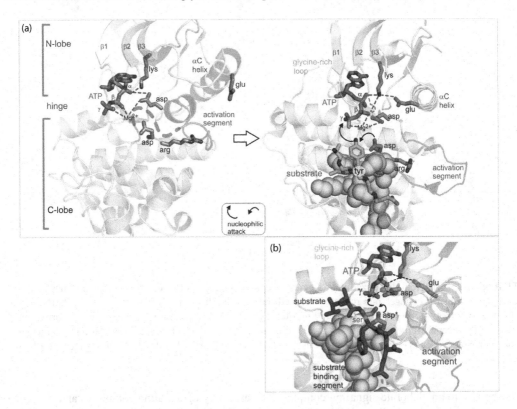

FIGURE 4.3 Conserved substructures within the consensus kinase fold involved in the phosphoryltransfer from ATP to substrate. (a) Dormant versus active tyrosine protein kinase. For clarity only a few molecular connections are shown, and one of the two Mg^{2+} atoms is omitted (situated between β- and γ-phosphate). Note the rather superficial binding of the substrate peptide in the right panel. This explains, in part, why serine and threonine are not good substrates; their hydroxyl group does not get close enough to both the γ-phosphate and the catalytic aspartate residue. Highlighted residues in the catalytic domain of the EGFR (right panel): Gly695-Val702 (glycine-rich loop); Lys721 (in β3 sheet); Glu738 (in αC helix); Arg812 (in VHRDLA motif); Asp813 (catalytic residue in VHRDLA motif); Asp831 (in DFG motif); Leu833-Gly850 (activation segment); Val852-Met859 (P+1 substrate binding residues in spheres in the right panel). (b) Active serine/threonine protein kinase (protein kinase B). Note that the substrate-peptide penetrates deeper into the cleft and that a short serine residue easily reaches both ATP and the catalytic aspartate. Highlighted residues in the catalytic domain of protein kinase B (PKB): Gly159-Lys165 (glycine-rich loop); Lys181 (in β3 sheet); Glu200 (in αC Helix); Asp275 (in RDI motif); Asp293 (in DFG motif); Leu296-Phe310 (activation segment); Gly312-Glu320 (P+1 substrate binding residues in spheres). **(See color insert following page 116.)**

interacts with ATP, orienting nucleotide phosphates through main-chain amide interactions; a lysine and a glutamic acid residue (in strand $\beta3$ and αC helix of the N-lobe respectively) forming ion pair interactions that facilitate lysine coordination and positioning of nucleotide α- and β-phosphate; an Asp-Phe-Gly (DFG) motif, of which aspartic acid coordinates the Mg^{2+} ion(s) and the nucleotide β- and γ-phosphate, and of which phenylalanine makes contact with a hydrophobic spine that establishes the relative positioning of important residues in the N- and C-lobe (not shown in figure); an activation segment, which contains residues that need to be phosphorylated for activation of the kinase (with the exception of the EGFR); and finally, a substrate interaction segment just C-terminal of the activation segment (referred to as "P+1 loop" because it interacts with the residue following the target hydroxyamino acid in the peptide substrate sequence). The resulting connections between the above-mentioned substructures direct the orientation of catalytic site residues, accommodate ATP and substrate binding, and lead to interdomain closure. The right conformation of the activation segment is often considered a primary endpoint of regulation of kinase activity.

With respect to the structural requirements for productive phosphate transfer, tyrosine kinases are not different but they do differ from other protein kinases in that they only phosphorylate tyrosine residues. This selectivity is explained, in part, by the observation that binding of the target amino acid occurs rather superficially. Serine and threonine are simply too short to let their hydroxyl group simultaneously approach the γ-phosphate of ATP and the catalytic aspartate residue (compare Figure 4.3b with Figure 4.3a). Tyrosine is much longer and, consequently, the phosphate accepting hydroxyl group penetrates further into the catalytic cleft. For more information we suggest an article by Kornev et al. (2006).

The illustrations in this chapter pretend that there are two unique conformations of receptor tyrosine kinases: an inactive one, in the absence of ligand, and an active one, when the receptor is engaged. It should be understood that protein kinases are rather flexible and can transit from one state to another even in the absence of "activating" modifications. Indeed, solution studies of IRK indicate that in the presence of millimolar quantities of ATP (comparable to cellular levels), the activation segment is actually in equilibrium between inhibiting, *gate-closed* conformations and *gate-open* conformations (in which the activation segment is displaced from the active site cleft). This, we believe, explains why two inactive kinases can phosphorylate each other when they are kept together long enough in a dimerized receptor complex. Allosteric changes brought about by activation segment phosphorylation or protein–protein interaction shift the equilibrium toward the active state, and this, of course, renders the receptor tyrosine kinase much more productive. Moreover, it should also be understood that all phosphorylation reactions occur against a background of phosphatase activity. These too warrant a low activation state of the nonengaged receptors. We will give an example for the insulin receptor, which is tightly controlled by the tyrosine phosphatase PTP1B.

4.3   COLOR ILLUSTRATIONS

To gain a better insight into the molecular mechanism of receptor activation, color illustrations are helpful. We have therefore prepared color versions of all figures in this chapter, and these are freely available in JPEG format on a special Web site dedicated to the teaching of signal transduction. You will find them in the "Receptor Pharmacology" section at: http://www.cellbiol.net/ste/book.php.

4.4   THE EPIDERMAL GROWTH FACTOR RECEPTOR

4.4.1   EXTRACELLULAR SEGMENT

The EGF receptor is member of a family of four receptors. The nomenclature of this family is confusing. We stick to the names EGFR (ERBB1), ERBB2 (Her2 or Neu), ERBB3 (Her3), and ERBB4 (Her4) and won't use the names in brackets. ERBB stands for avian erythroblastosis oncogene B, a gene carried by the avian erythroblastosis virus. A similar gene was found to be involved in the induction of neuroglioblastoma (neu) in the rat. Once the sequence of the human EGFR had been established, screening of cDNA libraries revealed the presence of human EGFR-related genes (Her2, 3, and 4). Only later it appeared that these were all members of the same family of EGF receptors and a more systematic naming deemed appropriate. However, once names have settled in the minds, they are hard to change.

The extracellular segment of the ERBB family is characterized by four domains; I, II, II, and IV. Domains I and III, stretching from amino acids 1–165 and 310–481, respectively, are structurally related, both having a β-helix or solenoid topology and consisting of numerous leucine-rich repeats (hence also named L1 and L2 domains). Domains II and IV, amino acids 166–309 and 482–618, respectively, both contain a succession of disulfide-bonded modules that comprise a rod-like structure (see Figure 4.4).

In the absence of ligand (or in the presence of ligand but under low pH conditions), extensive intramolecular contact occurs between domains and II and IV, and this keeps the extracellular segment in a *tethered* conformation. A prominent 20-residue β-hairpin/loop of domain II (residues 240–260)

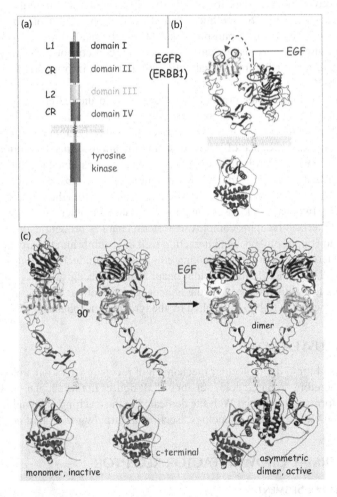

FIGURE 4.4 Modeled structures of the dimerization process of the extracellular domain of the EGFR: (a) Domain architecture of the EGF receptor. (b) Interaction between domain II and IV keeps the EGF receptor in a tethered conformation. EGF is bound to domain I but, because of acidic conditions, cannot make contact with domain III. (c) EGF binding leads to the adaptation of an extended configuration and liberates the dimerization finger in domain II. This now interacts with another domain II and forms an EGFR dimer.

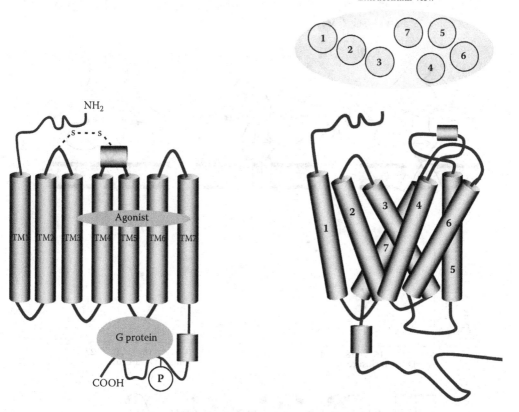

FIGURE 2.1 The molecular structure of rhodopsin-like 7-TM domain receptors. These receptors are characterized by the presence of seven membrane-spanning domains (TM1–TM7) with a short extracellular N-terminus and intracellular C-terminus shown in a two-dimensional schematic in (a). Agonist binding is predicted to be within the transmembrane domains. The extracellular structure is stabilized by a disulphide bond joining the first and second extracellular loops. The third intracellular loop is the main site of G-protein interaction, while both the third intracellular loop and carboxy tail are targets for phosphorylation by kinases responsible for initiating receptor desensitization and internalization. (b) Analysis of crystal structures has shown that the packing arrangement of the transmembrane domains is more complicated than that implied in (a) with transmembrane domains tilted to form the ligand binding pocket.

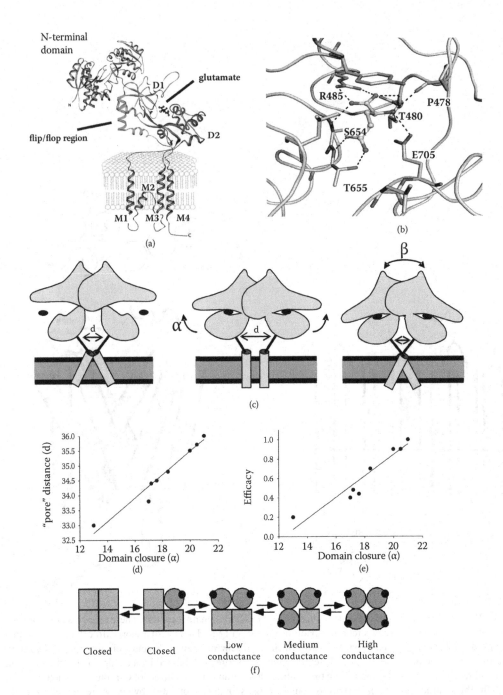

FIGURE 3.10 (a) A model of a glutamate receptor subunit. (b) Binding of glutamate at the GluR2 binding pocket. Glutamate interacts directly with residues in both domain 1 (R485, P478, and T480) and domain 2 (S654, T655, and E750), thereby stabilizing the domain closure. (c) Schematic illustration of the proposed model for subunit activation. Two subunits are shown. Agonist binding stabilizes a closed conformation of the lobes in the binding domain, thereby inducing an opening of the pore. Agonist stabilizing a high degree of domain closure (α) will subsequently induce a twist (β) between the subunits resulting in a conformational change that reduces the distance between the domains projecting to the pore. (d) Relationship between the degree of domain closure (α) and distance for the regions projecting to the pore (d) for eight agonists. (e) The relationship between efficacy, measured as the relative (to the full agonist glutamate) maximal response in a nondesensitizing mutant of the receptor and the domain closure. (f) Activation of the receptor is proposed to require activation of at least two subunits, and activation of more subunits opens the channels to a higher conductance level, that is, approximately 6 pS, 12 pS, or 17 pS, when 2, 3, or 4 subunits are activated, respectively.

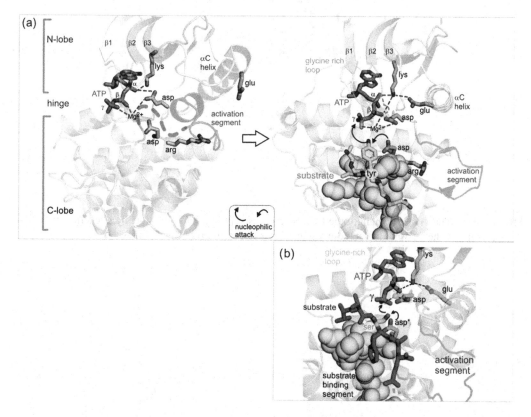

FIGURE 4.3 Conserved substructures within the consensus kinase fold involved in the phosphoryltransfer from ATP to substrate. (a) Dormant versus active tyrosine protein-kinase. For clarity reasons only a few molecular connections are shown, and one of the two Mg^{2+} atoms is omitted (situated between β- and γ-phosphate). Note the rather superficial binding of the substrate peptide in the right panel. This explains, in part, why serine and threonine are not good substrates; their hydroxyl group does not get close enough to both the γ-phosphate and the catalytic aspartate residue. Highlighted residues in the catalytic domain of the EGFR (right panel): Gly695-Val702 (glycine-rich loop); Lys721 (in β3 sheet); Glu738 (in αC helix); Arg812 (in VHRDLA motif); Asp813 (catalytic residue in VHRDLA motif); Asp831 (in DFG motif); Leu833-Gly850 (activation segment); Val852-Met859 (P+1 substrate binding residues in spheres in the right panel). (b) Active serine/threonine protein kinase (protein kinase B). Note that the substrate-peptide penetrates deeper into the cleft and that a short serine residue easily reaches both ATP and the catalytic aspartate. Highlighted residues in the catalytic domain of protein kinase B (PKB): Gly159-Lys165 (glycine-rich loop); Lys181 (in β3 sheet); Glu200 (in αC Helix); Asp275 (in RDI motif); Asp293 (in DFG motif); Leu296-Phe310 (activation segment); Gly312-Glu320 (P+1 substrate binding residues in spheres).

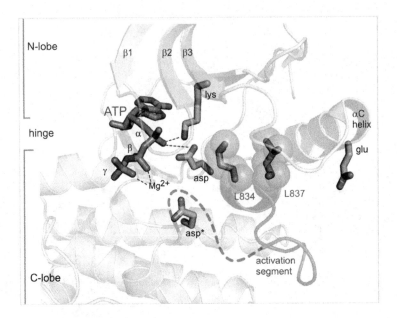

FIGURE 4.5 The kinase domain of the EGF receptor is kept in an inactive state by a leucine wedge that dislocates the αC-helix. Mutation of these residues leads to constitutive active kinases.

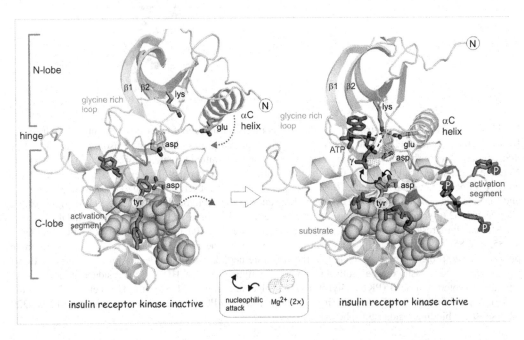

FIGURE 4.9 Molecular mechanism of insulin receptor kinase activation. In the inactive state, the activation segment occupies the site where normally substrate would bind to the kinase. Note that one of the tyrosines of the activation segment is even correctly orientated for phosphorylation. However, other important structures are not in the right configuration for accommodating ATP. Upon ligand binding the kinase domains phosphorylate each other at three tyrosine residues in the activation segment. This leads to a reorganization of the N-terminal lobe and to interdomain closure (compare the relative positions of lys, glu, and asp).

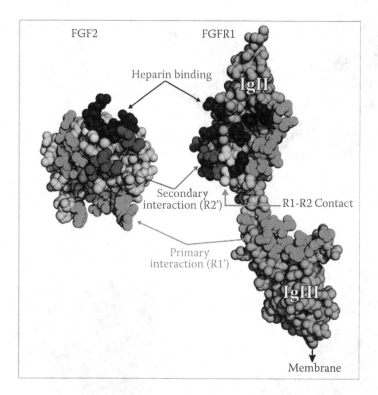

FIGURE 4.13 Multiple interaction sites between FGF2, FGFR1, and heparin sulphate. FGF interacts with two receptors. Its primary interaction is rather extensive, occurring with both Ig-domains II and III. The secondary interaction site is limited to domain Ig-II. It also has a binding site for heparin. Receptors interact with their ligand, with heparin, and with each other. Altogether, these interactions result in high-affinity binding, giving rise to stable dimers.

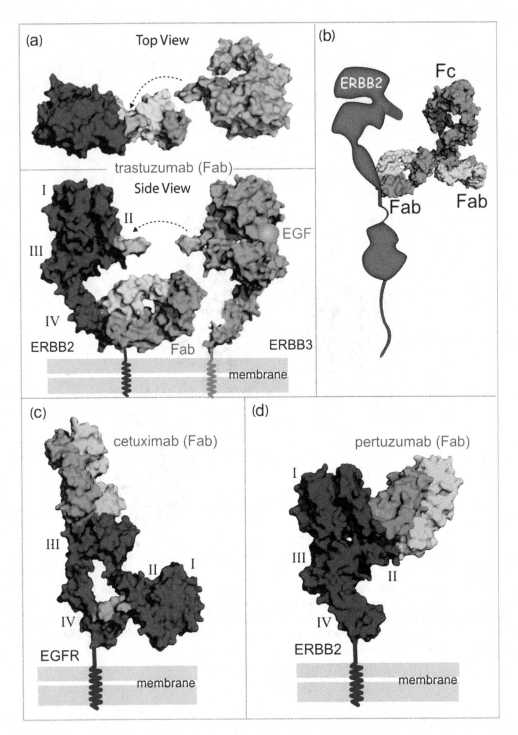

FIGURE 4.17 Overview of antibodies binding to EGFR or ERBB2. (a) Trastuzumab binds domain IV, and as shown from two perspectives (top and side views) it does not really hinder EGF binding. (b) The structural data show only the Fab fragment of the antibody, but realize that these are much bigger structures with an Fc segment that can interact with Fc-receptors carried by blood-borne cells. (c) Cetuximab binds domain III and does compete with EGF for binding. Notice that the receptor is in the tethered conformation, with its dimerization arm buried in domain IV. (d) Pertuzumab binds the dimerization arm (in green) and prevents its association with another receptor.

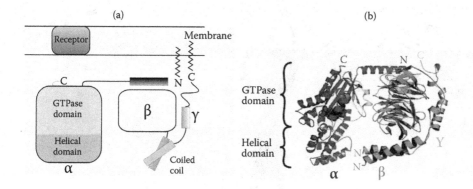

FIGURE 7.2 (a) Diagram to show G-protein α, β, and γ subunits attached to the outer cell membrane. (Adapted from Clapham, D. E., *Nature*, 379, 297, 1996.) (b) Ribbon model of Gα$_{t/i}$-GDP-β$_1$γ$_1$ with α in blue, β in green, and γ in gold. GDP is in red. (Adapted from Oldham, W. M., and Hamm, H. E., *Q. Rev. Biophys.*, 39, 117, 2006.)

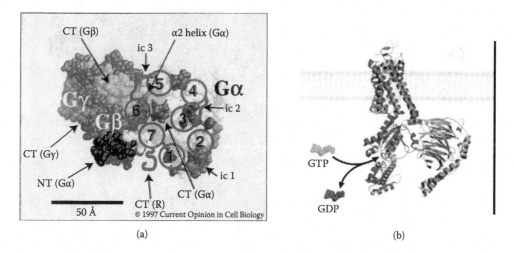

FIGURE 7.3 (a) Superposition of the seven transmembrane helices (numbered 1–7) of a GPCR on the outer surface of a G-protein. (Abbreviations: CT, C-terminus; NT, N-terminus; ic1, ic2, and ic3, first, second, and third intracellular loops of the GPCR.) (Adapted from Bourne, H. R., *Curr. Opin. Cell. Biol.*, 9, 134, 1997.) (b) Representation of the activated receptor–Gα$_o$βγ complex created by manually docking the G-protein onto an activated receptor model based on the crystal structure of rhodopsin. Color code same as Figure 7.2; magenta = rhodopsin. (Adapted from Oldham, W. M., and Hamm, H. E., *Q. Rev. Biophys.*, 39, 117, 2006.)

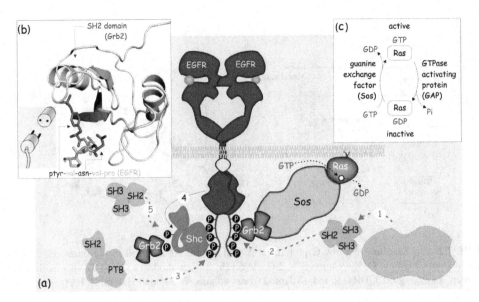

FIGURE 8.2 Recruitment of SH2- and PTB-containing proteins to activated tyrosine kinase receptors. (a) Receptor signaling complex formation through the binding of SH2- and PTB-containing proteins with the EGF receptor (adaptor proteins Grb2 and Shc, respectively). (b) Molecular detail of an SH2-binding sequence interacting with a peptide of the EGF receptor. The phosphotyrosine and asparagine bury themselves into the SH2 domain and constitute the key determinants of the interaction between the receptor and Grb2. The loss of phosphate weakens the interaction and causes separation of the two proteins. (c) Recruitment of Grb2/Sos results in activation of the GTPase Ras. Sos is a guanine exchange factor that facilitates the exchange of GDP for GTP. Ras is active in its GTP-bound state. Hydrolysis brings Ras back in its inactive GDP-bound state.

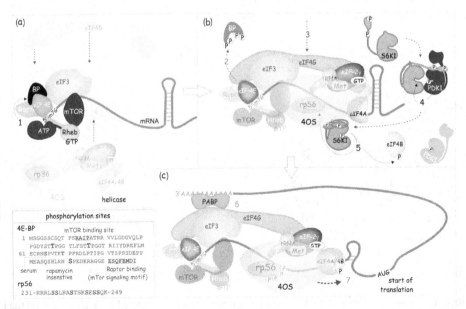

FIGURE 8.15 A series of ordered phosphorylation events facilitate the assembly of the translation initiation complex on the mRNA. (a) Activation and association of mTOR with the initiation complex causes the phosphorylation of 4E-BP (indicated as "BP") (1). Phosphorylated 4E-BP detaches from eIF-4E. (b) The dissociation of 4E-BP (2) permits the association of a big initiation factor eIF-4G that interacts with eIF-4E, eIF-3 and eIF-4A (3). Partly phosphorylated S6K1 is now fully activated by PDK1 through phosphorylation of its activation segment (4). S6K1 phosphorylates the ribosomal S6 protein (rbS6) and phosphorylates eIF-4B, a regulatory component of the RNA helicase that next joins the subunit eIF-4A (5). (c) The conditions are now favorable for binding of PABP (poly-A binding protein) which is attached to the 3'-poly A tail of the mRNA (6). The initiation complex now moves toward the start AUG codon (7) where it will be joined with the 60S ribosomal particle.

inserts between equivalent loops of domain IV (residues 561–585). The tethered conformation represents the monomeric and autoinhibited form of the receptor.

Upon binding of ligand, the tether is broken and the extracellular segment is fixed in an *extended* conformation. This exposes the 20 residue β-hairpin/loop, which now seeks contact with domain II of a homologous receptor, thus leading to the formation of a stable receptor dimer. This loop is therefore referred to as the *dimerization arm*. A similar mechanism of ligand-mediated "tethered-to-extended transition," applies for ERBB3 and ERBB4, although the relative orientation between domains I and III varies.

ERBB2 is different from the other members of the family for two reasons. Firstly, it lacks the interdomain contact (between II and IV) and occurs in a permanent extended-conformation. Secondly, no ligand has been found, and it qualifies as an orphan receptor. The permanent extended conformation allows it to interact with any of the three other ERBB receptors, once they are bound by ligand. ERBB2 does not form homodimers. Its primary role may be to act as a coreceptor that amplifies the ERBB signaling network (because two signaling complexes are formed, rather than one, with two EGF molecules). Its unique position within the ERBB family is also revealed by the observation that unlike the other receptors, its overexpression can cause cell transformation, even in the absence of added ligand for the other receptors. Indeed, the ERBB2 gene is found amplified or overexpressed in a subset of breast cancers and in some ovarian, gastric, and salivary cancers. These properties have made it a key target for cancer therapy (see later in this chapter).

4.4.2 Intracellular Segment

The purpose of EGF receptor-dimerization is to bring together, in juxtaposition, the two intracellular kinase domains. EGFR, ERBB2, and ERBB4 contain functional tyrosine kinase domains, whereas ERBB3 lacks an essential catalytic residue (aspartate replaced by asparagine in the highly conserved HRD motif). All four kinase domains can engage in the formation of homo- or heterodimers, which means that despite the lack of kinase activity, ERBB3 can nevertheless participate in signaling, either by acting as an activator (see below) or as a substrate to which, after tyrosine phosphorylation, adapter and effectors proteins bind.

Although the EGFR was the first receptor tyrosine kinase to be discovered, its mode of activation remained an enigma for quite some time. When tested in *in vitro* kinase assays, the isolated EGFR kinase, in solution as a monomeric protein, shows little activity. Surprisingly, the majority of crystal structures reveal an active configuration, with the activation segment nicely pushed out of the way and with the right positioning of the above mentioned conserved substructures. Only in the presence of the drug lapatinib (Tykerb) have crystals been obtained in which the kinase adopts an inactive conformation resembling that of inactive Src and cyclin-dependent kinases (CDKs). Moreover, unlike all other tyrosine kinases, the switch from inactive to active does not require a covalent modification; the activation segment does not need to be phosphorylated.

Added to this confusion came the finding that lung cancer in nonsmokers is frequently accompanied by EGFR mutations in which leucine-834 is replaced by arginine (L834R) or leucine-837 by glutamine (L837Q). Their replacement results in enhanced catalytic activity, despite the fact that they are surface-exposed amino acids that seem not to play an obvious role in the organization of the catalytic cleft. The answer to their role in kinase regulation came from a revision of structural analysis of Src-related protein tyrosine kinases in their inactive state. This analysis revealed that the equivalent of the above-mentioned leucine residues wedge into the interior of the kinase domain while buttressing a displaced orientation of the critical helix αC and preventing ion-pair interaction between glutamate and lysine (Figure 4.5). This suggested that leucine-834 and -837 keep the EGFR in a self-inhibited, inactive state. What led to the switch toward a competent conformation, as detected in crystal lattices and in EGF-treated cells, remained to be answered.

Close reexamination of the crystal lattice of the active form revealed an asymmetric dimer in which one kinase domain interacts with another in a manner analogous to that of a cyclin bound to

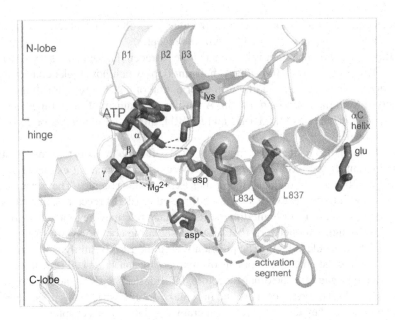

FIGURE 4.5 The kinase domain of the EGF receptor is kept in an inactive state by a leucine wedge that dislocates the αC-helix. Mutation of these residues leads to constitutive active kinases. **(See color insert.)**

cyclin-dependent kinase. The current understanding is that one of the kinases acts as an allosteric regulator of the other, much the same way as cyclin-A controls activity of CDK2 (Figure 4.6). Mutations of amino acids at the interface of the asymmetric dimer abrogate kinase activity. The monomers can swap positions easily and activate each other, leading to mutual phosphorylation of the tyrosine residues in the unstructured C-terminal tail (five tyrosine residues in between Y992 to

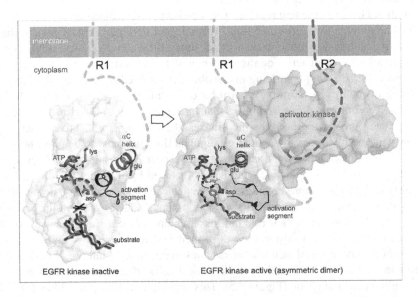

FIGURE 4.6 Allosteric regulation of the EGF receptor kinase domain by the formation of an asymmetric dimer. In this proposed model of kinase activation, one of the two protein kinases acts as the regulator of the other kinase domain (activator kinase), a mechanism of activation reminiscent of cyclin-mediated activation of cylin-dependent kinases.

Y1173). The phosphorylated tyrosine residues act as docking sites for adaptor and effector proteins (see Chapter 8), thus leading to the formation of a signaling complex.

4.5 THE INSULIN RECEPTOR

4.5.1 EXTRACELLULAR SEGMENT

The insulin receptor family comprises the insulin receptor (IR), the type-I insulin-like growth factor receptor (IGF-1R), and the insulin receptor-related (orphan) receptor (IRR). These normally are expressed at the cell surface as disulfide-linked homodimers but heterodimer hybrids are not excluded (IR/IGF-1R hybrids are detected). The insulin receptor, of which A- and B-isoforms exist, comprises two leucine-rich repeats (L1 and L2), separated by a cysteine-rich region (as in the EGFR), and followed by three fibronectin–type III domains. The second fibronectin domain houses an insert domain (IDα and -β) as well as a short C-terminal peptide (CT). The insertion domain contains a furin cleavage site that generates an extracellular α-chain and a transmembrane β-chain of the mature receptor (held together by extensive protein–protein contact and by a disulphide bond). Two insert regions of the α-chains (IDα), in turn, link to each other through four disulphide bonds (Figure 4.7). In this respect, the insulin receptor family differs from all other tyrosine kinase-containing receptors.

The insulin receptor dimer has an unexpected folded-over conformation that places the C-terminal surface of the first fibronectin-III domain in close juxtaposition to the L1 domain

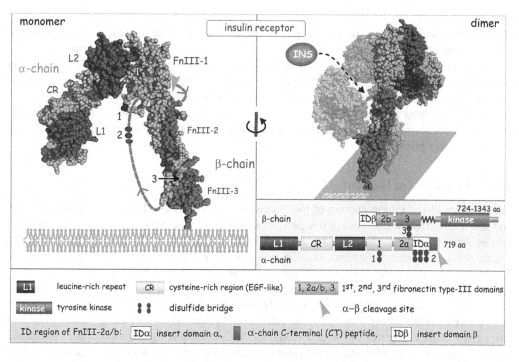

FIGURE 4.7 Insulin receptor structure. The insulin receptor is a homodimer. In the mature form, each component is present as two chains, α and β. The protein is organized in seven domains: L1 (leucine-rich region-1), CR (cysteine-rich region), L2, FnIII-1 (fibronectin-III-like domain 1), FnIII-2, FNIII-3, and the intracellular tyrosine kinase domain. Both the α and β chain contribute to the FnIII-2 domain. The long insert region (shown as a dotted line) separating FnIII-2a from -2b contains three disulphide bridges (position 2) that link the monomers. FNIII-1 provides a fourth disulphide bridge (position 1). A possible orientation between the two peptides is indicated in the right panel (dimer). The insulin-binding space is between the central β-sheet of L1 and the bottom loops of the FnIII-1 domain.

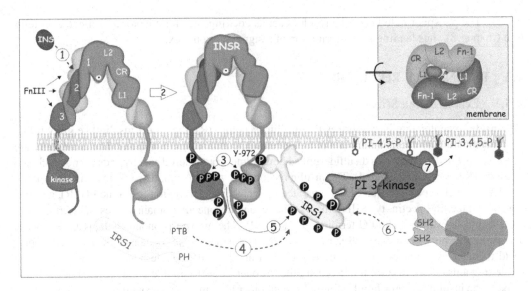

FIGURE 4.8 Insulin binding and possible consequence for receptor conformation. How binding of insulin leads to activation of the kinase domains remains to be elucidated. In this schematic representation we propose that the kinase domains approach each other due to a change in the relative position of the two receptors.

ligand-binding surface. High-affinity binding of insulin requires binding to domains L1, CR, and CT (of receptor 1) and to loops at the junction of the first and second Fn type-III domain (of receptor 2) (Figure 4.8). Although the dimer theoretically harbors two ligand-binding sites, high-affinity binding of insulin in one binding pocket appears to preclude binding to the second site (negative cooperativity). How insulin binding leads to tyrosine kinase activation remains to be discovered. Ligand binding either alters the receptor conformation or the relative position of the receptor subunits. It is possible that the disulphide bonds in the IDα domain act as a hinge around which the two insulin-receptors pivot.

4.5.2 INTRACELLULAR SEGMENT

The structure of the kinase domain of the inactive receptor has revealed an auto-inhibited state. This is witnessed by the observation that part of the activation segment occupies the substrate binding site. Note that one of the tyrosines even sits in the correct position for being phosphorylated (Figure 4.9, left structure). Furthermore, the amino acids that coordinate the binding of ATP are manifestly in total disarray: compare the position of asp, glu, and lys in the left and right kinases of Figure 4.9. Unlike the EGF receptor, rendering the insulin receptor catalytically competent does require posttranslational modification. Three tyrosine residues, Y1158, Y1162, and Y1163, have to be phosphorylated in order to bring the activation segment in an outward position. This conformational change liberates the substrate binding site, causes a reorganization of the N-terminal lobe, now ready to bind ATP, and leads to interdomain closure (Figure 4.9, right structure). Further phosphorylations then occur in tyrosine residues beyond the catalytic site; Y972, in an asparagine proline glutamate tyrosine (NPEY) motif of the juxtamembrane region, and Y1328 and Y1334 in the carboxy-terminal region. These three phosphotyrosines and their immediate amino acids form docking sites for SH2- or PTP-domain containing proteins.

A peculiarity of the insulin receptor is that it signals through the intervention of large docking proteins. These insulin receptor substrates (IRS-1 to -4) all possess pleckstrin homology (PH) and phospho tyrosine binding (PTB) domains but are otherwise rather unstructured (native disordered

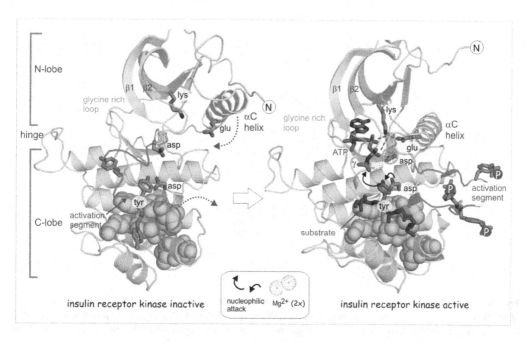

FIGURE 4.9 Molecular mechanism of insulin receptor kinase activation. In the inactive state, the activation segment occupies the site where normally substrate would bind to the kinase. Note that one of the tyrosines of the activation segment is even correctly orientated for phosphorylation. However, other important structures are not in the right configuration for accommodating ATP. Upon ligand binding the kinase domains phosphorylate each other at three tyrosine residues in the activation segment. This leads to a reorganization of the N-terminal lobe and to interdomain closure (compare the relative positions of lys, glu, and asp). **(See color insert.)**

proteins). The PTB domains bind directly to the tyrosine phosphorylated region of the receptor, which corresponds to pY972. Of the four docking proteins, IRS-1 and -2 are essential for insulin signaling: lack of IRS-1 is linked to a mild insulin resistance, which is compensated by increased insulin secretion. Absence of IRS-2 causes insulin resistance in the liver and skeletal muscle (among many other developmental defects) and results in type-2 diabetes because of a lack of β-cell compensation.

We elaborate further on IRS-2 because apart from its important role in relaying the insulin signal into the cell it also has an unexpected role in the regulation of the insulin receptor kinase. Phosphorylation of IRS-2 normally occurs in the YΦ(fi)XM motif (where Φ denotes a hydrophobic residue often, and X, any amino acid). There are 10 such sites, 9 of which recruit an important effector enzyme, phosphatidylinositol 3-kinase (PI 3-kinase), and one is the adaptor protein Grb2 (read further in Chapter 8). However, one phospho-acceptor tyrosine, Y628, is situated in a different sequence motif (yz-gly-asp-iso [YGDI]). Moreover, it is embedded in a protein segment that was initially discovered as a kinase regulatory loop-binding (KRLB) region. Although originally hailed as a novel protein–protein interaction domain, it now appears that this region is linear and most likely just acts as substrate. Surprisingly, the linear peptide containing Y628 (residues 621–634) folds over the C-lobe in a manner similar to the activation segment of the inactive kinase. However, due to a glycine at the P+1 position, the Y628 is slightly displaced relative to the tyrosines in the YΦ(Fi)XM motif, and this makes it a less good substrate. Importantly, a tyrosine residue at position P-7 sits with its side chain inserted in the ATP binding site and competes with its binding (Figure 4.10). As a consequence, the tyrosine kinase is effectively inhibited. This is a unique example of a very short negative feedback loop. A possible physiological role for IRS-2-mediated suppression of its own phosphorylation remains to be established.

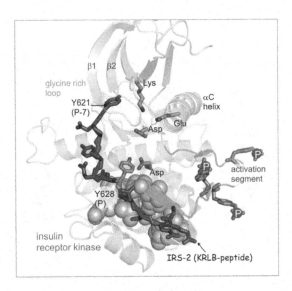

FIGURE 4.10   Inhibition of insulin tyrosine kinase by its substrate IRS-2. One of the phosphorylation sites of the IRS-2 substrate does not occur in the classic YΦXM motif but in a YGDI motif, in a segment of the protein that was originally designated a kinase regulatory loop binding region (KRLB). Because of the unusual motif, the orientation of the target tyrosine (Y628) is slightly distorted, thereby reducing the efficiency of phosphorylation. Moreover, a tyrosine seven residue downstream inserts into the ATP pocket and competes with binding. Altogether, these features make the IRS-2 protein not only a substrate but also an inhibitor of the insulin receptor tyrosine kinase.

4.5.3   TYROSINE PHOSPHATASE PTP1B CONTROLS THE PHOSPHORYLATION STATE OF THE INSULIN RECEPTOR

Perhaps the most spectacular example of a link between a phosphotyrosine phosphatase and human disease is type 2 (mature onset, insulin resistant) diabetes and obesity. Both genetic and biochemical studies provide good evidence for a role of tyrosine phosphatase in the signaling events downstream of the insulin and leptin receptors. Dephosphorylation of the insulin receptor by protein tyrosine phosphatases is critical in the control of the cellular response to insulin. Numerous studies have demonstrated that in humans and in animal models, the resistance to insulin in type 2 diabetes, and subsequent development of obesity, is accompanied by increases in tyrosine phosphatase activity and increases in the level of expression of defined members of the tyrosine phosphatase family; the receptor tyrosine phosphatase LAR and cytosolic tyrosine phosphatase PTP1B. However, disruption of the LAR gene in mice yields a complex phenotype consistent with having a postreceptor defect in insulin signaling but, surprisingly, associated with impaired activation of downstream signals such as PI 3-kinase (rather than the expected elevated signal). Matters are somewhat clearer for PTB1B. Here, insulin-induced activation of S6 kinase (regulation of protein synthesis) and transition through the G2/M phase checkpoint of the cell cycle is inhibited in Xenopus oocytes injected with the purified enzyme. When overexpressed in Rat1 fibroblasts, PTP1B reduces insulin-induced phosphorylation of its own receptor, the downstream phosphorylation of components of the signaling cascade, translocation of GLUT-4 (glucose transporter) to the membrane and glycogen synthesis. Conversely, loading of hepatoma cells with neutralizing antibodies to PTP1B enhances insulin-induced phosphorylation of its receptor and of the receptor substrate IRS-1.

An unequivocal link between insulin signaling and the tyrosine phosphatase was established through the use of PTP1B knock-out mice: these animals remained healthy and displayed an enhanced sensitivity to insulin. Moreover, when fed a high-fat diet, they failed to become obese and

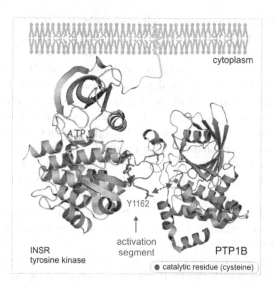

FIGURE 4.11 Dephosphorylation of the insulin receptor activation segment by PTP1B; PTP1B binds preferentially to the bis- or tris-phosphorylated activation segment of the insulin receptor. Residue pTyr-1162 is most readily recognized by the catalytic cleft of the phosphatase. Dephosphorylation renders the insulin receptor catalytically incompetent. Sequence comparison with other PTPs suggests that the features that confer the specificity of this reaction are unique to PTP1B and its close relative TCPTP.

retained their normal sensitivity to insulin (see Figure 4.11). By contrast, their wild-type (PTP1B$^{+/+}$) littermates suffered rapid weight gain and onset of insulin resistance, which coincided with a reduced level of tyrosine phosphorylation of the insulin receptor. All this suggests that the insulin receptor kinase-domain acts as a substrate of PTP1B. Surprisingly, the knock-out mice did not show any predisposition to cancer despite the potential of PTP1B to regulate growth factor receptor tyrosine kinase signaling and to counteract the transforming effects of the kinases Src and ERBB2. The activity of downstream protein kinases in the growth factor signaling network was only slightly enhanced (tested for ERK and PKB). A possible explanation comes from the finding that due to a lack of PTP1B, expression of RasGAP and phosphorylation of p62Dok are elevated and this leads to attenuation of the Ras-MAPK pathway. This is a good example of how feedback mechanisms prevent excess signaling (often referred to as the "robustness of the system").

4.6 FIBROBLAST GROWTH FACTOR

FGFs play important roles in all levels of animal development. Aberrant FGF signaling (due to mutations in the receptors) during limb and skeletal development leads to human dysmorphic syndromes: abnormal morphologic features such as dwarfism (hypochondroplasia, a more severe achondroplasia, or a lethal variant thanatophoric dysplasia) and premature closure of the skull sutures (craniosynostosis). Among other effects, an excess of fibroblast growth factor receptor (FGFR)-activity leads to a restrained proliferation of chondrocytes (bone-making cells). The role of FGF receptors has been particularly well studied in the development of the nervous system where they play a role in cell differentiation as well as in axon guidance and synaptogenesis.

4.6.1 EXTRACELLULAR SEGMENT

Four receptor tyrosine kinases, FGFR1–4, mediate the biological responses of FGFs, of which 22 members have been discerned. It should also be noted that several other ligands can bind FGF receptors, including a subset of neuronal cell adhesion molecules, including N-CAM, N-Cadherin, and L1. Each FGF receptor occurs in numerous isoforms because of alternative splicing. For instance, 18 named isoforms are produced of human FGFR1. These give rise to a bewildering array of different proteins ranging from just a change in one of the extracellular domains (version a, b, or c), a lack of expression of the first extracellular domain, an insertion into the C-terminal stretch of the kinase domain, to a complete loss of the intracellular segment (secreted protein).

The full-length receptors are composed of an extracellular segment comprising three immuno-globulin-like C2-type domains, IgI (residues 25–119), IgII (residues 158–246), and IgIII (residues 255–357). Of these, domains IgII and IgIII are involved in ligand binding. A short sequence of acidic amino acids, referred to as the acidic box, is inserted between IgI and IgII. FGF only poorly binds to purified receptors; and when it was found that it also binds to heparin sulphate proteogly-cans, it became clear that high-affinity binding requires a ternary complex of receptor, ligand and heparin sulphate motifs. The intimate relationship between heparin sulphate and FGF signaling is underscored by the observation that flies and mice with defects in heparin sulphate biosynthesis are phenocopies of those that have defects in the FGFR.

Structural analysis revealed that two FGF type-2 ligands, two FGF type-1 receptors, and two heparin oligosaccharides cooperate with each other to assemble into a symmetric functional dimeric unit (2FGF2 : 2FGF1R : 2 heparin-sulphate oligosaccharide [Figure 4.12]). High-affinity FGF bind-ing thus requires a high level of cooperativity between protein–protein and protein–heparin sul-phate interactions. Each FGF is bivalent and possesses a primary and secondary receptor binding site (in analogy with insulin). The primary ligand-binding site is large and encompasses regions in domains IgII and IgIII, whereas the secondary ligand-binding site is confined to IgII (Figure 4.13). A third protein–protein contact is made between two receptors. The symmetric juxtaposition of the

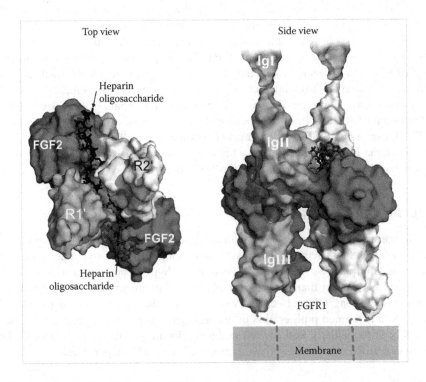

FIGURE 4.12 Top and side views of the FGF receptor bound to ligand and heparin sulphate oligosac-charides. Note that FGF2 binding to its receptor creates a canyon that nicely fits the heparin sulphate motifs. This surface illustration shows the multiple contacts between receptor, ligand, and the heparin sulphate oligosaccharides.

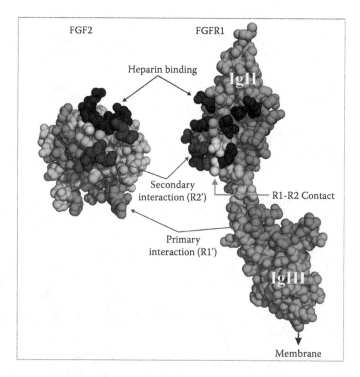

FIGURE 4.13 Multiple interaction sites between FGF2, FGFR1, and heparin sulphate. FGF interacts with two receptors. Its primary interaction is rather extensive, occurring with both Ig-domains II and III. The secondary interaction site is limited to domain Ig-II. It also has a binding site for heparin. Receptors interact with their ligand, with heparin, and with each other. Altogether, these interactions result in high-affinity binding, giving rise to stable dimers. **(See color insert.)**

two FGF-FGFR complexes creates a unique heparin-sulphate binding canyon, which recruits two heparin sulphate oligosaccharides. Simultaneous interactions of heparin sulphate with FGF and the IgII domain of the receptor fortify all above-mentioned protein–protein interactions and hence lead to sustained dimerization.

4.6.2 Intracellular Segment

The change in conformation between a dormant and an active receptor tyrosine kinase is difficult to discern for the FGFR. The activation segment undergoes relatively little change. Thanks to a number of gain-of-function mutations that were detected in the FGF2 receptor (for instance N549H, N549T, E565A, E565G, E565A, or K641R) of a subset of patients with craniosynostosis (premature fusion of skull sutures), a novel mechanism of regulation of tyrosine kinase activity has been revealed.

It was discovered that a molecular brake in the hinge region, constituted by a triad of amino acids, keeps the kinase in a catalytically inactive configuration (Figure 4.14a). In fact, a network of hydrogen bonds between Glu565 (in the hinge), Asn549 (in the loop between the αC helix and the β4 strand), and Lys641 (in the β8 strand of the C-lobe) inhibits the movement of the N-lobe toward the C-lobe, or in other words, inhibits interdomain closure. This, in turn, prevents the correct positioning of the highly conserved residues in the catalytic cleft (Figure 4.14b). Phosphorylation of the activation segment, on residues Y656 and Y657, leads to dissociation of the hydrogen-bond network and relaxes the N-lobe so that it rotates toward the C-lobe. A similar effect is obtained through mutations of any of these residues, for instance when Glu565 is replaced by glycine or Lys641 by arginine. These mutations cause gain-of-function of the FGF2 receptor, as detected in cells from a subset of patients with craniosynostosis.

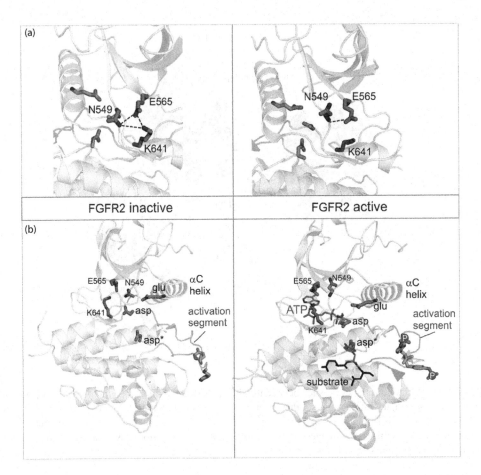

FIGURE 4.14 The molecular brake of the FGF receptor kinase family. (a) The FGF receptor kinase is kept in a dormant state through a network of hydrogen bonds, in between N549, E565, and K641, which prevents the right orientation of the N-lobe relative to the C-lobe. Phosphorylation of the activation segment breaks this inhibitory spell (right panel). (b) A classic view of the FGF tyrosine kinase shows the moderate shift of the overall structure between the inactive and active conformation. Compare the position of the essential residues glu, asp, and asp* in the left and right panes. This shift suffices to accommodate ATP and leads to phosphorylation of substrate.

All three residues of FGFR2 that mediate the inhibitory network of hydrogen bonds at the hinge region are fully conserved in all FGF receptors as well as in the PDGFR, VEGFR, KIT, CSF1R, FLT3, TEK, and TIE. This suggests that this mode of autoinhibition may be a common regulatory mechanism for these receptor tyrosine kinases. Detailed structural analysis has confirmed the presence of the same network and gain-of-function mutations that abrogate the triadic engagement have been reported for these receptor kinases.

4.7 ERYTHROPOIETIN RECEPTOR

Human erythropoietin is a haematopoietic cytokine required for the differentiation and proliferation of precursor cells into red blood cells. The erythropoietin receptors (EpoR) lack an intrinsic tyrosine protein kinase domain, but they signal nevertheless in a nearly identical fashion as the above-discussed receptor tyrosine protein kinases. As soon as the receptor is synthesized, in the rough endoplasmic reticulum, its cytosolic segment binds a cytosolic tyrosine protein kinase named JAK2 (Janus kinase-2).

In fact, without this association, the EpoR does not get processed in the Golgi and never reaches the cell surface. Instead it most likely ends its life prematurely inside a proteasome or a lysosome. Thus, with respect to receptor processing and signaling, EpoR and JAK2 are inseparable partners and, from a signaling point of view, JAK2 can be considered the equivalent of an intrinsic kinase domain.

The EpoR is a member of a subfamily of cytokine receptors that signal through JAK2. Other receptors are those that bind growth hormone, leptin, GM-CSH, prolactin, thrombopoietin, interleukin-3, or interleukin-5.

4.7.1 EXTRACELLULAR SEGMENT

The Epo receptor is composed of a short amino-terminal helix (residues 9–22) followed by two β-sandwich fibronectin-type III domains (FnIII), designated D1 and D2, each consisting of ~100 amino acids. The N-terminal helix is tucked away into the elbow formed by the D1 and D2 domains, in close proximity to the trp-ser-x-trp-ser (WSXWS) motif (residues 209–213) in D2 (Figure 4.15b). Alteration of the WSXWS sequence disrupts ligand binding and receptor signaling. The motif plays an essential role in folding, correctly positioning of the D1 and D2 domains relative to each other, and transport of the receptor to the cell surface. Loops connecting the β-strands in both D1 and D2 make extensive contact with erythropoietin.

Erythropoietin has a four-helical bundle topology and binds and correctly orientates two cell surface erythropoietin receptors. The receptor molecules are held together through two regions located on opposite faces of the erythropoietin. These ligand receptor interfaces have been identified as high affinity (Kd~1 nM) and low affinity (Kd~1μM) and are referred to as sites 1 and 2, respectively. Site 1 is composed of erythropoietin residues from helices A, B′, D, and part of the AB loop, whereas site 2 constitutes residues located in helix A and C (Figure 4.15b). Site 1 is characterized by a central hydrophobic binding pocket, flanked by hydrophilic interactions, covering a surface of 920 Å^2. The interactions at site 2 are less extensive, covering 660 Å^2, composed of a rather flat hydrophobic surface.

EpoR form homodimers at the cell surface, even in the absence of Epo, yet they do not signal. A rigid α-helix, comprising the transmembrane segment and a set of extracellular juxtamembrane residues, is thought to be responsible for locking the unliganded dimeric receptor in an inactive conformation. This lock is broken upon ligand binding. In comparing the structures of the receptor bound to the erythropoietin mimetic EMP1 with that of the natural protein it was revealed that the relative orientations of the D1 domains differ considerably. Viewed perpendicular to the membrane plane (top view), the D1 domains in the erythropoietin complex are positioned at 120° relative to each other, compared with 180° for the mimetic-containing complex. Moreover, in the case of the latter, the D2 domains are twisted away by 45°. This difference in orientation corresponds with a difference in signaling efficiency. Erythropoietin mimetics typically do not exceed 1/20 of the signal of the natural protein. These results indicate that signaling efficiency depends critically on the relative disposition of bound receptors and explains why the formation of a homodimer does not suffice. The 120° orientation somehow relieves an auto-inhibitory constraint imposed upon the appended JAK2 tyrosine kinases.

4.7.2 INTRACELLULAR SEGMENT

Members of the Janus family of nonreceptor tyrosine kinases are key mediators of cytokine receptor signaling and, consequentially, play a central role in hematopoiesis and immune responses. Humans express four Janus kinases: JAK1–3 and Tyk2. These tyrosine kinases contain seven highly conserved domains named JAK-homology (JH) domains 1–7 (Figure 4.15c). The C-terminal JH1 domain is a functional tyrosine kinase, whereas J2 is a pseudokinase (nonfunctional), which negatively controls its neighbor (mechanism not clear). The JH3 to JH7 domains mediate association of JAK with the membrane-proximal region of the cytokine receptor. Half of domain JH4 and extending to domain JH7 harbors a FERM motif, originally discovered in 4.1 protein of erythrocytes,

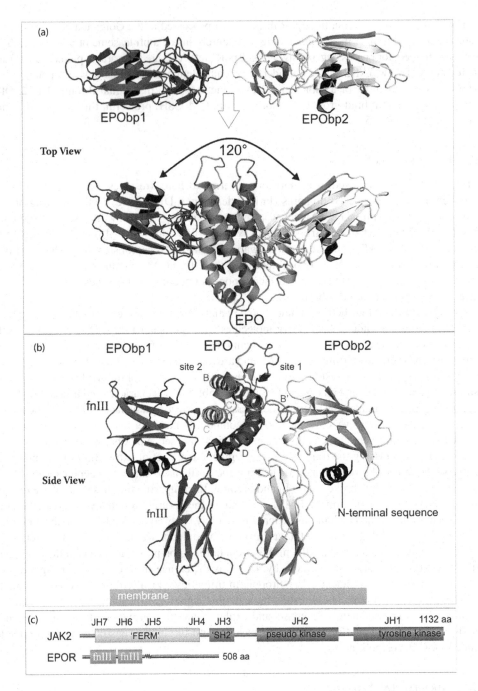

FIGURE 4.15 Structure of Epo bound to its receptors. (a) The Epo receptor occurs in dimers in the unliganded state but the relative orientation of the two receptors (here arbitrarily depicted as 180°) does not allow for kinase activation. Epo binding positions the first FnIII-domains of two receptors in a 120° orientation, which is commensurate with kinase activation. (b) A side view shows the structural role of the N-terminal sequence, which makes contacts with both the first and the second FnIII-domains. (c) Domain architecture of JAK2 and the Epo receptor. The FERM and SH2 are between quotation marks because they are related domains and do not fully match the signature sequences.

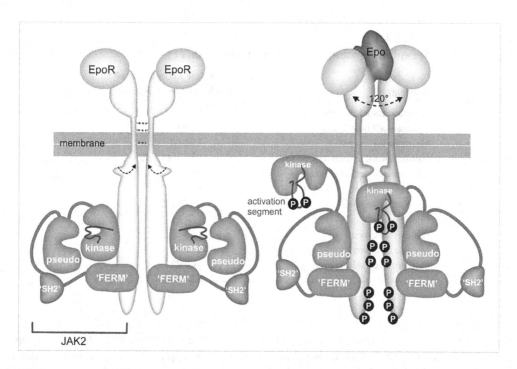

FIGURE 4.16 Model for Epo-mediated activation of JAK2. In the resting state, the pseudo kinase (JH2) maintains a strong interaction with the kinase domain (JH1), thus preventing its activity. Epo binding triggers the extracellular domains to adopt a 120° angular orientation, and this somehow relieves the inhibitory constraint of JH2. Phosphorylation in *trans* of the activation segments (on two tyrosine residues) leads to kinase activation and subsequent phosphorylation of tyrosine residues on the cytosolic segment of the Epo receptor. (Image adapted from Lu et al., *J Biol Chem*, 283:5258–5266, 2008.) **(See color insert.)**

where it plays a role in binding to cytoskeletal proteins. Its role in JAK2 is not clear. Furthermore, the stretch from JH3 to midway JH4 harbors an SH2-related domain, also of unknown function. Deregulation of JAK2 is implicated in several hematological malignancies. For instance, the majority of the Bcr-Abl-negative myeloproliferative disorders express a JAK2 mutant in which Val617, in the pseudokinase domain, is replaced by a phenylalanine. This leads to cytokine-independent activity of JAK2 but still requires the presence of homodimeric Epo receptors.

It is hypothesised that under resting conditions, the JH2 pseudokinase domain associates with the JH1 kinase domain and prevents transphosphorylation. The Epo-mediated change of the relative position of the receptor disconnects JH1 from JH2. The liberated JH1 domains find each other and after phosphorylation of the activation segment in *trans*, they phosphorylate the cytosolic segment of the Epo receptor (Figure 4.16). It is likely that the V617F mutation abrogates the inhibitory JH1–JH2 interaction, thus allowing transactivation without Epo. As mentioned earlier, an EpoR dimer is still vital; otherwise the two kinases would never meet.

The Epo receptor has eight potential phosphorylation sites between residues 368 and 504. The phosphotyrosine motifs recruit several SH2-containing proteins, amongst others: the transcription factor STAT5, the lipid kinase PI 3-kinase, and the tyrosine phosphatase SHP1.

4.8 RECEPTOR TYROSINE KINASES AS TARGETS FOR CANCER THERAPY

One of the major limiting factors in the classic chemotherapy approach to the treatment of cancer is, because of the adverse affects due to their indiscriminate nature, the extremely narrow time window during which antimitotic agents can be applied. This means that numerous cancer cells, not actually

TABLE 4.1
Receptor Tyrosine Kinases Involved in Cancer

Pathology	Tyrosine Kinase Receptor Involved (Mutated or Overexpressed)
Metastatic colorectal cancer	EGFR
Nonsmall-cell lung cancer	EGFR
Metastatic breast cancer	ERBB2
Gastrointestinal stromal tumors	KIT or PDGFR
Acute myeloid leukemia and Acute promyelocytic leukemia	FLT3
Juvenile hemangioma	VEGFR2/3
Glioblastoma	FGFR1
Endometrial cancer	FGFR2
Multiple myeloma	FGFR3
Bladder and cervical cancers	FGFR3

in the process of division during treatment, or hiding in a safe compartment of the body, escape. The demand for cancer cell–specific medicaments that can be applied for long periods of time is still largely unanswered, with the exception for the treatment of chronic myeloid leukemia. Receptor tyrosine kinases (or their ligands) are sought after targets for the development of the so-called magic bullets. Their activity is tightly controlled by default inhibitory structural constraints, but when mutated they may become potent oncoproteins. Indeed, elevated activity is often observed in transformed cells and it plays a driving role in cancer development. Examples of cancers in which receptor tyrosine kinases play a driving role are shown in Table 4.1.

Two approaches have reached the clinic: one concerns the application of humanized monoclonal antibodies (products ending with -*mab*) and the other, the application of small chemical compounds that bind in the catalytic cleft and compete with ATP (products ending with -*nib*). A few examples are shown in Table 4.2.

TABLE 4.2
Employment of Novel Anticancer Medicaments That Target Receptor Tyrosine Kinases or Their Ligands

Generic Name	Commercial Name	Target	Pathology Concerned
Trastuzumab	Herceptin	ERBB2	Metastatic breast cancer
Pertuzumab	Omnitarg	ERBB2	Metastatic breast cancer
Bevacizumab	Avastin	VEGF	Metastatic colorectal cancer
Cetuximab	Erbitux	EGFR	Metastatic colorectal cancer
Matuzumab	EMD72000	EGFR	Ovarian and peritoneal malignancies (in trial phase)
Imatinib	Gleevec/Glivec	KIT, PDGFR	Gastrointestinal stromal tumor
Gefitinib	Iressa	EGFR	Advanced nonsmall-cell lung cancer
Erlotinib	Tarceva	EGFR	Advanced nonsmall-cell lung cancer

4.8.1 Antibody Approach

The first evidence for a potential therapeutic role of monoclonal antibodies in the treatment of cancer dates back to 1984, when it was shown that mouse monoclonal antibodies, recognizing the neu oncogene (ERBB2), could block proliferation of human cancer cell lines. This finding has been translated into treatment, and since 1998, ERBB2-overexpressing metastatic breast cancers are treated with Trastuzumab. The majority of antibodies now being used in cancer treatment were developed prior to the era of structural exploration of the mode of activation of EGF receptors. A better understanding of where they bind and how they affect receptor signaling may help to improve the development of new antibodies with perhaps higher therapeutic efficacy. We will illustrate the binding site of four antibodies and explain their therapeutic benefit.

Trastuzumab binds domain IV of the ERBB2 receptor and, surprisingly, it interferes neither with ligand binding nor with receptor dimerization (Figure 4.17a,b). Yet it reduces EGF signaling. A number of theories as to the mode of action have been developed. Firstly, although the antibody does not prevent dimerization, it may affect the relative position of the cytosolic segments and hence affect signaling. The antibody may provoke receptor internalization and reduce the number of cell surface receptors. It may prevent proteolytic cleavage of the ERBB2 receptor and perhaps reduce the number of "free" cytosolic segments that appear to have constitutive kinase activity. Importantly, all treatment with antibodies provoke an innate immune response involving Fc receptor–mediated phagocytosis of the antibody-covered cells and, hence, destruction of ERBB2-expressing cells.

Cetuximab, too, binds domain III, but it does compete with EGF for binding to its receptor (Figure 4.17c). Pertuzumab binds the dimerization arm of ERBB2 and simply prevents association with other members of the ERBB family (Figure 4.17d). The cells have lost an important ally in growth factor signaling. Treatment with both of these antibodies could prove to be very efficient because it leaves little room to escape for the EGF receptor.

4.8.2 The Tyrosine Kinase Inhibitor Approach

The number of chemical compounds being tested in clinical trials is too high to comprehensively discuss in this chapter. The large majority binds the nucleotide-binding pocket with high affinity (of the order of 10^{-9} M) and competes with ATP. Some recently developed compounds against the EGFR are irreversible (for example, CI-1033). We will illustrate just one example, imatinib.

Imatinib will go into history as the first magic bullet of cancer chemotherapy. It emerged from a random screen of 2-phenylaminopyrimidine compounds, known to be inhibitors of PKC-α, in which they were tested as inhibitors of PDGF-R tyrosine kinase. The aim was to discover compounds that could suppress the growth of PDGF-R-activated cell lines. The test also included the oncogenic v-Abl (viral variant of c-Abl protein kinase) as a counter screen, because of its very distant sequence resemblance to PDGF-R. It came as a surprise, then, that the most potent inhibitor of PDGF-R kinase activity, CGP 531716, was also a potent inhibitor of v-Abl. Having new potential treatments in mind, it was further optimized for inhibition of c-Abl, the compound CGP 57148B, now widely known as imatinib (or Gleevec), coming out as the winner (Figure 4.18).

Imatinib binds in the catalytic cleft of c-Abl, acting as a competitive inhibitor of ATP binding (Figure 4.19). It binds most efficiently to the dormant kinase, in which the activation segment is not phosphorylated, and in doing so it effectively keeps the kinase in the dormant state. Importantly, imatinib shows selective and potent activity in cells possessing the Bcr-Abl oncogene, yet spares normal cells.

Bcr-Abl is the product of a somatic translocation between chromosomes 9 and 22, giving rise to a chimeric protein of which the tyrosine protein kinase component (a truncated c-Abl protein kinase) now manifests constitutive activity. The short chromosome that carries the Bcr-Abl fusion gene is named the Philadelphia chromosome. Bone marrow cells expressing the Philadelphia chromosome cause chronic myelogenous (or myeloid) leukemia.

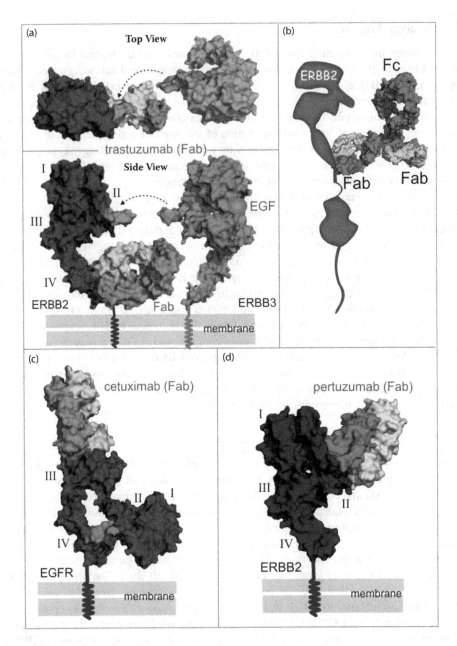

FIGURE 4.17 Overview of antibodies binding to EGFR or ERBB2. (a) Trastuzumab binds domain IV, and as shown from two perspectives (top and side views) it does not really hinder EGF binding. (b) The structural data show only the Fab fragment of the antibody, but realize that these are much bigger structures with an Fc segment that can interact with Fc-receptors carried by blood-borne cells. (c) Cetuximab binds domain III and does compete with EGF for binding. Notice that the receptor is in the tethered conformation, with its dimerization arm buried in domain IV. (d) Pertuzumab binds the dimerization arm (in green) and prevents its association with another receptor.

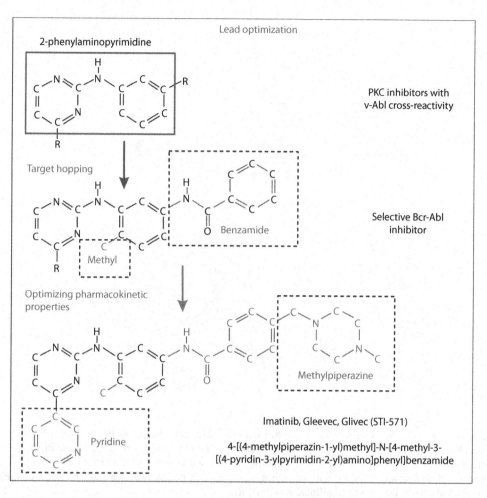

FIGURE 4.18 Optimization of imatinib as a chemotherapeutic agent. The discovery that 2-phenylamino-pyrimidine inhibitors of PKC also inhibit the unrelated v-Abl oncogene turned the attention to its potential use in the treatment of chronic myelogenous leukemia. Starting with the 2-phenylaminopyrimidine backbone, addition of the benzamidine group increased activity against tyrosine kinases, the methyl group reduced its activity against PKC. Addition of a 3'-pyridyl group improved the activity in cellular assays (bioavailability). Subsequent addition of N-methylpiperazine increased water solubility and oral bioavailability (surviving the stomach and entering the bloodstream).

Imatinib is recommended as first-line therapy in newly diagnosed patients with chronic myeloid leukemia. Not only does it drive the cancer into remission, clearing the blood and bone marrow of Philadelphia-expressing cells, it also has remarkably mild adverse effects, allowing prolonged treatment. Some patients involved in the early clinical trials have been taking it for more than 6 years. This prolonged treatment is deemed necessary because imatinib does not eradicate all Philadelphia-expressing cells. The fusion gene remains detectable in a sensitive PCR protocol.

Good activity was also found against PDGF-R, c-KIT, Lck, C-Raf, and the three VEGF receptors. Because of its strong inhibitory action on c-KIT (a tyrosine kinase receptor), it is also approved for the treatment of inoperable KIT-positive and metastatic gastrointestinal stromal tumors (GIST).

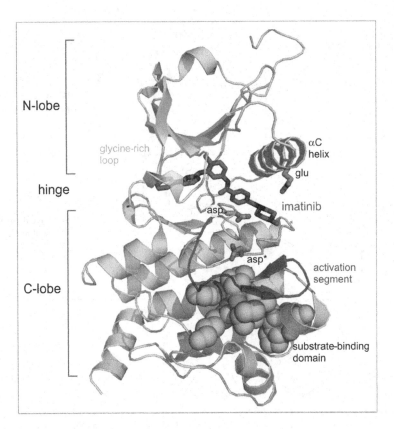

FIGURE 4.19 Binding of imatinib to the tyrosine kinase Abl. Only the catalytic domain of the tyrosine protein kinase Abl is shown. Note that imatinib binds the ATP-binding pocket of the kinase in its inactive conformation. The activation segment is not phosphorylated and covers the substrate binding site. In fact, imatinib prevents outward movement of the activation segment. Note also that Asp and Glu (in the αC-helix) are not in the correct position to coordinate ATP binding.

4.8.3 FUTURE DEVELOPMENTS

Certain patients are resistant to the treatment with imatinib, and a whole range of mutations has been detected that either concern amino acids directly involved in drug binding or that act at a distance from the catalytic site and have an allosteric influence on drug binding. They destabilize the auto-inhibited conformation of the Abl kinase to which the drug binds. This precludes drug binding but not ATP.

These discoveries provide a challenge for drug development because those drugs that act on protein kinases in their inactive conformation, while necessarily specific, may more easily suffer from resistance mutations. Remember that protein kinases adopt very different conformations in their inactive state and thus have a certain liberty to alter the amino acid sequence without affecting their catalytic potential. In contrast, drugs binding to active conformations are likely to be less specific but may offer the advantage that the kinase is less likely to escape inhibition. The general trend now is to shift attention away from single, highly selective inhibitors toward broader spectrum compounds or to cocktails of specific inhibitors acting in different ways. These approaches open up a range of new therapeutic promise but also the possibility of unacceptable adverse effects.

FURTHER READING

Textbooks

Gomperts BD, Kramer IM, Tatham PER. *Signal Transduction*. 2nd ed. Elsevier/AP, San Diego, CA, 2009.

Reviews

Burgess AW, Cho H-S, Eigenbrot C, Ferguson KM, Garrett TPJ, Leahy DJ, Lemmon MA, Sliwkowski MX, Ward CW, Yokoyama S. An open-and-shut case? Recent insights into the activation of EGF/ErbB receptors. *Mol Cell* 12:541–552, 2003.

Deininger M, Buchdunger E, Druker BJ. The development of imatinib as a therapeutic agent for chronic myeloid leukemia. *Blood* 105:2640–2653, 2005.

Gschwind A, Fischer OM, Ullrich A. The discovery of receptor tyrosine kinases: Targets for cancer therapy. *Nature Rev Cancer* 4:361–370, 2004.

Kornev AP, Haste NM, Taylor SS, Ten Eyck LF. Surface comparison of active and inactive protein kinases identifies a conserved activation mechanism. *PNAS* 103:17783–17788, 2006.

Shi Z, Resing KA, Ahn NG. Network for the allosteric control of protein kinases. *Curr Opin Struc Biol* 16:686–692, 2006.

Articles

Chen H, Ma J, Li W, Eliseenkova AV, Xu C, Neubert TA, Miller WT, Mohammadi M. A molecular brake in the kinase hinge region regulates the activity of receptor tyrosine kinases. *Mol. Cell* 27:717–730, 2007.

Klaman LD, Boss O, Peroni OD, Kim JK, Martino JL et al. Increased energy expenditure, decreased adiposity, and tissue-specific insulin sensitivity in protein-tyrosine phosphatase 1B-deficient mice. *Mol Cell Biol* 20:5479–5489, 2000.

Lu S, Jun-Shen Huang, Lodish HF. Dimerization by a cytokine receptor is necessary for constitutive activation of JAK2V617F. *J Biol Chem* 283:5258–5266, 2008.

McKern NM., Lawrence MC, Streltsov VA, Lou MZ, Adams TE et al. Structure of the insulin receptor ectodomain reveals a folded-over conformation. *Nature* 443:218–221, 2006.

Schlessinger J, Plotnikov AN, Ibrahimi OA, Eliseenkova AV, Yeh BK, Yayon A, Linhardt RJ, Mohammadi M. Crystal structure of a ternary FGF-FGFR-heparin complex reveals a dual role for heparin in FGFR binding and dimerization. *Mol. Cell* 6:743–750, 2000.

Syed RS, Reid SW, Li C, Cheetham JC, Aoki KH, Liu B, Zhan H, Osslund TD, Chirino AJ, Zhang J, Finer-Moore J, Elliott S, Sitney K, Katz BA, Matthews DJ, Wendoloski JJ, Egrie J, Stroud RM. Efficiency of signalling through cytokine receptors depends critically on receptor orientation. *Nature* 395:511–516, 1998.

Zhang X, Gureasko J, Shen K, Cole PA, Kuriyan J. An allosteric mechanism for activation of the kinase domain of epidermal growth factor receptor. *Cell* 125:1137–1149, 2006.

Section III

Ligand-Binding Studies of Receptors

5 Direct Measurement of Drug Binding to Receptors

Dennis G. Haylett

CONTENTS

5.1   INTRODUCTION

In this chapter, we look at ways in which the binding of ligands to macromolecules can be directly investigated. Although most interest centers on the interaction of drugs and hormones with receptors, the approach taken here can be applied to any similar binding process—for example, the combination of drugs with ion channels or membrane transport systems. The binding of ligands, including drugs, to plasma proteins has been studied for more than 50 years, but the study of binding to the much smaller amounts of protein (e.g., receptors) in cell membranes is more recent, having become feasible only when suitable radioactively labeled ligands became available. The first rigorous study of drug binding to receptors was that of Paton and Rang (1965), who investigated ^{3}H-atropine binding to muscarinic receptors in smooth muscle. The use of radiolabeled or fluorescently labeled drugs in binding studies is now common and for many pharmaceutical manufacturers forms an essential part of the screening process, providing a rapid means of determining the affinity of new drugs for a wide range of receptors. Labeling of drugs with radioisotopes or the introduction of fluorescent tags is attractive because very small quantities, often as low as 1 fmol, can be readily and accurately measured.

5.1.1   OBJECTIVES OF LIGAND-BINDING STUDIES

Ligand-binding studies include:

- *Measurement of dissociation equilibrium constants*, which is of particular value in receptor classification and in the study of structure/activity relationships, where the effects of changes in chemical structure on affinity (and efficacy) are explored.
- *Measurement of association and dissociation rate constants.*
- *Measurement of receptor density,* including changes in receptor density occurring under different physiological or pathological conditions. Examples include the reduction in β-adrenoreceptor density that occurs with the use of β-agonists in the treatment of asthma (downregulation) and the increase in β-adrenoreceptor numbers in cardiac muscle in response to thyroxine. The densities of receptors may be measured either directly in tissue samples or in intact tissues by quantitative autoradiography. Autoradiography, in which a picture of the distribution of the radiolabel in a section of tissue is obtained by placing a photographic film in contact with the tissue, has provided valuable information on the distribution of many receptors within the brain. Positron emission tomography (PET) and single-photon-emission computerized tomography (SPECT) utilizing ligands labeled with either positron emitters (e.g., ^{11}C) or gamma emitters are increasingly used to investigate receptor densities or occupancy of receptors by drugs *in vivo*.
- *Recognition and quantification of receptor subtypes*, which may be possible if subtype-selective ligands are available.
- *Use of radioligands in the chemical purification of receptors.* Here, the bound radioligand allows the receptors to be tracked through the various purification steps—for example, in the fractions eluting from separation columns. In such experiments, it is important for the radioligand to be irreversibly bound to the receptor.
- Finally, it may be possible to obtain some limited information on the *mechanisms of action of agonists* from the shapes of binding curves. For example, as discussed later, the binding of some agonists is affected by guanosine triphosphate (GTP), immediately suggesting the involvement of G-proteins in the transduction mechanism.

5.1.2 Nomenclature

Compared with the conventions adopted for discussing the relationship between drug concentration and response (Chapter 1), a rather different terminology has evolved for ligand-binding studies.

R: Binding site, most often a true receptor (but quite commonly the term *receptor* is applied indiscriminately to any binding site)

L: Labeled ligand whose binding is directly measured; L can be an agonist or antagonist or a molecule with a quite different action (e.g., a channel blocker)

I: An inhibitor of the binding of L; I can be an agonist or an antagonist

B: Often used to denote the amount of ligand bound; correspondingly B_{max}, is the maximum binding capacity

K_L, K_I: Dissociation equilibrium constants for binding of L and I (reciprocals of affinity constants)

K_d: Used more generally for the dissociation equilibrium constant of any ligand

5.1.3 Specificity of Binding

An all-important consideration in binding studies is the extent to which the measured binding of a labeled ligand represents association with the receptor or other site of interest. (In functional studies, this is not difficult, as the response can only be elicited by the binding of an agonist to the receptor and, for competitive antagonism, at least, it is likely that the antagonist also binds to the receptor.) Invariably in binding studies, uptake of the labeled ligand by other tissue components occurs (unless, of course, binding to a purified, soluble protein is under investigation). The binding to the receptor is normally termed *specific binding*, whereas the binding to nonreceptor tissue components is referred to as *nonspecific binding*. Nonspecific binding may be attributable to the following:

1. Ligand bound to other sites in the tissue (e.g., other receptors, enzymes, or membrane transporters). For example, some muscarinic antagonists will also bind to histamine receptors, and some adrenoreceptor ligands will also bind to the neuronal and extraneuronal uptake mechanisms for noradrenaline. Such uptake might be properly considered *specific*, but it is not the binding of primary interest to the investigator. Unlike other sources of nonspecific binding, this binding will be saturable, though it may be hoped that it will be of low affinity and so will increase in an approximately linear fashion over the concentration range of ligand used. If the characteristics of nonspecific binding of this sort are well established, it may be possible to eliminate it by the use of selective blockers (e.g., by the use of specific inhibitors of the uptake-1 process for noradrenaline).
2. Distribution of ligand into lipid components of the preparation (e.g., cell membranes) or uptake into intact cells or membrane vesicles.
3. Free ligand that is not separated from bound ligand during the separation phase of the experiment, including ligand bound to a filter or trapped in the membrane or cell pellet during centrifugation.

Unlike category 1 above, nonspecific binding arising from categories 2 and 3 will be nonsaturable and will increase linearly with ligand concentration. Nonspecific binding of types 1 and 2 and ligand trapped in pellets should increase in proportion to the amount of tissue used in the binding reaction; binding to filters and to the walls of centrifuge tubes should not. If the investigator is fortunate, in that nonspecific binding in category 1 is linear over the range of ligand concentrations used, then the bindings for all three categories simply combine to constitute a single, nonspecific, linear component. Nonspecific binding is usually estimated by measuring the binding of the ligand in the presence of an agent that is believed to bind selectively to the receptor at a concentration calculated to prevent virtually all specific binding without appreciable modification of nonspecific binding (further details are provided in Section 5.3.5).

5.2   TYPES OF LIGAND-BINDING EXPERIMENTS

Four kinds of ligand-binding studies will be discussed: (1) saturation, (2) kinetic, (3) competition, and (4) retardation.

5.2.1   SATURATION EXPERIMENTS

These experiments examine the binding of the ligand at equilibrium directly and can provide estimates of K_L and B_{max}. Initially, we consider the simple reaction:

$$L + R \underset{}{\overset{K_L}{\rightleftharpoons}} LR \tag{5.1}$$

This represents binding in isolation and would be applicable to the binding of a competitive antagonist (or a channel blocker) that produces insignificant structural change in the receptor. (The case for an agonist that must produce such a change, often an isomerization, to generate the active state is considered later.) The binding at equilibrium is given by the following equation (equivalent to Equation 1.2):

$$[LR] = R_{TOT} \frac{[L]}{K_L + [L]} \tag{5.2}$$

Alternatively,

$$B = B_{max} \frac{[L]}{K_L + [L]} \tag{5.3}$$

Typical units for B are pmol.mg protein^{-1}, pmol.mg dry tissue^{-1}, etc. A curve of B versus [L] has the form of a rectangular hyperbola, exactly equivalent to the curve describing receptor occupancy presented in Chapter 1, Figure 1.1.

It is convenient at this point to consider nonspecific binding. Ideally, nonspecific binding should be entirely independent of specific binding, so that the total uptake of labeled ligand by the tissue should be the simple sum of the two. If we can assume that the nonspecific binding is a linear function of the ligand concentration, then the observed binding will be given by:

$$B = B_{max} \frac{[L]}{K_L + [L]} + c[L] \tag{5.4}$$

where c is a constant. The relationship among total, specific, and nonspecific binding is indicated in Figure 5.1.

In practice, total and nonspecific binding are measured over a range of concentrations of L that will allow specific binding to approach saturation. The analysis of saturation experiments to obtain estimates of K_L and B_{max} is described later.

It is useful now to recall the Hill coefficient, which has been discussed in detail in Chapter 1. In binding studies, the Hill coefficient, n_H, is generally a convenient means of describing the steepness of the plot of specific binding against the logarithm of the ligand concentration, generally without any attempt to define the underlying mechanism. In the simplest case, a plot of specific binding against [L] is analyzed to provide a fit of the following equation (equivalent to Equation 1.6):

$$B = B_{max} \frac{[L]^{n_H}}{K_L^{n_H} + [L]^{n_H}} \tag{5.5}$$

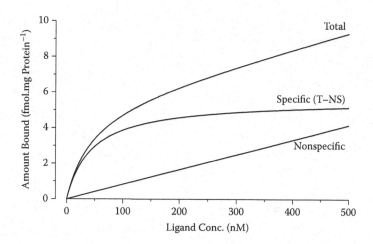

FIGURE 5.1 The binding of a labeled ligand to a receptor preparation normally involves a nonspecific component in addition to the specific receptor binding. In principle, at least, specific binding can be estimated from the total binding (T) by subtracting nonspecific binding (NS). (Curves are theoretical, with B_{max} = 5.6 fmol.mg protein^{-1}, K_L = 45 nM, and c = 0.0083 fmol·nM^{-1}.)

For a simple bimolecular reaction following the law of mass action, n_H would be unity. If n_H is greater than 1, the plot of specific binding against log [L] will be steep; if less than 1, it will be shallow. Under these circumstances, a Hill plot (see Chapter 1) would have slopes either greater or less than unity.

5.2.1.1 Multiple Binding Sites

It is, of course, quite possible that more than one kind of specific binding site exists for the labeled ligand. For example, receptor subtypes may be present (subtypes of 5HT receptors, adrenoreceptors, etc.), or the binding sites might be functionally quite different. For example, some receptor ligands may also be channel blockers (e.g., tubocurarine) or inhibitors of transmitter uptake (e.g., phenoxybenzamine). The question then arises as to whether or not the sites are interacting or noninteracting. In the case of only two sites that do not interact, an additional term can simply be added to the binding equation. For total binding,

$$B = B_{max1} \frac{[L]}{K_{L_1} + [L]} + B_{max2} \frac{[L]}{K_{L_2} + [L]} + c.[L] \tag{5.6}$$

where subscripts 1 and 2 specify the two sites (further terms can be added for additional components).

The curve for specific binding will no longer be a simple rectangular hyperbola, though whether distinct components can be distinguished by eye will depend on the difference in the K_L values and on the number of observations and their accuracy. Theoretical curves are shown in Figure 5.2. For relatively small differences in the K_L values of the two sites, the curve appears to have a single component, but analysis would show it to have a low Hill coefficient. The separate components are revealed more clearly when a logarithmic scale is used for the ligand concentration. Thus, two components are very apparent in the right panel of Figure 5.2.

5.2.1.2 Interacting Sites

For some receptors (for example, the nicotinic acetylcholine receptor), the binding site is duplicated on identical subunits incorporated into a multimeric protein, which allows for the possibility that ligand binding to one site may influence binding to the other. The two sites could in principle behave in an identical fashion, but it is more likely that incorporation of the subunits into an asymmetrical

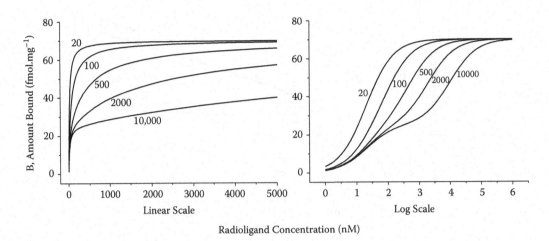

FIGURE 5.2 Theoretical curves for the specific binding of a labeled ligand to a preparation containing two classes of binding site. A high-affinity component with a B_{max} of 25 fmol·mg^{-1} has a fixed K_L of 20 nM. The second component, with a B_{max} of 45 fmol.mg^{-1} is given K_L values varying between 20 and 10,000 nM, as indicated. The K_L values for the two sites must differ considerably before the existence of two components becomes obvious. (Data are displayed using both linear and logarithmic concentration scales.)

multimer (a heteropentamer for the nicotinic receptor) introduces constraints that lead to different affinities for ligands. Of particular importance is the likelihood that occupation of one site by the ligand will increase or decrease the affinity for binding to the other (i.e., show positive or negative cooperativity). The following provides the simplest representation of this two-binding-site model:

$$L + R \xrightleftharpoons{K_1} LR + L \xrightleftharpoons{K_2} L_2R(\xrightleftharpoons{E} L_2R^*) \qquad (5.7)$$

This scheme is also discussed in Chapter 1 (in Appendix 1.2.3) and in Chapter 6. In this scheme, the two binding sites are considered initially identical (equilibrium constant = K_1). However, once one site is occupied, the affinity at the second site may change (equilibrium constant = K_2). L_2R^* is the active state produced when L is an agonist. The shape of the binding curve depends on the relative magnitudes of K_1 and K_2. When $K_1 > K_2$, positive cooperativity will occur (i.e., binding to the first site will increase affinity for the second); when $K_1 < K_2$, negative cooperativity will occur. Figure 5.3 illustrates the shapes of the binding curves predicted by Equation (1.14) for various ratios of K_1 to K_2.

In competition experiments, it is possible that the binding of the ligand is inhibited not by competition at a common site but by the inhibitor's affecting the binding remotely through interaction with a different part of the receptor molecule (i.e., by an allosteric action).

5.2.1.3 Agonists

The foregoing discussion of saturation experiments considered the binding step in isolation; however, for agonists to produce a tissue response, there must be some change (isomerization) in the receptor—for example, a conformational change to open an integral ion channel or to promote association with a G-protein. The complications arising with agonists will now be discussed.

5.2.1.3.1 The del Castillo–Katz Model of Receptor Activation
This model, represented below, has been discussed in Chapter 1, Sections 1.4.4 and 1.4.5.

$$A + R \xrightleftharpoons{K_A} AR \xrightleftharpoons{E} AR^* \qquad (5.8)$$

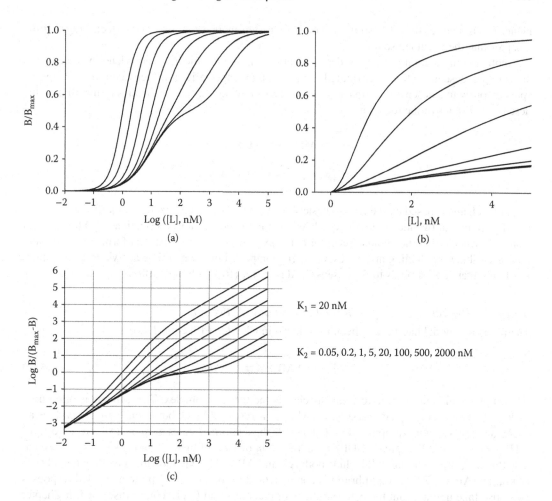

FIGURE 5.3 Binding of a radioligand to a receptor containing two identical binding sites (scheme shown in Equation 5.7 but ignoring the isomerization step). Binding of the first ligand molecule is given a K_1 of 20 nM. The K_2 value for binding of a second ligand molecule is given a range of values to represent varying degrees of cooperativity, from strongly positive (0.05 nM, left-most curve) to strongly negative (2000 nM, right-most curve). As illustrated in (a), for a logarithmic concentration scale, positive cooperativity steepens the curve, whereas negative cooperativity makes it shallower. Two components become quite evident for the larger values of K_2. In panel (b), the linear concentration scale has been expanded to show the S-shaped foot of the binding curve, indicative of positive cooperativity. The Hill plot, (c), shows that with a large degree of positive cooperativity n_H approaches 2 for intermediate concentrations of radioligand, becoming unity at either very high or very low concentrations (see Equation 1.15).

In a ligand-binding study, the measured binding includes AR^* as well as AR. The relevant equation, including both bound states, then is:

$$B_{(AR+AR^*)} = B_{max} \frac{[A]}{\left(\dfrac{K_A}{1+E}\right)+[A]} \tag{5.9}$$

In this equation, A has been used in preference to L to emphasize that an *agonist* is being considered. The equation retains the form of a rectangular hyperbola; 50% occupancy occurring when $[A] = K_A/(1 + E)$. $K_A/(1 + E)$ is thus an effective equilibrium constant and accordingly is referred to as K_{eff}. The important point to note is that binding measurements do not give an estimate of K_A

alone. K_{eff} is smaller than K_A, so the isomerization step increases affinity (in effect, dragging the receptor into the occupied state).

Another complication is receptor desensitization. Taking the nicotinic acetylcholine receptor as an example, desensitization is attributed to the receptor, especially in its activated form, changing spontaneously to a desensitized, inactive state. The following is a scheme incorporating all possible desensitized states of the receptor:

$$A+R \rightleftharpoons AR+A \rightleftharpoons A_2R \rightleftharpoons A_2R^*$$
$$\updownarrow \qquad \updownarrow \qquad\quad \updownarrow \qquad \updownarrow$$
$$A+R_D \rightleftharpoons AR_D+A \rightleftharpoons A_2R_D \rightleftharpoons A_2R_D^*$$

(This scheme is based on the Katz–Thesleff cyclic model of desensitization, modified to incorporate the binding of two molecules of acetylcholine and including an isomerization step.) It is evident from this scheme that the agonist–receptor complexes are of several different forms and the equations describing the binding are correspondingly complex. For the nicotinic acetylcholine receptor, it is found that agonist binds to the desensitized receptor (R_D) with high affinity.

5.2.1.3.2   The Ternary Complex Model of Receptor Activation
The following model has already been introduced in Chapter 1 (Section 1.4.6):

$$A + R \rightleftharpoons AR + X \rightleftharpoons ARX \tag{5.10}$$

ARX, the association of three reacting species, is the ternary complex. This scheme is often used to describe G-protein-mediated responses, when X is replaced by G, but in this case it clearly is an oversimplification. For example, it does not include the additional states introduced by the binding of GTP or guanosine diphosphate (GDP). From the point of view of ligand-binding studies, we need to note that measured binding will include both AR and ARX. The equation that gives the bound concentration (AR + ARX) at equilibrium is complex (and in the case of G-protein coupled responses must also take into account the concentrations of receptors and G-protein, as discussed in Chapter 1, and of GTP and GDP). A particular feature of the binding of agonists to receptors that couple to G-proteins is that the concentration of GTP will affect the binding curve. The binding of agonists often exhibits components with high and low affinities, and GTP is found to increase the proportion in the low-affinity state. This will be considered further when discussing competition experiments.

5.2.2   Kinetic Studies

Both the onset of binding, when a ligand is first applied, and the offset, when dissociation is promoted, can be studied directly. The relevant kinetic equations relating to the simple bimolecular interaction of ligand with receptor are presented in Chapter 1, Section 1.3.

5.2.2.1   Measurement of the Dissociation Rate Constant, k_{-1}
To measure the dissociation rate constant, all that is necessary, in principle, is first to secure a satisfactory occupancy of the receptors by the ligand and then to prevent further association, either by adding a competing agent in sufficient concentration or by lowering [L] substantially by dilution. The amount of drug bound to the receptors is measured at selected times after initiating net dissociation and, for the simple model considered in Sections 1.2 and 1.3 of Chapter 1, will show an exponential decline.

$$LR \xrightarrow{\;k_{-1}\;} L + R \tag{5.11}$$

$$B_t = B_0 e^{-k_{-1}t} \tag{5.12}$$

$$\log_e B_t = \log_e B_0 - k_{-1}t \tag{5.13}$$

B_0 and B_t are the amounts bound initially (at $t = 0$) and at specific times (t) after initiating dissociation. A plot of $\log_e B_t$ against t is linear with a slope of $-k_{-1}$; k_{-1} may thus be estimated directly from the slope of this plot or may be obtained by nonlinear least squares curve fitting to Equation (5.12). It is always desirable to plot $\log_e B_t$ against t to detect any nonlinearity that might reflect either the presence of multiple binding sites or the existence of more than one occupied state of the receptor.

5.2.2.2   Measurement of the Association Rate Constant, k_{+1}

For the simple bimolecular reaction involving a single class of binding site, the onset of binding should also contain an exponential term. Thus,

$$B_t = B_\infty(1 - e^{-k_{on}t}) \tag{5.14}$$

where B_t is the binding at time t, B_∞ is the binding at equilibrium, and k_{on} is the observed onset rate constant. However, as shown in Chapter 1, k_{on} is not a simple measure of k_{+1}; rather:

$$k_{on} = k_{-1} + k_{+1}[L] \tag{5.15}$$

Equation (5.14) can be converted into a linear form:

$$\log_e\left(\frac{B_\infty - B_t}{B_\infty}\right) = -k_{on}t \tag{5.16}$$

and k_{on} can be obtained from the slope of the plot of the left-hand side of the equation against t.

Once k_{on} is known, k_{+1} can be estimated in at least two different ways. First, an independent estimate of k_{-1} can be obtained from dissociation studies as described above, where, from Equation (5.15), $k_{+1} = (k_{on} - k_{-1})/[L]$. Second, k_{on} can be measured at several different concentrations of L and a plot of k_{on} against [L] constructed in which, according to Equation (5.15), k_{+1} is given directly by the slope. This plot will also provide an estimate of k_{-1} (intercept). Additionally, it is possible to perform a simultaneous nonlinear least squares fit of a family of onset curves (obtained by using different concentrations of L), the fitting routine providing estimates of k_{+1}, k_{-1}, and B_{max}. (Problem 5.2 provides an opportunity to calculate binding rate constants.)

In the case of multiple binding sites or if the ligand–receptor complex isomerizes, the onset and offset curves will be multiexponential. It is generally assumed that nonspecific binding will occur rapidly, and this should certainly be so for simple entrapment in a membrane or cell pellet. If, however, specific binding is very rapid or nonspecific binding particularly slow (possibly reflecting uptake of the ligand by cells), then the time course of nonspecific binding also must be determined to allow an accurate assessment of the onset of specific binding. Note, too, that the onset of ligand binding will be slowed in the presence of an inhibitor, a phenomenon that is employed in *retardation* experiments (discussed in Section 5.2.4).

5.2.3   COMPETITION EXPERIMENTS

Saturation experiments are, of course, only possible when a labeled form of the ligand of interest is available. Competition experiments, on the other hand, are particularly useful in allowing the determination of dissociation constants for unlabeled drugs that compete for the binding sites with a ligand that is available in a labeled form. This approach has been widely adopted by the pharmaceutical industry as a rapid means of determining the affinity of novel compounds for a particular receptor for which a well-characterized labeled ligand is available.

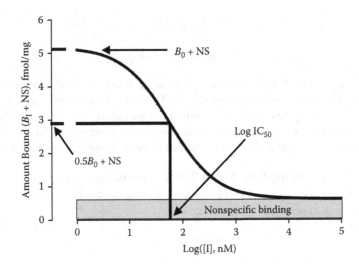

FIGURE 5.4 In this illustration of a competition experiment, a fixed concentration of radioligand, in the absence of inhibitor, produces specific binding of B_0. The specific binding in the presence of a competitive inhibitor is denoted by B_I. A constant amount of nonspecific binding is assumed to be present. The concentration of inhibitor that reduces specific binding by 50% is referred to as the IC_{50}.

In competition experiments, a fixed amount of a labeled ligand, generally at a concentration below K_L, is equilibrated with the receptor preparation in the presence of a range of concentrations of the unlabeled inhibitor I. In these studies, the amount of ligand bound is usually plotted against log[I]. Figure 5.4 provides an example for the simple case where the ligand and inhibitor compete reversibly for a single class of site. In this illustration, the constant level of nonspecific binding has not been subtracted, whereas in most published studies it would be. The amount of nonspecific binding could, of course, be defined by applying high concentrations of the inhibitor itself; but if the competing agent is expensive or in short supply, it is possible to employ another well-characterized inhibitor for the same purpose. The two main features of this curve are its position along the concentration axis and its slope. The position along the concentration axis is conventionally indicated by the IC_{50}, the concentration of inhibitor that reduces the specific binding by 50%. The predicted relationship (see also Equation 1.48) between the amount of specific binding in the presence of I (B_I) and [I] is given by:

$$B_I = B_{max} \frac{[L]}{K_L\left(1+\dfrac{[I]}{K_I}\right)+[L]} \tag{5.17}$$

Provided that a value for K_L is available, it is possible to use this equation to obtain a value for K_I, the dissociation equilibrium constant for the inhibitor, by nonlinear least squares analysis of the displacement curve. Alternatively, K_I can be calculated from the IC_{50}, which may be obtained by simple interpolation by eye, from a Hill plot, or by fitting a curve to an equation of the type:

$$B_I = B_0 \frac{IC_{50}}{IC_{50}+[I]} \tag{5.18}$$

where B_0 is the specific binding observed in the absence of competing ligand.

5.2.3.1 Relationship between K_I and IC_{50}

B_0 is given by Equation (5.3):

$$B_0 = B_{max} \frac{[L]}{K_L + [L]}$$

and, by definition, when $[I] = IC_{50}$, $B_I = 0.5B_0$, therefore binding in the presence of the IC_{50} concentration of the inhibitor:

$$B_{IC_{50}} = 0.5.B_{max} \frac{[L]}{K_L + [L]} \tag{5.19}$$

Also from Equation (5.17):

$$B_{IC_{50}} = B_{max} \frac{[L]}{K_L \left(1 + \dfrac{IC_{50}}{K_I}\right) + [L]} \tag{5.20}$$

Equating the two expressions for $B_{IC_{50}}$:

$$B_{max} \frac{[L]}{K_L \left(1 + \dfrac{IC_{50}}{K_I}\right) + [L]} = 0.5.B_{max} \frac{[L]}{K_L + [L]}$$

by cancellation and rearrangement:

$$K_I = IC_{50} \frac{K_L}{K_L + [L]} = \frac{IC_{50}}{\left(1 + \dfrac{[L]}{K_L}\right)} \tag{5.21}$$

The term $1 + ([L]/K_L)$ is often referred to as the Cheng–Prusoff correction. It is clear from this analysis that the IC_{50} does not give a direct estimate of K_I unless $[L]$ is very low, when IC_{50} tends to K_I. Just as with saturation experiments, the situation will be complicated by the presence of different classes of binding sites (e.g., receptor subtypes) and by the involvement of G-proteins in agonist binding.

5.2.3.2 Multiple Binding Sites

The effect of multiple binding sites on competition curves will be determined by the relative affinities of the labeled ligand and displacing agent for the various sites. Considering the simple situation where the ligand exhibits the same affinity for each of two sites (e.g., propranolol for β_1 and β_2 adrenoreceptors), the displacement curve for an inhibitor will show two components only if the K_I values for the binding of the inhibitor to the two sites are sufficiently different and if the measurements of displacement are accurate and made over an adequate range of concentrations of I (see also Figure 5.2 and Section 5.4.4).

5.2.3.3 G-Protein Linked Receptors

As already mentioned, GTP affects binding of agonists to G-protein coupled receptors, and this has been much studied because of the light it can throw on the mechanism of action of such receptors. These receptors often exhibit two states that bind agonists with different affinities. The interactions of G-proteins with receptors are discussed in Chapter 7, and here it is only necessary to note that the high-affinity form of the receptor is coupled to the G-protein. In the simplest model, when GTP replaces GDP on the α subunit, the G-protein splits to release the α-GTP and $\beta\gamma$

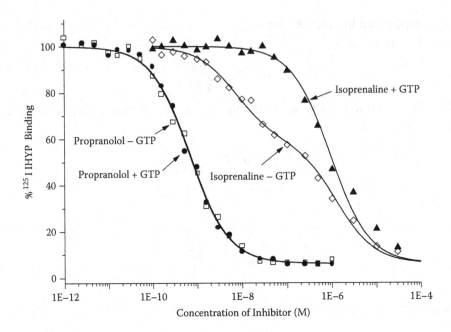

FIGURE 5.5 Effect of GTP on the competition binding curves of isoprenaline and propranolol. Membranes prepared from L6 myoblasts were incubated with ^{125}I-iodopindolol (50 pM) in the presence of either (–)-isoprenaline or (–)-propranolol with or without 100 μM GTP for 90 min at 25°C. GTP has no effect on the binding of the antagonist but shifts the curve for displacement by the agonist to the right (by abolishing the high-affinity component of binding). (Redrawn using data of Wolfe, B. B. and Molinoff, P. B., in *Handbook of Experimental Pharmacology,* Trendelenburg, U., and Weiner, N., Eds., Springer-Verlag, Berlin, 1988, Chapter 7.)

subunits, which mediate the cellular effects of the agonist. The receptor then dissociates from the G-protein, reverting to the low-affinity state. Hence, in the absence of GTP, a significant proportion of the receptors will be in the high-affinity state, but in its presence most will adopt the low-affinity state. The resulting *GTP shift* is illustrated in Figure 5.5. Note that it applies only to the binding of agonists, as antagonists do not promote coupling of receptors to the G-protein. If there is a relatively low concentration of G-protein, so that it is depleted by association with the receptor, then the competition curve for an agonist in the absence of GTP may exhibit two components, as in Figure 5.5.

5.2.4 RETARDATION EXPERIMENTS

It is useful to consider a particular variant of competitive binding experiment that has been used especially to investigate the nicotinic acetylcholine receptor. In essence, it is possible to determine the dissociation equilibrium constant for a reversible competitive inhibitor by the reduction it produces in the rate of binding of an irreversible radioligand (e.g., α-bungarotoxin). In practice, the time-course of binding of the irreversible ligand is studied in the absence and presence of the inhibitor. The expected outcome is shown in Figure 5.6.

When the irreversible ligand is applied by itself, the change in the proportion of sites occupied, p_{LR}, with time will be given by:

$$\frac{dp_{LR}(t)}{dt} = k_{+1}[L]\{1 - p_{LR}(t)\} \tag{5.22}$$

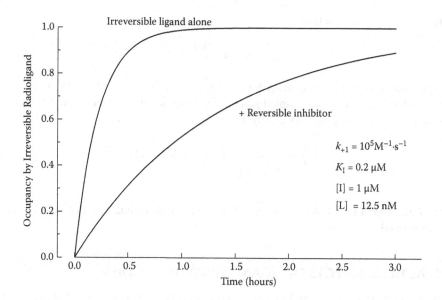

FIGURE 5.6 Retardation experiment. A reversible inhibitor will slow down the rate of association of an irreversible ligand with its receptor. These curves have been constructed according to Equation (5.27) using the numerical values indicated in the figure. These have been chosen to illustrate the effect of an antagonist, such as tubocurarine, on the binding of α-bungarotoxin to the nicotinic receptor of skeletal muscle.

where $(1 - p_{LR}(t))$ is the proportion of receptors remaining free and available to bind with L. If $p_{LR} = 0$ at $t = 0$, the solution is:

$$p_{LR}(t) = 1 - e^{-k_{+1}[L]t} \qquad (5.23)$$

This equation is the application of Equation (1.22) to an irreversible ligand (i.e., $k_{-1} = 0$), and in the long run all of the receptors will be occupied so that $p_{LR}(\infty)$ is unity. The rate constant for equilibration is thus given by $k_{+1}[L]$. For the case where binding is studied in the presence of an inhibitor, Equation (5.22) becomes:

$$\frac{dp_{LR}(t)}{dt} = k_{+1}[L]\{1 - p_{LR}(t) - p_{IR}(t)\} \qquad (5.24)$$

where p_{IR} is the proportion of receptor sites occupied by the inhibitor. The rate of association is slowed because the free concentration of binding sites has been reduced through occupation by I. If we assume that I equilibrates rapidly with the available sites, then the occupancy by I at any given time can be estimated using the appropriate form of the Hill–Langmuir equation (Equation 5.3):

$$p_{IR}(t) = \{1 - p_{LR}(t)\}\frac{[I]}{K_I + [I]} \qquad (5.25)$$

Substituting in Equation (5.24):

$$\frac{dp_{LR}(t)}{dt} = k_{+1}[L]\left\{1 - p_{LR}(t) - (1 - p_{LR}(t))\frac{[I]}{K_I + [I]}\right\}$$

$$= k_{+1}[L](1 - p_{LR}(t))\left(1 - \frac{[I]}{K_I + [I]}\right) \qquad (5.26)$$

The solution for $p_{LR} = 0$ at $t = 0$ is:

$$p_{LR}(t) = 1 - e^{-k_{+1}[L]\left(1 - \frac{[I]}{K_I + [I]}\right)t}$$

(5.27)

The onset rate constant (see Equation 5.23) is reduced by the factor $1 - [I]/(K_I + [I])$. If the rate constants for binding of the irreversible ligand are determined in the absence and presence of the inhibitor and denoted k_0 and k_I, respectively, then:

$$\frac{k_0}{k_I} = \frac{k_{+1}[I]}{k_{+1}[L]\left(1 - \frac{[I]}{K_I + [I]}\right)} = \frac{[I]}{K_I} + 1$$

(5.28)

Thus, from the ratio of k_0 to k_I for a given concentration of I, an estimate of its equilibrium constant can be determined.

5.3 PRACTICAL ASPECTS OF LIGAND-BINDING STUDIES

Until relatively recently, ligand-binding studies have used exclusively radiolabeled ligands. The use of radioisotopes was dictated by the need to measure accurately the very small quantities of ligand associated with the receptor preparation. Considerable effort has now led to the design of fluorescent moieties that can be attached to ligand molecules and that have sufficiently large fluorescent signals to permit the measurement of the fluorescence changes that occur when the ligand binds to very small quantities of receptor. The majority of radioligand-binding studies estimate the amount of binding by the separation of bound from free ligand, using either centrifugation or filtration, followed by measurement of the quantity bound. This separation stage, however, can be avoided in scintillation proximity assays (SPAs). These assays are applicable to ligands containing radioisotopes (e.g., tritium) that produce low-energy β-particles that travel only a very short distance (less than 10 μm) in aqueous solution. In one form of SPA, the receptor preparation is immobilized on microbeads containing scintillant molecules. The scintillant molecules are able to detect β-radiation emanating from radioligand bound to the receptors on the bead surface (and thus in close proximity) but will not respond to radiation from the relatively remote radioligand molecules free in the aqueous solution. For this technique to work, it must be possible to couple the receptor preparation to the bead in a way that does not interfere with the binding of the ligand. Provided this can be done, scintillation proximity counting provides a simple method of detecting binding and can, furthermore, be used to follow the time-course of binding while the reaction mixture remains in the scintillation counter. Techniques employing fluorescently labeled ligands (e.g., fluorescence polarization and fluorescence resonance energy transfer methods) can also avoid the need to separate bound from free ligand. The use of fluorescently labeled ligands has the additional advantage of avoiding the hazards associated with the use and disposal of radioisotopes. Both SPAs and fluorescence polarization assays are amenable to high-throughput screening using multiwell plates.

5.3.1 RECEPTOR PREPARATIONS

Most receptors (a notable exception being the steroid receptors that influence DNA transcription) are located on the cell surface, and purified cell membranes are thus an obvious choice of preparation. When a tissue is homogenized, however, any membrane fraction isolated may well contain membranes from intracellular organelles in addition to cell membranes from all the cell types present in the tissue. Thus, a membrane preparation from the brain will contain membranes not only from neurons but also from glia, as well as the smooth muscle and endothelial cells of blood vessels. It may, however, be possible to prepare membranes from pure cell preparations (e.g., cell lines in culture or cells obtained by disaggregation of the tissue with enzymes and subsequently subjected to purification by differential centrifugation). Increasingly, binding studies are performed on membranes from cell lines transfected with cloned human receptor genes, and a wide range of such cloned receptors is now commercially available for routine drug screening.

A feature of cell disruption is that it may expose receptors that were not originally on the cell surface. Some of the receptors will have been in the process of insertion while others may have been endocytosed. This would lead to an overestimate of the cell-surface receptor density. On the other hand, cell membranes may form vesicles that can have either an outside-out or inside-out orientation. Cell-surface receptors in inside-out vesicles will not bind the ligand unless they can penetrate the vesicle. It is usually necessary to wash membrane preparations thoroughly to remove endogenous material that might affect the binding (e.g., proteolytic enzymes, endogenous ligands). One important advantage of cell membranes is that often the preparation can be stored deep-frozen for many weeks without any change in binding properties.

The use of cell membranes can be criticized on the grounds that the receptors have been removed from their natural environment and will no longer be subject to cellular control mechanisms; for example, the phosphorylation of intracellular domains may be modified. These problems can be avoided by using intact cells for binding studies. Tissue slices (e.g., brain, heart) are used, as are cells isolated from dissected tissue by collagenase or trypsin digestion. Permanent cell lines in culture can also be used. However, the possibility that application of proteolytic enzymes to aid the disaggregation of tissues might modify the receptors is of some concern. When using intact cells, it is also possible that some ligands will be transported into the cells, leading to a higher nonspecific binding. Furthermore, some cells may contain enzymes that metabolize the ligand. On the other hand, because cells must be maintained under physiological conditions to remain viable, binding results are, perhaps, more likely to reflect the true *in vivo* situation. Studies on purified, soluble receptors are much less common and subject to the uncertainty that removal from the lipid environment of the cell membrane may modify binding.

5.3.2 LABELED LIGANDS

The ligand that is chosen to be labeled should ideally have significant *selectivity* for the prime receptor of interest since although nonlinear least squares methods allow complex binding curves to be analyzed, single-component curves will yield more precise estimates of the binding parameters. If it is not possible to avoid multiple binding components, the curves will be more satisfactorily analyzed if the individual components exhibit substantially different dissociation equilibrium constants. A *high affinity* is also desirable, as it allows the binding to be studied at a low ligand concentration, which, other things being equal, will reduce nonspecific binding. A high ratio of specific to nonspecific binding will reduce the errors in the estimated parameters. A high affinity, however, also has consequences for the rate at which the binding reaches equilibrium. The association rate constant, k_{+1}, has an upper limit, determined by collision theory, of about $10^8 \, M^{-1}sec^{-1}$, from which it follows that ligands with high affinities must have very low k_{-1} values. From Equations (5.12) and (5.15), it is seen that this will lead to both a slow onset (at the low concentrations of L being used) and a slow offset of binding. A slow rate of offset is advantageous in the separation of bound from free ligand by filtration, where it is important to ensure that the washing steps do not cause significant dissociation.

5.3.2.1 Radioligands

Radioligands should have a *high specific activity* so that very small quantities of bound ligand can be accurately measured. The specific activity, simply defined as the amount of radioactivity, expressed in becquerels (Bq) or curies (Ci) per mole of ligand, is dependent on the half-life of the isotope used and on the number of radioactive atoms incorporated into the ligand molecule. A radioisotope with a short half-life decays rapidly so that for a given number of atoms many disintegrations occur in unit time, resulting in a high specific activity. The isotopes used most frequently for labeling are ^{125}I and ^3H, with half-lives of 60 days and 12.3 years, respectively (labeling with ^{14}C, with a half-life of

5760 years, would result in a low specific activity). Ligands labeled with single atoms of either ^{125}I or ^{3}H will have maximum specific activities of 2200 and 29 Ci per mmol, respectively. A basic difference exists between labeling with ^{3}H and with ^{125}I. With ^{3}H, the radioisotope can replace hydrogen atoms in the molecule with only insignificant changes in the chemical properties; indeed, it would be possible to replace several H with ^{3}H without a significant change in chemical properties but with a useful gain in specific activity. In contrast, most natural ligands and nearly all drugs do not contain an iodine atom that can be replaced by ^{125}I. Instead, it is necessary to produce an iodinated derivative; this *will* have different chemical properties and quite likely a different affinity for the receptor. (For this reason, it is usual to incorporate only one atom of ^{125}I in each ligand molecule.) It is necessary to check that the radioiodinated derivative retains the desired properties of the parent compound. With radioiodine, it is possible to achieve 100% isotopic labeling, as it is possible to obtain pure ^{125}I and to separate the labeled ligand from both unincorporated ^{125}I and noniodinated parent compound. It is obviously important to ensure that the label is associated only with the intended ligand. Potential problems include the possibilities that contaminating substances might also have been labeled and that the radioligand may have suffered chemical modification during storage. Highly radioactive ligands can suffer radiation damage, and the presence of radioactive impurities will almost certainly lead to a reduction in the ratio of specific to nonspecific binding.

For many receptors, both hydrophilic and hydrophobic radioligands are available. In some cases, the hydrophobic ligands have been found to give higher estimates of B_{max}, suggesting that they have access to receptors within the cell that are denied to hydrophilic ligands. This is exemplified by the greater B_{max} values observed (in neuroblastoma membranes) for the muscarinic receptor ligand ^{3}H-scopolamine (tertiary amine) compared with ^{3}H-N-methylscopolamine (quaternary ammonium). These differences in access to receptors can actually be exploited to study receptor internalization.

5.3.2.2 Fluorescently Labeled Ligands

The most commonly used fluorescence method is fluorescence polarization. For this it is necessary that the fluorescent label exhibits polarization to light. The excitation beam will only excite dye molecules that have the appropriate orientation. If now the labeled ligand rotates rapidly with respect to the polarization lifetime, the excited molecules will quickly become randomly orientated and the emitted light will show little polarization. On the other hand, ligand bound to a large receptor molecule/preparation rotates much more slowly, and the fluorophore has insufficient time to rotate appreciably between excitation and emission, resulting in a larger degree of polarization. The change in polarization allows the amount of ligand bound to receptor to be determined. The measurements can be made in multiwell plates. In this technique it is important that a high percentage of the labeled ligand is bound. This, of course, means that the free concentration of ligand is lowered and the analysis must allow for this depletion. (See Section 5.3.3.4.) Several suitable fluorescent labels have been identified including flourescein and the BODIPY® (Molecular Probes (Invitrogen), Eugene, Oregon) range of fluorophores.

5.3.3 INCUBATION CONDITIONS

5.3.3.1 Incubation Medium

Binding to intact living cells must of necessity be performed in a physiological solution, and the results obtained are hence quite likely to correlate with functional studies. It would be wise to avoid the inclusion of protein (e.g., albumin), as protein may well bind the labeled ligand to a significant extent and lower the relevant free concentration. This would not be detected by measurement of the total concentration in the supernatant obtained by centrifugation. Binding to membranes, by contrast, is quite often performed in a simple buffer solution (e.g., 20- or 50-mM Tris or HEPES buffers). It is clear, however, that the affinity of some ligands for receptors is increased in solutions of low ionic strength. This effect has been clearly demonstrated for muscarinic cholinergic receptors. In principle, it could be avoided by including sufficient NaCl to make the incubation medium isotonic

TABLE 5.1

Effect of Temperature on the Kinetics of [^{3}H]-Flunitrazepam Binding to Rat Brain Homogenates

Temp. (°C)	k_{+1} (M^{-1}.s^{-1})	k_{-1} (s^{-1})	K_D (nM)
0	7.3×10^5	7.3×10^{-4}	1.0
22	4.6×10^6	1.0×10^{-2}	2.2
35	1.1×10^7	5.9×10^{-2}	5.3

Source: Speth, R. C. et al., *Life Sci.*, 24, 351, 1979. (Reprinted by permission of the publisher. Copyright 1979 by Elselvier Science Inc.)

with the appropriate physiological solution. Particular ions have been shown to have effects on certain receptor systems. Mg^{2+}, for example, commonly affects binding to G-protein coupled receptors, which is in keeping with its known effects on G-protein activation. The ionization of weakly acidic or basic groups in both receptor and ligand will be affected by pH and is likely to modify binding. Accordingly, binding studies should be done at physiological pH, if at all possible.

5.3.3.2 Temperature

Temperature has effects on both the rates of reaction and dissociation equilibrium constants. A rise in temperature will increase the rates of both association and dissociation, as shown in Table 5.1 for the binding of ^{3}H-flunitrazepam to rat brain membranes. The effect on the dissociation equilibrium constant is less because the changes in k_{+1} and k_{-1} are in the same direction. It has been found for some receptors that the effect of temperature on affinity is greater for agonists than for antagonists.

Table 5.2 illustrates the results for binding to β-adrenoreceptors obtained by Weiland et al. (1979). It was suggested that the difference in the effect of temperature on agonist as compared with antagonist binding reflected the structural changes in the receptor (isomerization) that occur with agonists but not antagonists. More recent investigations of this issue have not, however, confirmed the generality of this conclusion.

TABLE 5.2

K_I Values for Inhibition of ^{125}I-Iodohydroxybenzylpindolol Binding to β-Adrenoreceptors in Turkey Erythrocyte Membranes at 1°C and 37°C

	K_I (nM) 37°C	K_I (nM) 1°C	$\dfrac{K_I (37°C)}{K_I (1°C)}$
Agonists			
Isoprenaline	254	11	23.3
Noradrenaline	2680	48	55.5
Adrenaline	5230	326	16
Antagonists			
Propranolol	1.6	0.59	2.6
Pindolol	4.5	1.5	2.95
Atenolol	5300	2530	2.09

Source: Weiland, G. A. et al., *Nature*, 281, 114, 1979.

Note: The binding curves for both agonists and antagonists were unaffected by GTP.

In the light of these results, it might seem best to measure binding only at the relevant physiological temperature; however, conducting the incubation at low temperature has some advantages. For example, proteolytic damage to the receptor and breakdown of the ligand, if it is chemically unstable, will be reduced during very long incubations (though this advantage may be offset by the longer incubation time required for equilibration).

5.3.3.3   Duration of Incubation

Equilibrium studies clearly require an incubation period that is long enough to allow equilibration to be achieved. As discussed above, the time required will be longer at lower temperatures. It is critically dependent on the affinity of the ligand for the receptor. As outlined earlier, the rate constant for the onset of binding is given by $k_{-1} + k_{+1}[L]$. If k_{+1} is given a value of $10^7 \text{ M}^{-1}\text{sec}^{-1}$, it can be estimated that to achieve 97% of equilibrium for a ligand with a K_L of 100 pM, at relevant concentrations, would require about 1 hour at 37°C and as much as 58 hours at 0°C. The effect of a competing drug is to slow the rate of equilibration. These considerations demonstrate the desirability of conducting pilot kinetic studies before any detailed equilibrium measurements are made.

5.3.3.4   Amount of Tissue

The aim should be to employ sufficient material to give a good ratio of specific to nonspecific binding without causing significant *depletion* of the labeled ligand. Nonspecific binding associated with binding to a filter is likely to be a fixed amount at any given ligand concentration, so increasing the amount of receptor present should increase the signal-to-noise ratio. A large concentration of receptor may, however, bind a substantial fraction of the ligand present and so reduce the free concentration. Such depletion is an important consideration. If the free ligand concentration can be measured directly, this should be done, and the concentration so obtained is applicable to the equations presented in this chapter. An alternative, if [L] cannot be measured, is to derive equations that allow for depletion arising from both specific and nonspecific binding. Such equations have been presented by Hulme and Birdsall (1992), but some of the assumptions made are necessarily oversimplifications. It is preferable to try to design the study so that depletion is kept to an insignificant level (say, <5%) and so can be ignored.

5.3.4   Methods of Separating Bound from Free Ligands

For particulate receptor preparations (intact cells or membranes), it is usual to separate bound from free ligand by either centrifugation or filtration. (For soluble receptor preparations, equilibrium dialysis, using a semipermeable membrane, or gel filtration can be employed.)

5.3.4.1   Filtration

At the appropriate time, the reaction mixture is either tipped or drawn by suction onto the filter and the supernatant immediately filtered under vacuum. The filter, often made of glass fiber, must retain all of the receptor preparation, while at the same time allowing a rapid separation. It is also necessary to check for binding of ligand to the filter. Several examples of "specific," saturable binding of radioligand to filters can be found in the literature. The receptor preparation retained by the filter is normally washed two or three times with a small volume of incubation buffer that does not contain the ligand in order to remove superficial labeled compound. It is essential to minimize any dissociation of bound ligand during these washes. This can be achieved by using only a few, rapid washes and by washing with buffer at a low temperature. Commercially available filtration systems now allow many samples to be handled simultaneously. Commonly used filtration equipment does not, however, allow the supernatant to be collected for the determination of the free ligand concentration.

5.3.4.2   Centrifugation

Incubation is often performed in small plastic tubes, which can be centrifuged directly to form, within seconds, a cell or membrane pellet. The supernatant can then be either tipped off or removed by suction. The radioactivity of the supernatant can be measured to determine the free ligand concentration. Any supernatant remaining on the surface of the pellet or tube can be reduced by washing, again using cold buffer. Most receptors will be within the pellet and will not be exposed to the wash solution, so dissociation should be limited. It is obviously important that washing does not disturb the pellet, causing loss of receptors. In some experiments using intact cells, separation has been achieved by conducting the incubation over a layer of oil of appropriate density. At the desired time, the cells are centrifuged through the oil layer, with virtually all of the supernatant remaining on top. Supernatant and oil are then removed by suction, and no washing step is needed. If plastic tubes are used, the tip of the tube containing the pellet can be cut off, so reducing further any counts due to radioligand attached to the tube wall. Finally, the bound radioligand (on the filter or in the pellet) is quantified using standard methods for measuring radioactivity (usually scintillation counting).

5.3.5 DETERMINATION OF NONSPECIFIC BINDING

Nonspecific binding is estimated by setting up additional incubation mixtures, which, in addition to the labeled ligand, also include enough of a displacing agent to virtually eliminate the specific receptor binding. Because most of the displacing agents employed to define nonspecific binding act competitively, it is necessary to use a concentration that is 100 to 1000 times larger than its K_d to ensure that higher concentrations of the ligand do not overcome the inhibition. It is also important to check that the displacing agent does not reduce nonspecific binding. This is likely to be more of a problem if a nonlabeled form of the ligand itself is used; therefore, preference should be given to a chemically distinct displacing agent. Extra reassurance can be obtained if similar values for nonspecific binding are estimated using more than one displacing agent. This is often the case in competition experiments where several competing drugs produce an identical maximal inhibition of binding, thus providing a reliable estimate of the residual nonspecific binding.

5.4 ANALYSIS OF BINDING DATA

The analysis of binding experiments essentially has two steps:

1. Preliminary inspection and analysis of the data to try to establish a model that adequately describes the binding. For example, multiple components or cooperativity may be identified.
2. Estimation of the model parameters (e.g., B_{max}, K_L) with some indication of the errors associated with the estimates.

It is always desirable to plot the data in terms of the amount of ligand bound as a function of either the ligand concentration (saturation experiments) or the inhibitor concentration (competition experiments). A logarithmic concentration scale usually provides a clearer picture of the relationship, with deviations from a simple monotonic curve being more obvious. It is also common to use linearizing transformations of the binding curves, both to reveal binding complexities and to provide initial estimates of binding parameters. Various linear transformations have been used to analyze saturation experiments, as will now be outlined.

5.4.1 SCATCHARD PLOT

Equation (5.3) can be rearranged to give:

$$\frac{B}{[L]} = \frac{B_{max}}{K_L} - \frac{B}{K_L}$$

(5.29)

The Scatchard plot is bound over free (B/[L], y-axis) versus bound (B, x-axis) (the Eadie–Hofstee plot is bound versus bound/free). If this equation is applicable (i.e., the binding represents a simple bimolecular interaction), the data points will fall on a straight line, the slope will be $-K_L^{-1}$, and the intercept on the x-axis (when B/[L] = 0) will give B_{max}. (See Figure 5.10 for a Scatchard plot of the data provided in Problem 5.1.) Curved Scatchard plots can indicate positive or negative cooperativity or the presence of sites (e.g., receptor subtypes) with different affinities for the ligand. The Scatchard plot, in the past, has been the primary means of obtaining estimates of K_L and B_{max}, but it is only reliable if the data are very good and a straight line is obtained. It should be noted that simple linear regression should not be applied to the Scatchard plot, as B with its associated error occurs in both x and y values. Linear regression of Scatchard plots systematically overestimates K_d and B_{max}. Because nonlinear Scatchard plots are even more difficult to handle, there is often a strong temptation to fit straight lines to plots that clearly are not straight. Nonlinear least square methods (see Section 5.4.5 below) are much to be preferred for the estimation of parameters with their confidence limits.

5.4.2 Lineweaver–Burk Plot

This double-reciprocal plot is based on another rearrangement of Equation (5.3):

$$\frac{1}{B} = \frac{K_L}{B_{max}} \cdot \frac{1}{[L]} + \frac{1}{B_{max}} \tag{5.30}$$

A plot of $1/B$ versus $1/[L]$ will give a straight line providing that Equation (5.3) applies; when $1/B = 0$, then $1/[L] = -1/K_L$, and when $1/[L] = 0$, then $1/B = 1/B_{max}$. A Lineweaver–Burk plot is shown in Figure 5.10, where it may be compared with the Scatchard plot of the same data. The double-reciprocal plot spreads the data very poorly and is inferior to the Scatchard plot.

5.4.3 Hill Plot

This plot has already been discussed in detail in Chapter 1 and earlier in this chapter. Yet another rearrangement of Equation (5.3) gives:

$$\frac{B}{B_{max} - B} = \frac{[L]}{K_L} \tag{5.31}$$

$$\log\left(\frac{B}{B_{max} - B}\right) = \log[L] - \log K_L$$

The Hill plot is log (B/($B_{max} - B$)) versus log [L]. As noted earlier, the slope of the Hill plot (the Hill coefficient, n_H) is of particular utility. If the equation holds, a straight line of slope = 1 should be obtained. A value greater than 1 may indicate positive cooperativity, and a slope less than 1 either negative cooperativity or commonly the presence of sites with different affinities. The data of Problem 5.1 are also presented as a Hill plot in Figure 5.10.

5.4.4 Analysis of Competition Experiments

Equation (5.18), which describes competitive binding, can also be transformed into the form of a Hill plot:

$$\log\left(\frac{B_I}{B_0 - B_I}\right) = \log IC_{50} - \log[I] \tag{5.32}$$

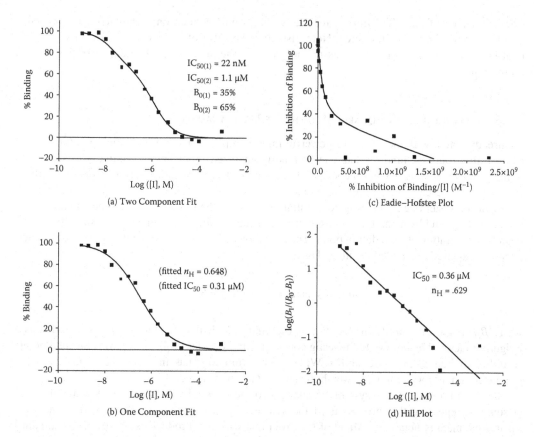

(a) Two Component Fit

(b) One Component Fit

(c) Eadie–Hofstee Plot

(d) Hill Plot

FIGURE 5.7 Analysis of a competition experiment in which the binding of a radiolabeled β-adrenoreceptor antagonist (^{125}I-iodopindolol) is inhibited by a $β_2$ selective antagonist. The four panels indicate various ways in which the data can be analyzed (see text). (The data for the figure have been extracted from Figure 4, Chapter 7, of Wolfe, B. B. and Molinoff, P. B., in *Handbook, of Experimental Pharmacology*, Trendelenburg, U. and Weiner, N., Eds., Springer-Verlag, Berlin, 1988.)

For simple competitive interaction at a single class of site, a plot of $\log (B_I/(B_0 - B_I))$ versus $\log[I]$ will be linear with a slope of -1 and intercept on the x-axis of $\log (IC_{50})$. This estimate of IC_{50} can be used to derive a value for K_I as discussed earlier. A different plot, equivalent to the Eadie–Hofstee plot for saturation experiments, has also been used to reveal more complex binding characteristics in competition experiments.

Figure 5.7 provides an example of the analysis of a competition study in which two sites are indicated. A plot of B versus $\log[I]$ (Figure 5.7a,b) might initially suggest two components, but the scatter of the observations would counsel caution. The Hill plot (Figure 5.7d) reveals a slope (by linear regression) of -0.629 (significantly different from -1), which is not consistent with simple 1:1 competition at a single binding site but is instead suggestive of multiple binding sites or negative cooperativity. An Eadie–Hofstee plot (Figure 5.7c) is clearly nonlinear. Nonlinear least squares analysis of the data (see next section) is shown in Figure 5.7a,b. In Figure 5.7b, a single component is fitted using Equation (5.18), but with the terms raised to the power n_H. The fit is quite reasonable and yields an n_H of -0.648, close to the value from the Hill plot. A closer fit (Figure 5.7a) (predictably) is obtained with a two-component model (in which n_H is constrained to one) according to:

$$B_I = B_{0(1)}\left(\frac{IC_{50(1)}}{IC_{50(1)} + [I]}\right) + B_{0(2)}\left(\frac{IC_{50(2)}}{IC_{50(2)} + [I]}\right) \tag{5.33}$$

The conversion of each IC_{50} into K_I for the two sites will depend on a knowledge of the affinity of the radioligand for the sites. Note also that the ratio of $B_{0(1)}$ to $B_{0(2)}$ will only give the relative proportions of the two sites in the tissue if the sites have identical affinities for the radioligand.

5.4.5 NONLINEAR LEAST SQUARES METHODS OF DATA ANALYSIS

As already noted, with the advent of powerful microcomputers and software incorporating appropriate fitting routines, binding data can be readily analyzed by means of nonlinear least squares fitting procedures. It is beyond the scope of these notes to give a full description of this method. In essence, however, the procedure first requires the selection of an expression that is believed to represent the system being investigated. Initial guesses are then made of the unknown parameters (e.g., K_L, B_{max}), and by using these guesses the expected binding is calculated corresponding to the ligand concentration at each datum point. The deviations of the observed points from the calculated points are squared and added together. Thus,

$$\text{Sum of squares} = \sum w(B_{obs} - B_{calc})^2 \tag{5.34}$$

where B_{obs} is the measured binding, B_{calc} is the binding calculated using the guesses, and w is a weighting factor. This allows the investigator to give more or less weight to particular data points according to their perceived reliability. Where each datum point has an associated standard error, it is quite common, for example, to weight inversely with the variance.

The program then makes systematic changes to the guessed values and recalculates the sum of squares, repeating this process until the sum of squares reaches a minimum (i.e., the least squares estimate is obtained). Many of the programs will also produce estimates of the standard deviation of the estimated values. The process is described in more detail in Colquhoun's textbook *Lectures on Biostatistics*, and its application to binding studies has been considered specifically by Wells (see the "Further Reading" section at the end of the chapter). SigmaPlot® (Systat Software) and Origin® (OriginLab®) are examples of commercially available graphing and curve-fitting programs. Prism® (GraphPad Software) is particularly well-suited for the analysis of ligand-binding experiments.

Closer least squares fits can obviously be obtained by adopting more complicated models involving extra parameters. The use of more complicated models can, of course, be more readily justified if there is independent supporting evidence available (e.g., knowledge of multiple binding sites from functional studies).

5.5 RELEVANCE OF RESULTS FROM BINDING STUDIES

Binding studies are done independently of any biological response, and it is obviously desirable to have some check to ensure that the binding is occurring at a relevant or identifiable site. Thus, wherever possible, the binding results should be compared with results from functional studies. This can be achieved most easily for competitive antagonists. In this case, Schild plots (see Chapter 1) can provide an estimate of affinity from the shift of concentration–response curves that should correspond to the K_d obtained in binding studies. Hulme and Birdsall (1992) provide an excellent illustration of such a correlation for muscarinic receptors, and a further example is provided in Figure 5.8, which compares functional and binding studies of potassium channel blockers. It will clearly be more difficult to establish such relationships when there are subtypes of a receptor in a tissue. In these circumstances, the availability of agents that exhibit selectivity for subtypes will assist the interpretation.

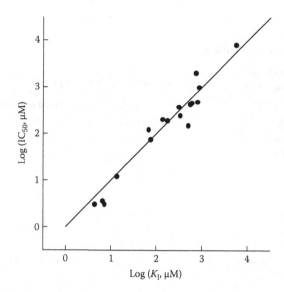

FIGURE 5.8 Correlation between the abilities of various compounds to inhibit ^{125}I-monoiodoapamin binding to guinea-pig hepatocytes (K_I values, abscissa) and their abilities to inhibit the K^+ permeability increase induced by angiotensin II in these cells (IC_{50} values, ordinate). The straight line is that expected for direct equivalence. The measurements are highly correlated, suggesting that the compounds do indeed produce their effects by binding to the apamin-sensitive K^+ channels. (Data from Cook, N. S. and Haylett, D. G., *J. Physiol.*, 358, 373, 1985.)

PROBLEMS

These problems are provided to afford an opportunity for the reader to analyze binding data of different sorts. The problems do not require nonlinear least squares analysis, but this would be recommended to those with access to appropriate facilities. It must be emphasized that, while linearizing transformations allow binding data to be clearly visualized, parameter estimation should utilize nonlinear least squares fits of the untransformed data. The analysis of each set of data is discussed in detail below in "Solutions to Problems."

PROBLEM 5.1: SATURATION BINDING

The data in Table 5.3 are from an experiment measuring ^{125}I-monoiodoapamin binding to guinea-pig hepatocytes. Conditions were such that depletion of radioligand was negligible over the entire concentration range studied.

1. Plot specific (inhibitable) binding against [L]. Make initial estimates of K_L and B_{max} from this graph.
2. Construct a Scatchard plot of the data and derive new estimates of K_L and B_{max}.
3. Construct a Hill plot ($\log(B/(B_{max} - B))$) vs. log [L]. What can be concluded from the slope of this plot?

PROBLEM 5.2: KINETICS

The onset of binding of radiolabeled apamin to guinea-pig hepatocytes was studied for three concentrations of the ligand over a 200-second period and provided the results in Table 5.4.

These data are plotted in Figure 5.9 and indicate how the rate constant for onset of binding increases with the ligand concentration. For each set of results the expected binding is given by:

$$B_t = B_\infty(1 - e^{-(k_{-1}+k_{+1}[L])t})$$

(5.35)

Estimate k_{+1} and k_{-1} from the data (see Section 5.2.2.2).

TABLE 5.3
Data for Problem 5.1

Radioligand Concentration [L] (pM)	Amount Bound (fmol · mg Dry Tissue⁻¹)	
	Total	Noninhibitable
20	0.110	0.018
50	0.224	0.046
100	0.351	0.071
150	0.495	0.143
200	0.557	0.180
300	0.708	0.275
500	0.942	0.462
1000	1.530	0.900
1500	1.920	1.310

TABLE 5.4
Data for Problem 5.2

Time (sec)	Specific Binding (fmol/mg Dry Tissue)		
	[L] = 30 pM	[L] = 100 pM	[L] = 300 pM
5	.025	.071	.165
10	.029	.112	.294
15	.041	.135	.340
20	.063	.166	.392
30	.063	.218	.460
50	.098	.257	.481
100	.102	.260	.503
200	.112	.270	.488

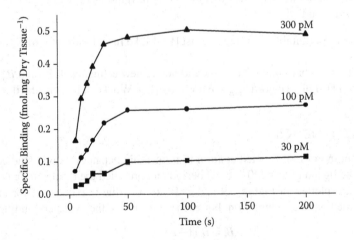

FIGURE 5.9 Plot of the data for Problem 5.2.

TABLE 5.5
Data for Problem 5.3

[Sotalol] (M)	Total Binding (fmol/mg Protein)		
	[IHYP] = 30 pM	[IHYP] = 100 pM	[IHYP] = 300 pM
0.0	34.0	56.2	75.1
1.0×10^{-8}	33.8	57.0	74.0
3.2×10^{-8}	32.5	55.3	74.6
1.0×10^{-7}	31.0	55.0	73.8
3.2×10^{-7}	26.2	51.8	69.6
1.0×10^{-6}	20.0	42.6	67.0
3.2×10^{-6}	9.7	26.3	50.6
1.0×10^{-5}	4.2	13.0	35.0
3.2×10^{-5}	3.0	7.9	22.5
1.0×10^{-4}	1.9	5.0	12.5
3.2×10^{-4}	1.4	3.8	11.9
1.0×10^{-3}	1.2	3.5	10.0

PROBLEM 5.3: COMPETITION EXPERIMENT

The binding of three concentrations of ^{125}I-labeled iodohydroxybenzylpindolol (IHYP) to membranes from turkey erythrocytes was studied in the absence and presence of a range of sotalol concentrations. Table 5.5 presents the results. Plot the total amount of IHYP bound against log [sotalol], and draw smooth curves by eye through each set of points. Estimate the IC_{50} for each curve. Given that the K_L for IHYP is 37 pM, calculate K_I from each IC_{50} (see Equation 5.21). Tabulate the specific binding for each set of data, and construct Hill plots (Equation 5.32). Are the results consistent with a single population of receptors? Compare each IC_{50} from these plots with your previous estimates.

SOLUTIONS TO PROBLEMS

PROBLEM 5.1: SATURATION DATA

The raw data are plotted in Figure 5.10a. The top two points of the specific data might suggest that B_{max} has been reached by about 1000 pM, with a value between the measured values at 1000 and 1500 pM, say 0.62 fmol/mg dry wt. An estimate of K_L can be obtained by reading from the graph the ligand concentration that produces binding of 0.5 B_{max} (i.e., 0.31 fmol/mg dry wt.; see Equation 5.3). This estimate will depend on how the curve has been drawn but is likely to be around 120 pM.

A Scatchard plot of the data is shown in Figure 5.10c. For convenience, the fitted line is the regression of B/F on B (though, as noted earlier, this is statistically unsound) and provides an estimate for B_{max} (x-intercept) of 0.654 fmol/mg dry wt. and an estimate for K_L (−1/slope) of 132 pM. A Lineweaver–Burk (double-reciprocal) plot is provided for comparison in Figure 5.10d. Linear regression gives another estimate for B_{max} (1/y-intercept; see Equation 5.30) of 0.610 fmol/mg dry wt. The estimate of K_L from this plot (slope × B_{max}) is 114 pM.

To construct the Hill plot (Figure 5.10e), it was assumed that B_{max} was 0.654 fmol/mg dry wt., the Scatchard value. The slope of the plot is 1.138 with a standard deviation of 0.12, so it would not be unreasonable to suppose n_H was indeed 1 and so consistent with a simple bimolecular interaction. Figure 5.10b shows a nonlinear least squares fit of Equation (5.3) to the specific binding data (giving all points equal weight). The least squares estimates are 0.676 fmol/mg dry wt. for B_{max} and 150 pM

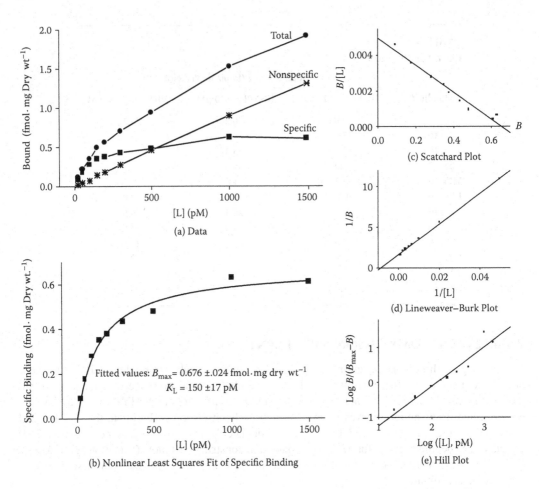

FIGURE 5.10 Analysis of the saturation data provided for Problem 5.1 (see accompanying text).

for K_L. (Estimates of the standard errors of these values are noted in the figure.) A nonlinear least squares fit of the *total* binding data to Equation (5.4) gave B_{max} = 0.686 fmol/mg dry wt. and K_L = 151 pM. The data for Problem 5.1 was in fact generated by setting the points randomly about a curve with B_{max} = 0.68 fmol/mg dry wt. and K_L = 150 pM. Both the Scatchard and double-reciprocal plots, in this case, underestimate both parameters, the latter plot being particularly inaccurate.

PROBLEM 5.2: KINETIC DATA

A graphical analysis, which allows the determination of k_{+1} and k_{-1} from the given data, is described in Section 5.2.2.2. For each set of data, it is necessary to determine k_{on}. These values can be obtained from the semilogarithmic plots of $\ln((B_\infty - B_t)/B_\infty)$ versus t (see Equation 5.16). But what value should be taken for B_∞? Estimates can be made by eye from the data, and for Figure 5.11c the B_∞ for 30 and 100 pM have been taken as the highest recorded values and for 300 pM as the mean of the values at 100 and 200 sec.

In plotting Figure 5.11c, the points beyond 50 seconds have been ignored because the errors in $(B_\infty - B_t)$ become proportionally very large. Linear regressions have been fitted to the three lines, giving k_{on} estimates of 0.0377 sec^{-1} (30 pM), 0.0572 sec^{-1} (100 pM), and 0.0765 sec^{-1} (300 pM). Nonlinear least squares fits, using Equation (5.14), were also made of each set of data (using Origin), and the fitted curves are shown in Figure 5.11a. The fitted values for B_∞ were 0.110 ± 0.005,

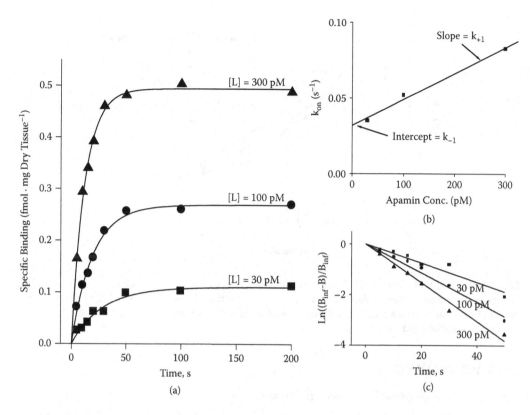

FIGURE 5.11 Analysis of the kinetic data provided for Problem 5.2 (see accompanying text).

0.269 ± 0.006, and 0.494 ± 0.006 fmol · mg dry wt.$^{-1}$ and for k_{on} 0.0351 ± 0.004, 0.0518 ± 0.003, and 0.0828 ± 0.003 sec^{-1}. These latter values have been plotted against [L] in Figure 5.11b, and linear regression gives a slope ($\equiv k_{+1}$) of 1.72×10^{-4} pM^{-1} sec^{-1} (= 1.7×10^{8} M^{-1} sec^{-1}) and y-intercept ($\equiv k_{-1}$) of 0.032 sec^{-1}. (All three curves were also fitted simultaneously to Equations 5.14 and 5.15 using a nonlinear least squares program [D. Colquhoun, unpublished] and provided values for k_{+1} and k_{-1} directly: $k_{+1} = 1.63 \times 10^{-4}$ pM^{-1} sec^{-1}, $k_{-1} = 0.034$ sec^{-1}.)

PROBLEM 5.3: COMPETITION DATA

The individual plots of the data will produce curves equivalent to that in Figure 5.4, the nonspecific binding, of course, increasing with radioligand concentration. The IC$_{50}$ can be read from the curves directly (taking account of nonspecific binding) or can be obtained from Hill plots for specific binding (see Equation 5.32). Hill plots of the data are presented in Figure 5.12, the points for concentrations outside 3×10^{-8} to 3×10^{-4} M being excluded because of the large errors associated with them. The lines are seen to be straight, and linear regression indicates slopes not significantly different from –1. The fitted lines have therefore been constrained to have a slope of –1. The x-intercepts corresponding to the IC$_{50}$ are 1.43 μM, 2.48 μM, and 5.74 μM. (Compare these with estimates obtained by direct interpolation on the plots of the raw data.) Nonlinear least squares fits of each set of data to Equation (5.18) provided IC$_{50}$ estimates of 1.20 ± 0.07 μM, 2.51 ± 0.13 μM, and 6.17 ± 0.45 μM. The K_I can be obtained from the IC$_{50}$ using Equation (5.21). Taking K_L as 37 pM gives K_I values of 0.66, 0.68, and 0.68 μM, respectively, which as expected are very similar. The data for this problem were actually generated using a starting value for K_I of 0.68 μM.

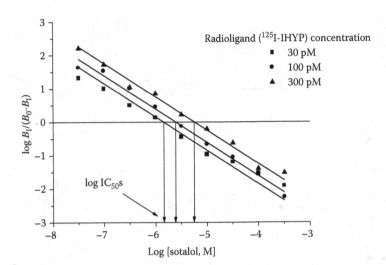

FIGURE 5.12 Hill plots of the results of the competition experiment used for Problem 5.3. The fitted lines have been constrained to have a slope of –1. IC_{50} values are given by the x-intercepts and can be used to determine K_1 for the binding of sotalol (see accompanying text). The IC_{50} values, as expected from Equation (5.21), increase with radioligand concentration.

FURTHER READING

FIRST RIGOROUS STUDY OF RADIOLIGAND BINDING

Paton, W. D. M. and Rang, H. P., The uptake of atropine and related drugs by intestinal smooth muscle of the guinea-pig in relation to acetylcholine receptors, *Proc. Roy. Soc. London Ser. B*, 163, 1, 1965.

SCINTILLATION PROXIMITY METHOD

Udenfriend, S., Gerber, L., and Nelson, N., Scintillation proximity assay: A sensitive and continuous isotopic method for monitoring ligand/receptor and antigen/antibody interactions, *Anal. Biochem.*, 161, 494, 1987.

EFFECT OF IONIC STRENGTH ON LIGAND BINDING

Birdsall, N. J. M., Burgen, A. S. V., Hulme, E. C., and Wells, J. W., The effects of ions on the binding of agonists and antagonists to muscarinic receptors, *Br. J. Pharmacol.*, 67, 371, 1979.

COMPREHENSIVE TREATMENT OF THEORETICAL AND PRACTICAL ASPECTS OF RADIOLIGAND BINDING EXPERIMENTS

Hulme, E. C., and Birdsall, N. J. M., Strategy and tactics in receptor binding studies, in *Receptor–ligand interactions: A practical approach*, Hulme, E. C., Ed., IRL Press, Oxford, 1992, chap. 4.
Limbird, L.E. Cell surface receptors: A short course on theory and methods, Kluwer Academic Publishers 3rd ed., 2004.
Keen, M. (Ed.), Receptor binding techniques, *Methods in molecular biology*, Vol 106, Humana Press, 1999.

PARAMETER ESTIMATION INCLUDING NONLINEAR LEAST SQUARES METHODS

Colquhoun, D., *Lectures on Biostatistics*, Clarendon Press, Oxford, 1971.
Wells, J. W., Analysis and interpretation of binding at equilibrium, in *Receptor–Ligand Interactions: A Practical Approach*, Hulme, E. C., Ed., IRL Press, Oxford, 1992, chap. 11.

Section IV

Transduction of the Receptor Signal

6 Receptors Linked to Ion Channels

Mechanisms of Activation and Block

Alasdair J. Gibb

CONTENTS

6.1   INTRODUCTION

Many measurements in pharmacology rely on a chain of events following receptor activation to produce a measurable response: for example, contraction of the smooth muscle of a piece of guinea-pig ileum in response to muscarinic receptor activation by acetylcholine. This means that the relationship between receptor occupancy and response is likely to be complex, and mechanisms of drug action in such systems are often difficult to define.

In contrast to this, agonist responses at ligand-gated ion channels and drug effects at ion channel receptors are often more amenable to mechanistic investigation because the response (ionic current through open ion channels when measured with voltage or patch-clamp techniques) is directly proportional to receptor activation. This is a great advantage and has allowed electrophysiological techniques to be used to study receptor activation and drug block of ion channel receptors in great detail.

This chapter deals mainly with information that can be obtained from equilibrium, or at least steady-state recordings of ion channel receptor activity. However, a great deal of information has also been obtained from kinetic studies of ion channels where the aim has been to determine values for the rate constants in a receptor mechanism. In general, only equilibrium constants can be determined from equilibrium studies.

6.1.1   THE RESPONSE TO RECEPTOR ACTIVATION

Activation of a ligand-gated ion channel receptor causes opening of the ion channel, which forms a central pore through the receptor structure. Ions such as Na^+ and K^+, and often also Ca^{++}, depending on the ionic selectivity of the channel, flow through cationic channels that are formed by nicotinic acetylcholine receptors (AChRs), ionotropic glutamate receptors, $5HT_3$ receptors, or P2X ATP receptors. These ionic currents are generally excitatory and lead to depolarization of the cell. Chloride ions, with some contribution from HCO_3^- ions, are the main charge carriers through $GABA_A$ and glycine receptor channels, and these currents are generally, but not always, inhibitory.

The ligand-gated ion channel receptors mediate fast synaptic transmission at the neuromuscular junction and throughout the central and peripheral nervous systems. These receptors are also located presynaptically on nerve terminals at many synapses where their activation affects transmitter release. In addition, where the receptor-channels are permeable to Ca^{2+}, they are involved in the control of the intracellular Ca^{2+} concentration and hence feed into many of the transduction mechanisms that involve Ca^{2+} as a second messenger. Ca^{2+} influx through glutamate receptors of the NMDA (N-methyl-D-aspartate) subtype is of particular importance in the processes of synaptogenesis and control of the strength of synaptic connections in the brain, while excess Ca^{2+} influx through NMDA receptor channels is thought to be the main cause of neuronal cell death during hypoxia or ischemia in the brain.

Over the past 50 years, the development of electrophysiological techniques has allowed the effects of agonists and antagonists at the ligand-gated ion channel receptors to be studied with great precision. This has been particularly useful in studies of the mechanism of action of drugs because the result of receptor activation (current through the ion channel) can be measured directly, and channel opening is directly linked to receptor activation. Thus, it should be no surprise that the first physically plausible mechanism for receptor activation was the result of electrophysiological studies of AChR activation. Those experiments were performed by Katz and coworkers in the Biophysics Department at University College London more than 50 years ago.

6.2   AGONIST MECHANISMS

The simplest agonist mechanism that can be used to describe activation of the ligand-gated ion channel receptors is that first suggested by del Castillo and Katz (1957) for activation of nicotinic AChRs at the neuromuscular junction.

$$A + R \underset{k_{-1}}{\overset{k_{+1}}{\rightleftharpoons}} AR \underset{\alpha}{\overset{\beta}{\rightleftharpoons}} AR^* \tag{6.1}$$

This mechanism makes the vital point that receptor activation must represent a distinct step (most likely several steps) subsequent to agonist binding (see also Chapter 1). However, this mechanism does not allow for the fact that there is now considerable functional, biochemical, and structural evidence that there are two acetylcholine (ACh) binding sites on nicotinic acetylcholine receptors of muscle and electric organs, and it is probably the case that other four-transmembrane domain subunit receptors (see Egebjerg, Chapter 3, this volume) such as the glycine and GABA receptors also require binding of two agonist molecules for efficient activation of the receptor. At present, the mechanism most commonly used to describe AChR activation is as follows:

$$A + R \underset{k_{-1}}{\overset{2k_{+1}}{\rightleftharpoons}} AR + A \underset{2k_{-2}}{\overset{k_{+2}}{\rightleftharpoons}} A_2R \underset{\alpha}{\overset{\beta}{\rightleftharpoons}} A_2R^* \tag{6.2}$$

Here the microscopic association and dissociation rate constants for each step in the receptor activation mechanism are given, where k_{+1} and k_{+2} refer to agonist binding, k_{-1} and k_{-2} agonist dissociation, and β and α are the rate constants for channel opening and closing respectively. The factor of 2 before k_{+1} and k_{-2} occurs because the mechanism *assumes* that either of the two agonist binding sites can be occupied or vacated first. In addition, note that the two sites are assumed to be equivalent before agonist binding.

6.2.1 EVIDENCE FOR NONIDENTICAL AGONIST BINDING SITES

The AChR agonist binding sites on the receptor are some distance from the ion channel and outside the membrane. They are in pockets formed at interfaces between each α-subunit and an adjacent ϵ or δ subunit. The environment of the two binding sites cannot, in principle, be identical because of the nonidentical adjacent subunits and the fact that the receptor is a pentamer. However, functional evidence demonstrating nonequivalance of the two binding sites has not been consistent between species.

The best evidence that the binding sites are different comes from studies of the *Torpedo* AChR where both binding studies of native receptors and patch-clamp studies of cloned receptors expressed in fibroblasts suggest that there is on the order of a 100-fold difference in affinity for ACh between the two sites. Similar experiments on the BC3H1 mouse cell line and on recombinant human receptors suggest that there is also heterogeneity of the agonist binding sites on mammalian muscle AChR. In contrast, some experiments have found no evidence for a large difference between ACh binding at the two sites on frog endplate AChRs (Colquhoun and Ogden, 1988). For mammalian nAChRs (nicotinic acetylcholine receptors) competitive antagonists have been discovered that are selective between the two sites, such as tubocurarine and the α-conotoxins. There is little evidence of cooperativity between the two agonist binding sites (in the sense that affinity at one site alters when the other site is occupied) and cooperativity of the AChR response results from the large increase in probability of channel opening that occurs when two agonist molecules are bound, compared with when one or no agonist is bound.

It should be noted that the presence on a receptor of two agonist/antagonist binding sites, which may be different, adds considerably to the complexity of the results expected from binding studies or dose-ratio experiments such as the Schild method as described later in this chapter. It can also be noted here that homomeric receptors (such as the neuronal nicotinic α-7 receptor or homomeric AMPA receptor: see Egebjerg, Chapter 3) will have equivalent agonist binding sites before agonist binding. A further interesting point is that if the glutamate receptor subunit stoichiometry is tetrameric, then heteromeric non-NMDA receptors composed of, for example, two GluR1 and two GluR2 subunits will, in principle, have nonidentical binding sites on the equivalent subunits if the subunits are adjacent to each other in the molecule, but will have equivalent binding sites when the GluR1 and GluR2 subunits alternate in position around the central ion channel. These are very good examples of how information on receptor structure can be indispensable in interpreting the results of functional studies of drug action.

6.2.2 Application of the Two-Binding-Site Mechanism

Equation (6.2) has proved to be a good description of AChR activity in a wide range of experimental situations (reviewed by Edmonds et al., 1995) and more recently has been used as a starting point in developing mechanisms to describe the activation of other ligand-gated ion channels such as glutamate receptors, $5HT_3$ receptors, and $GABA_A$ receptors.

Expressions relating the equilibrium occupancy of any state in this mechanism to agonist concentration can be derived as described in Chapter 1. If we define the equilibrium constants for agonist binding as $K_1 = k_{-1}/k_{+1}$ and $K_2 = k_{-2}/k_{+2}$ and a constant E describing the efficiency of channel opening (equivalent to *efficacy*) as $E = \beta/\alpha$, then the equilibrium occupancy of the open state (A_2R^*), equivalent to the channel open probability, p_{open}, will be

$$p_{A_2R^*} = \frac{[A]}{[A] + \dfrac{1}{E}\left\{[A] + K_2\left(2 + \dfrac{K_1}{[A]}\right)\right\}} \tag{6.3}$$

It is instructive to write this equation in the form analogous to that for a single agonist binding site mechanism

$$p_{A_2R^*} = \frac{[A]^2}{\dfrac{K_1 K_2}{E}[A]\left\{[A] + \dfrac{[A]}{E} + \dfrac{2K_2}{E}\right\}} \tag{6.4}$$

since this form illustrates the low-concentration dependence of p_{A2R^*} on the square of the agonist concentration, which steepens the dose-response curve. The maximum $p_{A2R^*} = E/(1+E)$, and the half maximum, or $[A]_{50}$ concentration, of the dose-response curve are given by:

$$[A]_{50} = \frac{K_2 + \sqrt{K_2^2 + K_1 K_2(1+E)}}{1 + E} \tag{6.5}$$

The equilibrium occupancy of the open state of an ion channel is usually referred to as the p_{open} and is the fraction of time that a single channel is open or, equally, the fraction of a population of channels that are open at equilibrium. For a two-binding site agonist mechanism, the relationship between the p_{open} and the agonist concentration (p_{open} curve) has the familiar sigmoid shape (when the agonist concentration is plotted on a logarithmic scale) of a dose-response curve, but is steeper than for a single binding site mechanism.

6.2.3 Hill Coefficients and Cooperativity

In Chapter 1 (Appendix 1.2.3) the Hill equation and the Hill coefficient, n, are described. Hill coefficients greater than or less than unity are often interpreted as indicating positive or negative cooperativity, respectively, in the relationship between receptor occupancy and response. For example, positive cooperativity could arise due to amplification in a transduction mechanism mediated by G-proteins and changes in cell calcium concentration.

If the receptor has two agonist binding sites, the question arises as to whether binding of agonist at one site can influence the binding of the agonist at the other site. This is referred to as *cooperativity between agonist binding sites*. Binding at one site that reduces the affinity at the second site is referred to as *negative cooperativity*, and binding at one site that increases the affinity at the second site is termed *positive cooperativity*. Note that there may be cooperativity between agonist binding sites even although the unoccupied sites have the same affinity for the agonist. It is also possible that the two agonist binding sites are different before agonist binding occurs (on average, one site is then more likely to be occupied before the other), and in this case it is still possible for the binding of agonist at one site to influence binding at the other site.

$$n = 2\left(\frac{1+[A]/K_1}{1+2[A]/K_1}\right) \tag{6.6}$$

The slope of the p_{open} curve for Equation (6.2) is more complex than for a single agonist binding site: Equation (6.4) does not have the same form as the Hill–Langmuir equation, and the Hill plot is not a straight line (as mentioned in Chapter 1, Appendix 1.2.3). This is because for the two-agonist binding site mechanism the Hill coefficient n depends on the agonist concentration.

When $[A] \ll K_1$, then $n = 2$ but falls to $n = 1$ when $[A] \gg K_1$. In a study of AChR activation at the frog endplate, estimates were made of $EC_{50} = 15\mu M$, $K_1 = K_2 = 77\mu M$ and $n = 1.6$ at the EC_{50} concentration. An approximation to the Hill plot is often used with agonist-response data for ligand-gated ion channels to suggest a lower limit for the number of agonist binding sites on the receptor. It turns out that, for many (but not all) mechanisms, if $[A] \ll K_A$, then the slope of a plot of log(response) versus log[A] approaches the number of agonist binding reactions required for receptor activation. Figure 6.1 illustrates this using data recorded from a *Xenopus* oocyte expressing embryonic mouse muscle AChR receptors. In this example, the response being measured is the summed current

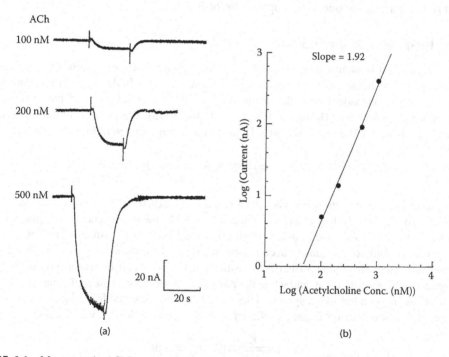

(a)

(b)

FIGURE 6.1 Macroscopic AChR responses and the Hill slope for AChR activation. (a) Current through AChR ion channels in response to increasing concentrations of ACh was recorded from *Xenopus* oocytes that had been injected 3 days previously with cRNA for the α, β, γ, and δ subunits of the mouse muscle AChR. (Courtesy of Prof. S.F. Heinemann, Salk Institute.) An inward current through the AChR ion channels is shown as a downward deflection of the trace. Small artifacts on the trace indicate the time when the solution flowing into the bath was changed from control to the indicated ACh concentrations, and then back to control. Currents were recorded with a two-microelectrode voltage clamp. The membrane potential was −60 mV and the recordings were made at room temperature. (b) The response (in nA) to increasing concentrations of ACh is plotted against ACh concentration (in nM) on log–log scales. The slope of the line (1.92) is an approximation to the Hill coefficient (when receptor occupancy is small) and suggests that two agonist molecules must bind to the receptor to produce efficient receptor activation.

flowing through many thousands of open receptor channels in the oocyte membrane. At these low agonist concentrations ($[A] \ll K_A$), the slope of the plot (in this case 1.92) suggests that the binding of two ACh molecules is necessary for receptor activation, and this correlates well with the known subunit stoichiometry of muscle AChRs of $\alpha_2\beta\gamma\delta$ where the ACh binding sites are known to be formed by the α subunits (see Egebjerg, Chapter 3).

6.2.4 HILL COEFFICIENT FOR HOMOMERIC RECEPTOR CHANNELS

Several functional receptors have been described in expression systems where the receptor is expressed from a single receptor subunit. Receptor subunits that form functional homomeric channels include the neuronal nicotinic $\alpha7$ subunit, the $5HT_3$ receptor subunit, some non-NMDA receptor subunits, the embryonic glycine receptor α subunit, and the P2X ATP receptor subunits. Based on analogy with the known structure of Torpedo AChRs, it is assumed that AChRs, $5HT_3$ receptors, and glycine receptors have a pentameric structure of five subunits surrounding a central ion channel pore. Such a structure suggests that there will be five agonist binding sites on a homomeric receptor. What then should we expect the Hill coefficient to be for these receptors? Hill coefficients for these receptors are generally found to be in the range from 1 to 3. Such measurements are complicated by receptor desensitization (see Section 6.2.5). However, these results can be interpreted as indicating that where there are five agonist binding sites on the receptor, perhaps only two need be occupied for full receptor activation (see also Chapter 3, Problem 3.1).

6.2.5 RECEPTOR DESENSITIZATION

Desensitization can be defined as the tendency of a response to wane, despite the presence of a stimulus of constant intensity (e.g., constant agonist concentration). In the case of the nicotinic ACh receptor there is good evidence that desensitization results from a change in receptor conformation to an inactive refractory state (Rang and Ritter, 1970). To describe this in terms of the AChR activation mechanism we could add a desensitized state to the scheme shown in Equation (6.2) to give

$$A + R \underset{k_{-1}}{\overset{2k_{+1}}{\rightleftharpoons}} AR + A \underset{2k_{-2}}{\overset{k_{+2}}{\rightleftharpoons}} A_2R \underset{\alpha}{\overset{\beta}{\rightleftharpoons}} A_2R^* \underset{k_{-D}}{\overset{k_{+D}}{\rightleftharpoons}} A_2R_D \qquad (6.7)$$

Here k_{+D} and k_{-D} are the rate constants for entry into and exit from the desensitized state A_2R_D. Investigation of the applicability of a range of mechanisms like the linear scheme in Equation (6.7) to AChR desensitization (Katz and Thesleff, 1957; Rang and Ritter, 1970) provided good evidence that linear schemes could not adequately account for AChR desensitization. In particular, it was noted that onset was often slower than offset of desensitization at agonist concentrations producing around 50% steady-state desensitization, and while the rate of onset was dependent on the nature of the agonist, offset was independent of the agonist. These results are not expected from linear schemes like in Equation (6.7). It was concluded that a cyclic scheme such as the following was necessary:

$$A + R \overset{K_A}{\rightleftharpoons} AR \underset{a}{\overset{b}{\rightleftharpoons}} A_2R^*$$

$$\Big\Updownarrow K'_D \qquad \Big\Updownarrow K_D \qquad (6.8)$$

$$A + R_D \overset{K'_A}{\rightleftharpoons} AR_D$$

Here the equilibrium constants for each reaction are given, and only a single agonist binding step is shown for simplicity.

The desensitized state of the receptor has very high affinity for the agonist ($K'_A \ll K_A$), and receptors are more likely to desensitize when occupied by agonist ($K_D \ll K'_D$). These observations have important consequences for radioligand binding studies utilizing ligand-gated ion channel receptor agonists. Generally, because desensitization is fast relative to the time scale of a binding experiment, what is measured will be dominated by the equilibrium constant for binding of the agonist to the desensitized state of the receptor, and this may be of higher affinity by several orders of magnitude than the affinity of the agonist for the resting, nondesensitized receptor. This is simply another case of the results developed in Chapter 1 showing that, in general, the *apparent* affinity of agonists estimated by methods such as radioligand binding will be a function of all the equilibrium constants in the receptor mechanism.

Desensitization is probably a quite general receptor phenomenon, although it varies widely in extent and rate of onset and offset. The scale and time course of AChR desensitization is illustrated in Figure 6.2, which shows responses of a patch of cell membrane containing several AChRs to increasing concentrations of ACh. Two things are obvious: first, during each ACh application, the response rises rapidly to a peak and then wanes to a level where the trace can be seen stepping between single channel current levels. Second, it can be seen that with increasing ACh concentration,

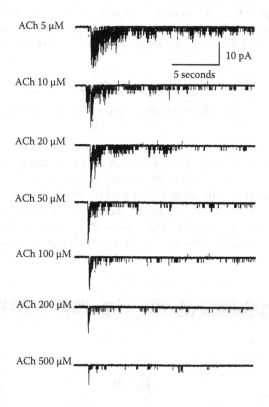

FIGURE 6.2 Activation of single AChR channels in an outside-out membrane patch. Responses to increasing concentrations of ACh of a membrane patch containing several AChRs. A small artifact near the beginning of each trace indicates the time when the solution flowing into the recording chamber was changed to solution containing the indicated concentration of ACh. With increasing ACh concentration, it can be seen that the channels are activated more rapidly and that receptor desensitization becomes increasingly more rapid such that the peak response is reduced at the higher ACh concentrations. Once the response to agonist has reached a steady state, probably more than 90% of the receptors in the patch are desensitized. It is then possible to see individual clusters of channel openings, which reflect periods when single AChRs briefly exited from a desensitized state and underwent repeated activation by the agonist ACh before reentering the desensitized state again. Identification of these clusters provides a means of directly observing and measuring the p_{open} for the receptor at high agonist concentrations as illustrated in Figure 6.3.

the peak response does not simply become greater. Instead, it first increases and then decreases due to the increasing rate of onset of desensitization.

6.2.6 DETERMINATION OF THE P_{OPEN} CURVE

Due to the occurrence of desensitization, the shape of the full relationship between agonist concentration and response cannot be determined from experiments like that illustrated in Figure 6.1. In practice, the most accurately determined part of the macroscopic dose-response curve is often at the low concentration limit where the effects of desensitization on the dose-response curve are small.

Single channel recording provides a way around the problem of desensitization because periods when all the receptors in the membrane patch are desensitized are obvious at high agonist concentrations as long stretches of recording where no channel openings occur. Desensitization has therefore been used to provide a means of obtaining groups of successive openings, all due to the activity of a single AChR, referred to as *clusters* (a cluster being a group of closely spaced bursts of openings). The desensitized periods are simply discarded, and the channel p_{open} is measured during the clusters of activity between desensitized periods.

In each trace in Figure 6.2, after several seconds of exposure to ACh it becomes possible to identify individual clusters of AChR channel openings. Analysis of these clusters of channel openings as illustrated in Figure 6.3 allows the relationship between ACh concentration and p_{open} to be determined.

$$p_{open} = \frac{charge\ passed\ during\ cluster\ (pC)}{single\ channel\ current\ (pA)\ \times\ cluster\ duration\ (secs)} \tag{6.9}$$

Figure 6.3 shows an example of a cluster of AChR channel openings recorded from an outside-out membrane patch in the presence of 10 µM ACh. The p_{open} during the cluster is, in principle, simple to calculate: The fraction of time the channel is open is the total time spent in the open state, divided by the duration of the cluster. However, the limited bandwidth of any recording system means that some short openings will be too short to be measured. It is, therefore, preferable to measure the charge passed during the cluster (since charge is not lost with filtering) and use the accumulated charge (the integral of the current during the cluster) to calculate the p_{open}.

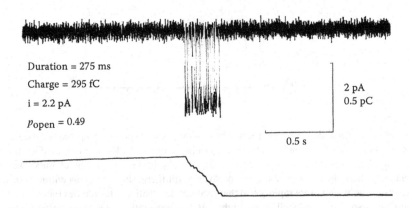

FIGURE 6.3 Measurement of receptor p_{open} during clusters of AChR channel openings. An outside-out patch expressing mouse muscle AChR as described for Figure 6.1. The upper trace shows a single cluster of AChR channel openings activated by 10 µM ACh. The lower trace shows a trace of the output from an analog integrator circuit. The duration of the cluster is 275 ms and the charge passed was 295 fC. The average single-channel current was 2.2 pA, giving a p_{open} for this cluster of 0.49.

Using the method of integrating the charge passed during each cluster of channel activity, it is possible to determine accurately the p_{open} curve at high agonist concentrations. However, notice that this method depends on identification of clusters of channel openings where each cluster can be assigned unambiguously as resulting from the activity of a single receptor channel: At low p_{open} it is possible for two channels to be active during a cluster without giving any clear double openings but, of course, giving about double the true p_{open} for a single receptor. Therefore, the lower part of the p_{open} curve cannot be determined in this type of experiment. Ideally, the whole p_{open} curve should be determined from experiments where there is only one receptor present in the patch of membrane being recorded from. In practice, this is extremely difficult to achieve because the density of receptors is too high in most cell membranes and there is no way to tell how many receptors are in the patch (on the other hand, in some expression systems, e.g., transfected HEK cells, it is possible to control the density of receptors to achieve occasional patches containing a single receptor).

Figure 6.4 shows an example of a cluster of AChR channel openings and the p_{open} curve obtained from the same patch. It was possible to identify clusters clearly when the p_{open} was greater than about 0.4. The results are complicated by the presence of open channel block of the AChR channel by the agonist ACh (see Section 6.3.3 and Equation 6.25). This causes the p_{open} to gradually decrease at high agonist concentrations, particularly above 1mM. The maximum p_{open} for the patch illustrated in Figure 6.4a was 0.83 ± 0.01 ($n = 45$ clusters) and occurred at 200 µM ACh (Figure 6.4b). How

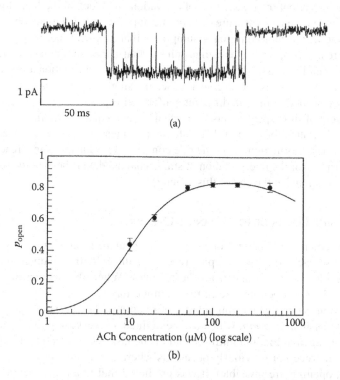

(a)

(b)

FIGURE 6.4 p_{open} curve for mouse muscle AChR expressed in *Xenopus* oocytes. (a) Shows a cluster of AChR channel openings activated in response to 200 µM ACh. The cluster p_{open} = 0.87. (b) Shows the relationship between cluster p_{open} and ACh concentration. The data points show the mean ± s.e. ($n = 8$–82 clusters) at each ACh concentration. The solid line shows the fit of the reaction mechanism given in Equation (6.25) to the data, where the agonist can both activate the receptor and block the open ion channel. The equilibrium constants for agonist binding to the two binding sites on the receptor were assumed to be equal (K_A) and were estimated to be 22 µM, the ratio of channel opening to closing rate constants (β/α) was 7.9, and the equilibrium constant for open channel block (K_B) was 4.9 mM. (Adapted from Gibb et al., 1990, *Proceedings of the Royal Society* 242, 108–112.)

should these results be interpreted? The p_{open} curve in Figure 6.4b was fitted with the relationship between p_{open} and ACh concentration predicted for the two agonist binding site mechanism extended to allow for block of the open ion channel by ACh (Equation 6.35). This fitting allows estimates to be made for each of the equilibrium constants in the reaction mechanism.

There is, however, one difficulty with interpreting the results of fitting the p_{open} curve. The difficulty is that when the maximum p_{open} approaches unity, increasing β/α or decreasing K_A has a very similar effect on the p_{open} curve, both changes simply shifting it to the left. Thus β/α and K_A cannot be estimated independently ($E = \beta/\alpha$ and K_A are correlated) when the maximum p_{open} is high. One solution to this is to estimate β/α separately and then fix this value when fitting the p_{open} curve to estimate K_A. Fortunately, estimates of β and α can be obtained from the analysis of bursts of single channel openings recorded at low agonist concentrations as described below. A *burst* of openings is defined as the openings that occur during a single occupancy by the agonist—for endplate AChR, typically there may be two or three openings in a burst separated by gaps of around 10–100 microseconds in duration.

6.2.7   ANALYSIS OF SINGLE-CHANNEL RECORDINGS

Development of the single channel recording technique was an enormous advance for studies of ion channel receptor function (Neher and Sakmann, 1976). For the first time it became possible to ask detailed questions about the mechanism of activation and block of the ligand-gated ion channel receptors. It became possible to measure directly the duration of ion channel openings and closings and so avoid some of the most limiting assumptions that had been necessary when interpreting macroscopic current records. An interesting point is that although single channel recordings are generally made at equilibrium, it is possible to obtain detailed information about the rates of channel opening and closing. This is because, in a sense, any single molecule is never at equilibrium but spends randomly distributed times in different conformational states.

The mean length of time spent in any individual state is equal to the inverse of the sum of the rates of all possible routes for leaving that state, and so measurement of channel open times and closed times provides information about the rate constants for transitions in a reaction mechanism. A complete description of the interpretation of single channel data is beyond the scope of this chapter (see "Further Reading" at the end of this chapter).

6.2.8   ANALYSIS OF BURSTS OF ION CHANNEL OPENINGS

Equation (6.2) predicts that channel openings will occur in groups or *bursts*. Bursts of openings occur because each time the receptor reaches state A_2R, the channel may either open or an agonist molecule can dissociate from the receptor. When the agonist dissociation rate k_{-2} is similar to the channel opening rate β, the channel may open and close several times before agonist dissociation occurs, generating a burst of openings. The burst of openings and closings is also referred to as an *activation*, which can be defined as everything that occurs from the first opening following agonist binding until the end of the last opening before all agonist molecules dissociate from the receptor (obviously occasions where the agonist binds and then dissociates without channel opening are invisible). It was predicted that ligand-gated ion channel receptor activation would result in bursts of channel openings given what was known about fast synaptic transmission (reviewed by Edmonds et al., 1995), and this idea has been used to interpret data from single channel recordings of AChR channel openings at the frog neuromuscular junction (Colquhoun and Sakmann, 1985).

From Equation (6.2) the mean open time is predicted to be the reciprocal of the rate constant for channel closing ($\tau_{open} = 1/\alpha$). For bursts recorded at very low agonist concentrations, the mean closed time within bursts, $\tau_g = 1/(\beta + 2k_{-2})$, and the mean number of gaps per burst, $N_g = \beta/2k_{-2}$. Using these two simultaneous equations it is then possible to calculate β and k_{-2}.

From recordings of bursts of recombinant embryonic mouse muscle AChR channel openings at low concentrations of ACh (less than 1 μM), the duration of openings and closings and the number of closings per burst were measured. On average $\tau_{open} = 3.0$ ms, $\tau_g = 94$ μs, and $N_g = 0.86$, giving $\alpha = 333$ s^{-1}, $\beta = 4919$ s^{-1} and $k_{-2} = 2860$ s^{-1}. If we assume $k_{+2} = 2 \times 10^8$ M^{-1}s^{-1}, then $K_A = 14$ μM. Thus $\beta/\alpha = 15$, and the maximum $p_{open} = \beta/(\alpha+\beta) = 0.94$. These values are consistent with those obtained from fitting the p_{open} curve in Figure 6.4. The ratio $\beta/(\alpha + \beta)$ indicates that ACh is a high-efficacy agonist while the large value for β indicates that a high ACh concentration will very rapidly (within a few hundred μs) activate the channel, as is observed during neuromuscular transmission.

6.3 ANTAGONISM OF ION CHANNEL RECEPTORS

The use of the Schild method for estimation of the dissociation equilibrium constant of a competitive antagonist is described in detail in Chapter 1. The great advantage of the Schild method lies in the fact that it is a null method: Agonist *occupancy* in the absence or presence of antagonist is assumed to be equal when *responses* in the absence or presence of the antagonist are equal. Even when the relationship between occupancy and response is complex, the Schild method has been found to work well.

6.3.1 COMPETITIVE ANTAGONISM AND THE SCHILD EQUATION

Using the procedures outlined in Chapter 1, it is straightforward to show that the Schild equation is also obtained for competitive antagonism of ion channel receptors if there is a single agonist binding site. However, where there are two agonist binding sites to consider, the situation is more complicated, as several new questions about the mechanism must be answered:

- Is the antagonist affinity for both binding sites equal? It is quite possible that even if the agonist has the same affinity for both sites, an antagonist will not.
- Can two antagonist molecules occupy the receptor at the same time?
- Does binding of the antagonist at one site influence the affinity of the other site for either agonist or antagonist?

The situation can be simplified by assuming that—

- agonist affinity at each site is the same.
- antagonist affinity at each site is the same.
- occupancy of one site by either agonist or antagonist does not influence the affinity of the second site for either agonist or antagonist.

Even with these simplifying assumptions a mechanism to describe the simultaneous action of both agonist and antagonist at a two-binding-site receptor is complex:

$$B+R+A \underset{k_{-A}}{\overset{2k_{+A}}{\rightleftharpoons}} B+AR+A \underset{2k_{-A}}{\overset{k_{+A}}{\rightleftharpoons}} A_2R \underset{\alpha}{\overset{\beta}{\rightleftharpoons}} A_2R^*$$

$$k_{-B} \Big\Vert 2k_{+B} \qquad k_{-B} \Big\Vert k_{+B} \tag{6.10}$$

$$B_2R \underset{k_{+B}}{\overset{2k_{-B}}{\rightleftharpoons}} B+BR+A \underset{k_{-A}}{\overset{k_{+A}}{\rightleftharpoons}} BRA$$

An expression for the equilibrium occupancy of p_{A2R*} can again be obtained using the methods outlined in Chapter 1. A potential complication is that this mechanism contains a cycle and so the product of the reaction rates in both clockwise and counterclockwise directions should be equal in order to ensure the principle of microscopic reversibility is maintained. In this case microscopic reversibility is maintained. Thus:

$$2k_{+A} \cdot k_{+B} \cdot k_{-A} \cdot k_{-B} = 2k_{+B} \cdot k_{+A} \cdot k_{-B} \cdot k_{-A} \tag{6.11}$$

In the presence of both agonist, A, and antagonist, B, p_{A2R*} depends on both the agonist and antagonist concentration in quite a complicated fashion. However, the relationship is essentially an extension to Equation (6.3) and is arrived at as follows:

1. The proportions of all forms of the receptor must add up to 1.

$$p_{B2R} + p_{BR} + p_{BRA} + p_R + p_{AR} + p_{A_2R} + p_{A_2R*} = 1 \tag{6.12}$$

2. When the system is at equilibrium, each individual reaction step in Equation (6.10) can be used to write down expressions for each form of the receptor in terms of the active form of the receptor, A_2R^*.

$$p_{A_2R} = \frac{1}{E} p_{A_2R*}, \quad p_{AR} = \frac{2K_A}{[A]E} p_{A_2R*}, \quad p_R = \frac{K_A^2}{[A]^2 E} p_{A_2R*} \tag{6.13}$$

$$p_{BAR} = \frac{2[B]K_A}{K_B[A]E} p_{A_2R*}, \quad p_{BR} = \frac{[B]K_A^2}{2K_B[A]^2 E} p_{A_2R*}, \quad p_{B2R} = \frac{[B]^2 K_A^2}{K_B^2[A]^2 E} p_{A_2R*} \tag{6.14}$$

The relationship between p_{A2R*} and both agonist and antagonist concentration can then be written as:

$$p_{A_2R*} = \frac{[A]}{[A] + \dfrac{1}{E}\left\{[A] + K_A\left[2 + \dfrac{2[B]}{K_B} + \dfrac{K_A}{[A]}\left(1 + \dfrac{[B]}{K_B}\right)^2\right]\right\}} \tag{6.15}$$

It is clear from comparison of Equation (6.15) with Equation (6.3), reproduced below as Equation (6.16) with $K_A = K_1 = K_2$,

$$p_{A_2R*} = \frac{[A]}{[A] + \dfrac{1}{E}\left\{[A] + K_A\left(2 + \dfrac{K_A}{[A]}\right)\right\}} \tag{6.16}$$

that there is now no simple expression relating dose ratio to antagonist concentration. After equating occupancies in the absence and presence of the blocker and multiplying the agonist concentration in Equation (6.15) by the dose ratio, then r can be found from the expression

$$\left(2 + \frac{K_A}{[A]}\right) = \frac{1}{r}\left[2 + \frac{2[B]}{K_B} + \frac{K_A}{r[A]}\left(1 + \frac{[B]}{K_B}\right)^2\right] \tag{6.17}$$

This expression can be rearranged to give a quadratic equation in r

$$\frac{2[A]}{K_A} + 1 = \frac{1}{r}\left(\frac{2[A]}{K_A} + \frac{2[A][B]}{K_A K_B}\right) + \frac{1}{r^2}\left(1 + \frac{[B]}{K_B}\right)^2 \tag{6.18}$$

and this can be rearranged to have the standard form

$$r^2(a) + r(b) + (c) = 0 \tag{6.19}$$

whose two solutions are found from the equation

$$r_1, r_2 = \frac{-b \pm \sqrt{b^2 - 4ac}}{2a} \tag{6.20}$$

One solution is negative and the other is (perhaps surprisingly) the familiar Schild equation.

$$r = \frac{[B]}{K_B} + 1 \tag{6.21}$$

More directly, it may be seen by inspection of Equations (6.15) and (6.16) that

$$\left(2 + \frac{K_A}{[A]}\right) = 2\left(\frac{1 + [B]/K_B}{r}\right) + \frac{K_A}{[A]}\left(\frac{1 + [B]/K_B}{r}\right)^2 \tag{6.22}$$

and so for the right and left sides of this equation to be equal

$$\frac{1 + [B]/K_B}{r} = 1 \tag{6.23}$$

and so the Schild equation applies.

Thus, if we *assume* that the two binding sites are identical and independent, then the Schild equation holds for the two binding site mechanism. If however, the antagonist binds with different affinity to each site, then the dose ratio becomes a complex function of both agonist and antagonist concentrations and equilibrium constants (Colquhoun, 1986). It is therefore not surprising that a parallel shift of the p_{open} curve with increasing concentration of antagonist is predicted not to be observed when the binding sites are different, and so the dose ratio will depend on the response level at which it is measured. However, some simplifying assumptions can still be made. If the p_{open} is small ($[A] \ll K_A$), then an approximately parallel shift of the dose-response curve occurs and the dose ratio is

$$r \approx \sqrt{\left(1 + \frac{[B]}{K_{B1}}\right)\left(1 + \frac{[B]}{K_{B2}}\right)} \tag{6.24}$$

where K_{B1} and K_{B2} are the equilibrium constants for the blocker at the two sites. In this situation the Schild plot is not linear: It has a slope of less than unity at antagonist concentrations around K_B (where $K_B = (K_{B1}K_{B2})^{1/2}$) and tends to unity at high or at low antagonist concentrations (Colquhoun, 1986).

An example of the use of the Schild plot in examining the action of the antagonist tubocurarine on AChRs at the frog neuromuscular junction (Colquhoun, Dreyer, and Sheridan, 1979) is shown in Figure 6.5. This figure illustrates an experiment where the net inward current measured in response to different concentrations of carbachol is plotted first in the absence (control) and then in the presence of increasing concentrations of tubocurarine. Recordings were made at two different membrane potentials, and then the Schild plot for each membrane potential was constructed. The results illustrate that at −70 mV the Schild plot is linear and has a slope close to unity, suggesting competitive antagonism (without any distinction between binding sites for the antagonist). However,

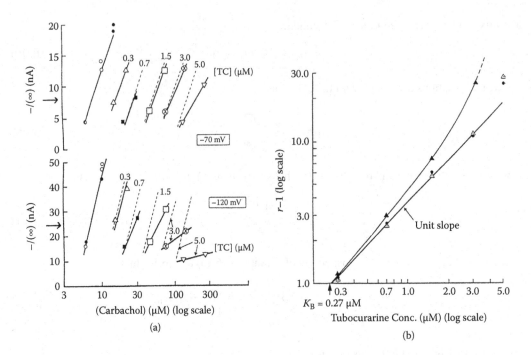

FIGURE 6.5 Use of the Schild method for estimation of the K_B of a competitive antagonist. (a) Shows log concentration-response curves for the equilibrium net inward current ($-I_{(\infty)}$) evoked by carbachol in the presence of increasing concentrations of tubocurarine (TC) at a membrane potential of –70 mV (upper panel) and at a membrane potential of –120 mV (lower panel). It can be seen that, except for the highest concentration of tubocurarine (5 μM), at –70 mV this antagonist produces an approximately parallel shift of the carbachol dose-response curve as expected for competitive antagonism. However, in the same experiment at a membrane potential of –120 mV, the shift of the dose-response curves is far from parallel. This is because the positively charged tubocurarine molecule is being attracted into the AChR channel when the inside of the cell is made more negative. The dashed lines in the upper and lower panels show the responses predicted for pure competitive antagonism with $K_B = 0.27$ μM. Dose ratios were calculated at a response level of –8 nA at –70 mV and –24 nA at –120 mV. (b) Shows the Schild plot of log(r – 1) against log(tubocurarine concentration). The filled circles show equilibrium dose ratios at –70 mV, filled triangles show equilibrium dose ratios at –120 mV, and open triangles show the peak response at –120 mV. Because open channel block by tubocurarine is relatively slow to develop, when the peak response is measured, mainly competitive antagonism is seen and the Schild slope is close to unity. The fact that both curves coincide at low antagonist concentrations (small dose ratios) suggests that the K_B for competitive binding to the receptor is independent of the membrane potential, as might be expected if the agonist binding site is outside the membrane potential field. (Adapted from Colquhoun et al., 1979, *Journal of Physiology*, 293, 247–284.)

at a membrane potential of –120 mV the Schild plot is nonlinear and has a slope steeper than unity. This occurs because tubocurarine also blocks the open ion channel of the endplate AChR and when the membrane potential is made more negative, the positively charged tubocurarine molecule is attracted into the ion channel, resulting in a noncompetitive block of the receptor as discussed in the next section.

6.3.2 ION CHANNEL BLOCK

The ion channel blocking mechanism has been widely tested and found to be important in both pharmacology and physiology. Examples are the block of nerve and cardiac sodium channels by local anesthetics, or block of NMDA receptor channels by Mg^{2+} and the anesthetic ketamine.

The channel block mechanism was first used quantitatively to describe block of the squid axon K^+ current by tetraethylammonium ions (TEA). The effects of channel blockers on synaptic potentials and synaptic currents were investigated, particularly at the neuromuscular junction, and the development of the single channel recording technique allowed channel blockages to be observed directly for the first time.

6.3.3 A MECHANISM FOR CHANNEL BLOCK

The idea that drugs could act by directly blocking the flow of ions through ion channels probably started, like any hypothesis, as some sort of abstract idea without any physical basis. It is easy to draw a cartoon with something like the plug in a sink, blocking the flow of water down the plughole (ion channel). However, to be useful it is necessary to convert the cartoon into a mechanism that is both physically plausible (i.e., does not contravene any of the accepted laws of physics) and provides quantitative predictions that can be tested experimentally.

Ideally, the aim would be to estimate the association and dissociation rate constants for the channel blocking drug. This would then give the dissociation equilibrium constant (K_B) for drug binding. Just as in the use of the Schild method to quantify competitive antagonism, a quantitative estimate of the K_B for channel block allows comparison of different drugs and a pharmacological classification of the ion channels they bind to.

We could say that when an ion channel is open, the drug binding site is exposed. If a drug binds to that site, flow of ions through the channel is blocked. We might further suppose that the drug has to unblock before the channel can close normally. A standard mechanism used to describe channel block of ligand-gated ion channel receptors is then:

$$A + R \underset{k_{-1}}{\overset{2k_{+1}}{\rightleftharpoons}} AR + A \underset{2k_{-2}}{\overset{k_{+2}}{\rightleftharpoons}} A_2R \underset{\alpha}{\overset{\beta}{\rightleftharpoons}} A_2R^* + B \underset{k_{-B}}{\overset{k_{+B}}{\rightleftharpoons}} A_2RB \qquad (6.25)$$

where β and α are the channel opening and closing rates and k_{+B} and k_{-B} are the microscopic association and dissociation rate constants for blocking the channel by the drug B. Here, B is indicated on the transition into the blocked state to remind the reader that the rate of this reaction depends on B. Notice that this mechanism does not take into account the possibility that a drug could bind to the channel in the closed (occupied *or* unoccupied) conformation.

With mechanisms like these it is often possible to simplify the analysis of the action of a channel blocker by assuming agonist binding is much faster than channel opening and closing and then combining several closed states together so that the mechanism approximates a three-state system.

$$A_2R \underset{\alpha}{\overset{\beta'}{\rightleftharpoons}} A_2R^* + B \underset{k_{-B}}{\overset{k_{+B}}{\rightleftharpoons}} A_2RB \qquad (6.26)$$

Notice that the channel opening rate is now denoted β'. Since the channel can only open from the A_2R state, the effective opening rate β' is obtained by multiplying the real opening rate β by the equilibrium occupancy of A_2R.

$$\beta' = p_{A_2R}\beta \qquad (6.27)$$

6.3.4 MACROSCOPIC KINETICS: RELAXATIONS, SYNAPTIC CURRENTS, AND NOISE

Measuring the occupancy of the open channel state of the receptor as a function of time ($p_{A2R*}(t)$) during the response to a perturbation of the receptor equilibrium can be used to obtain information about the rates' channel gating and interaction of drugs with ion channel receptors. The system is said to *relax* toward a new equilibrium. The time course of the *relaxation* is used to measure rates from the average behavior of many ion channels in a recording, while *noise analysis* uses the frequency of the moment-to-moment fluctuations in occupancy of the open channel state at equilibrium to provide information about the rates in the receptor mechanism.

For k states, a relaxation (or noise spectrum) will contain $k-1$ exponential (or Lorentzian) components. Thus, the mechanism in Equation (6.26) above will have two states in the absence of blocker and so give rise to relaxations (or noise spectra) that can be fitted with single exponential (or Lorentzian) functions. Addition of the blocker creates an extra state (the blocked state) giving $k = 3$. For $k = 3$, the occupancy of the open state as a function of time will be described by two exponentials

$$p_{A_2R^*}(t) = p_{A_2R^*}(\infty) + w_1 \exp\left(-\frac{t}{\tau_1}\right) + w_2 \exp\left(-\frac{t}{\tau_2}\right) \tag{6.28}$$

The reciprocals of the *time constants*, τ_1 and τ_2, are the *rate constants* λ_1 and λ_2. The weights of the exponentials (w_1 and w_2) are complicated functions of the transition rates in Equation (6.26). However, the rate constants are *eigenvalues* found by solving the system of differential equations that describe the above mechanism. λ_1 and λ_2 are the two solutions of the quadratic equation

$$\lambda^2 + b\lambda + c = 0 \tag{6.29}$$

where

$$-b = \lambda_1 + \lambda_2 = \alpha + \beta' + [B]k_{+B} + k_{-B} \tag{6.30}$$

and

$$c = \lambda_1\lambda_2 = \alpha k_{-B}\left[1 + \frac{\beta'}{\alpha}\left(1 + \frac{[B]}{k_{-B}/k_{+B}}\right)\right] \tag{6.31}$$

Notice that when β' is small (i.e., when the occupancy of A_2R is very small, as it will be if the agonist concentration is low) then

$$\lambda_1 + \lambda_2 = \alpha + [B]k_{+B} + k_{-B} \tag{6.32}$$

and

$$\lambda_1\lambda_2 = \alpha k_{-B} \tag{6.33}$$

With the simplifying assumption of a small β', the *sum* and the *product* of the rate constants measured in an experiment can be used to calculate k_{-B} and k_{+B} if α is known from experiments in the absence of the blocker. This is simply done by plotting the sum or the product of the measured rate constants against blocker concentration. From Equation (6.33) above, the product of the rate constants should be independent of blocker concentration with a value equal to αk_{-B}, while the sum of the rate constants (Equation 6.32) will give a straight line with slope equal to k_{+B} and intercept of $\alpha + k_{-B}$. If the experimental data is consistent with these predictions, then the data points plotted in this way should lie on a straight line and this is then good evidence that the mechanism of action of the drug is to block the open ion channel.

The assumption that β' is very small has been used when studying the effects of channel blockers on synaptic currents since the transmitter concentration (and hence p_{A2R}) is probably small during the decay phase of the current. During noise analysis experiments a low agonist concentration is used so that again, under these conditions β' should be small.

6.3.5 CHANNEL BLOCK AT EQUILIBRIUM

The relationship between p_{open} ($p_{control}$) and agonist concentration for the two-agonist binding site mechanism is given in Equation (6.4) and reproduced below in a slightly different form.

$$p_{control} = \frac{1}{1 + \dfrac{1}{E} + \dfrac{2K_2}{[A]E} + \dfrac{K_1K_2}{[A]^2E}} \tag{6.34}$$

When an open channel blocker is added, the p_{open} in the presence of the blocker ($p_{blocker}$) given above is a function of both agonist (A) and blocker (B) concentration.

$$p_{blocker} = \frac{1}{1 + \dfrac{1}{E} + \dfrac{2K_2}{[A]E} + \dfrac{K_1K_2}{[A]^2E} + \dfrac{[B]}{K_B}} \tag{6.35}$$

Taking the ratio of $p_{control}/p_{blocker}$ gives this simple result:

$$\frac{p_{control}}{p_{blocker}} = 1 + \frac{p_{control}}{K_B}[B] \tag{6.36}$$

Since the current recorded in a voltage clamp experiment is directly proportional to the channel p_{open}, the ratio of current in the absence of blocker to that in the presence of increasing concentrations of blocker can be used to calculate K_B. The experimental design is to obtain a fairly large response to agonist alone, and then to calculate the ratio of this control response to responses to the same concentration of agonist in the presence of increasing concentrations of channel blocker. The ratio $p_{control}/p_{blocker}$ when plotted against [B] will be a straight line that intercepts the y-axis at 1 and has a slope of $p_{control}/K_B$. If $p_{control} = 1$, then the slope $= 1/K_B$. If $p_{control}$ is known for a particular agonist concentration, then obviously K_B can still be estimated. If we *assume* $p_{control} = 1$, then the calculated K_B will be greater than the true K_B: for example, by a factor of 2 if $p_{control} = 0.5$, by a factor of 10 if $p_{control} = 0.1$. Another way to look at this is to note that if the control p_{open} is known ($p_{control}$) then the IC$_{50}$ for the blocker is $K_B/p_{control}$ so K_B can be obtained from the IC$_{50}$.

6.3.6 SINGLE-CHANNEL ANALYSIS OF CHANNEL BLOCK

Below is an outline of some of the information that can be obtained from single channel data using fairly simple measurements such as the mean open time and mean shut time. This analysis is illustrated in Figure 6.6 for the block of NMDA receptor channels by Mg^{2+} ions.

6.3.6.1 Open Times

Channel blockers will produce a reduction of the mean open time from

$$\tau_o = \frac{1}{\alpha} \tag{6.37}$$

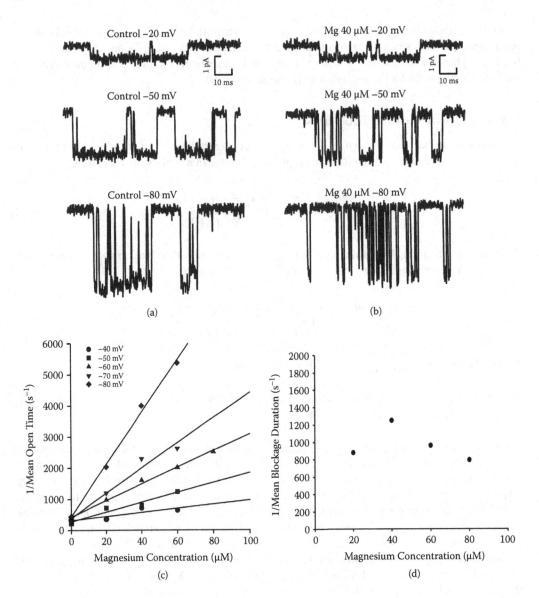

FIGURE 6.6 Single channel analysis of ion channel block. Representative recordings of single channel currents through NMDA receptor channels recorded are illustrated at membrane potentials of –20 mV, –50 mV, and –80 mV in control recordings (a) and in the presence of 40 μM magnesium (b). The rapid blocking and unblocking of the channel are particularly evident at more negative voltages. The inverse mean open time and inverse mean duration of the additional channel closings caused by Mg^{2+} are plotted against Mg^{2+} concentration in (c) and (d). These results confirm the linear relationship between Mg^{2+} concentration and inverse mean open time and the lack of Mg^{2+} concentration-dependence of the channel blockages predicted by the simple open channel block mechanism. The solid lines in (c) illustrate linear regression of the data recorded at each membrane potential. The slopes of these lines give estimates of the value of k_{+B} of 6.6, 15.7, 26.6, 40.4, and $84.0 \times 10^6\ M^{-1}s^{-1}$ at –40, –50, –60, –70, and –80 mV membrane potential.

in control to Equation (6.38) in the presence of blocker.

$$\tau_o = \frac{1}{\alpha + k_{+B}[B]} \tag{6.38}$$

This is calculated from the rule that the mean lifetime of any state is equal to the reciprocal of the sum of the rates for leaving that state (Colquhoun and Hawkes, 1982). A plot of $1/\tau$ against [B] should therefore give a straight line of slope k_{+B}. This is illustrated in Figure 6.6c where for a range of membrane potentials and Mg^{2+} concentrations the inverse NMDA channel mean open time follows this linear relationship, giving k_{+B} values in the range 6.6×10^6 $M^{-1}s^{-1}$ at -40 mV to 8.4×10^7 $M^{-1}s^{-1}$ at -80 mV.

6.3.6.2 Closed Times

Closed periods due to channel blockages have, from the same rule, a mean lifetime of

$$\tau_g = \frac{1}{k_{-B}} \tag{6.39}$$

Note the durations of channel blockages are predicted to be independent of the blocker concentration, and this is illustrated in Figure 6.6d, where the blockage duration shows no clear dependence on Mg^{2+} concentration.

6.3.6.3 Blockage Frequency

The frequency of blockages, per second of open time, is $k_{+B}[B]$, and so the mean *number* of blockages in each channel opening is simply the blockage frequency multiplied by the mean open time.

$$N_g = \frac{k_{+B}[B]}{\alpha} \tag{6.40}$$

6.3.6.4 Bursts of Openings

Where the channel blocker converts single openings into obvious bursts (e.g., local anesthetic block of nicotinic channels), the mean number of openings per burst is of course one more than the mean number of gaps (blockages).

$$N_o = 1 + \frac{k_{+B}[B]}{\alpha} \tag{6.41}$$

Notice that the mean total open time per burst will be:

$$N_o\tau_o = \left(1 + \frac{k_{+B}[B]}{\alpha}\right)\frac{1}{\alpha + k_{+B}[B]} \tag{6.42}$$

$$N_o\tau_o = \left(\frac{\alpha + k_{+B}[B]}{\alpha}\right)\frac{1}{\alpha + k_{+B}[B]} \tag{6.43}$$

$$N_o\tau_o = \frac{1}{\alpha} \tag{6.44}$$

This is an important result. The simple open channel block mechanism predicts that the total open time per burst is the same as the mean open time in the absence of blocker (Neher, 1983), even although openings are now chopped up by channel blockages. In fact for channels that give bursts of openings in control recordings, the total open time per burst is constant in the presence or absence of blocker.

This result is also of importance because it shows that simple open channel blockers do not reduce the charge passed by the channel during each activation and so they will not reduce the charge injected at a synapse by a synaptic current. Instead, what they do is prolong the time over which the charge is injected, which can have quite dramatic effects on synaptic transmission.

6.3.6.5   Burst Length

The mean burst length is found as shown below.

$$\tau_b = \frac{1}{\alpha} + N_g \cdot \tau_g \tag{6.45}$$

$$\tau_b = \frac{1}{\alpha} + \frac{1}{k_{-B}} \cdot \frac{k_{+B}[B]}{\alpha} \tag{6.46}$$

$$\tau_b = \frac{1}{\alpha}\left(1 + \frac{[B]}{K_B}\right) \tag{6.47}$$

Thus, a plot of the mean burst length versus [B] will give a straight line of intercept $1/\alpha$ and slope $1/(\alpha K_B)$:

$$\tau_b = \frac{1}{\alpha} + \frac{1}{\alpha K_B} \cdot [B] \tag{6.48}$$

6.3.7   The Time Scale of Channel Block

Channel blockers are often divided into *slow, intermediate,* or *fast* blockers. This classification is based on the very wide range of values that have been found for the microscopic dissociation rate constant of different channel blockers.

Nearly all channel blockers have been found to have microscopic association rate constants (k_{+B}) in the range around 10^7 M^{-1} s^{-1}. In contrast, microscopic dissociation rate constants (k_{-B}) range over several orders of magnitude from around 10^5 s^{-1} (e.g., block of nicotinic receptor channels by ACh) to $0.01 s^{-1}$ for MK-801 (dizocilpine) block of NMDA channels. The mean lengths of the blockage gaps can therefore range from 10 μs up to 100 seconds. It is only when the blockages are in the *intermediate* range, of the order of 1 ms in duration, that the gaps are easily detected in single channel recordings. If the blocker is a *slow* blocker with very long blockage gaps, the data record looks as though the frequency of channel openings has decreased. If the blocker is *fast,* the single channel amplitude appears decreased because the blocking and unblocking is too fast to be resolved.

6.3.8   Use Dependence of Channel Blockers

It follows from the fact that the blocker is assumed to bind only to the activated state of the channel that the degree of block will be not only concentration-dependent but also *use-dependent*: In other words, the more the channels are activated, the more they become blocked.

It follows from the above discussion on the time scales of channel block that the degree of use dependence will be critically dependent on the microscopic dissociation rate constant, k_{-B}. *Slow* blockers show extreme use-dependence, and this is augmented with blockers that display the *trapping* phenomenon. Trapping occurs when the channel can close, and the agonist dissociate, with the blocker still bound in the channel. The blocker is then trapped in the channel until the next time the receptor is activated. Important examples of trapping block are the action of hexamethonium at autonomic ganglia and the block of the NMDA receptor channel by MK-801 or the anaesthetic ketamine or memantine, a drug used to treat Alzheimer's disease.

6.3.9 Voltage Dependence of Channel Block

One of the interesting results from early voltage clamp experiments with channel blocking drugs is that the potency of the blocker is dependent on the membrane voltage. In contrast, this was found not to be the case for competitive antagonism at endplate nicotinic receptors (Figure 6.5). These results were interpreted as indicating that the acetylcholine binding site on the receptor (and therefore competitive block at that site by tubocurarine) is not influenced by the potential difference across the membrane, whereas if binding is affected by the membrane potential, then the binding site must be at a region of the protein that is part of the way across the electric field of the membrane.

Binding of a charged drug at a site within an electric field will be influenced by both chemical interactions (hydrogen bonding, etc., common to all drug-receptor interactions) and also by the electric field and charge on the drug.

The microscopic rate constants for association and dissociation at a site within an electric field (for block by charged drugs) are exponential functions of the membrane voltage:

$$k_{+B}(V) = k_{+B}(0)\exp\left(\frac{-\delta zFV}{RT}\right) \tag{6.49}$$

$$k_{-B}(V) = k_{-B}(0)\exp\left(\frac{\delta zFV}{RT}\right) \tag{6.50}$$

Here δ refers to the fraction of the membrane voltage that the blocking drug senses at the binding site, and the sign on the δ is determined by whether the blocking drug approaches the binding site from the inside or outside of the membrane. As expressed here, these equations describe the rate constants for block from the outside. The valence of the blocking drug is given as z; and F, R, and T are the Faraday constant (9.65×10^4 C mol^{-1}), the gas constant (8.32 JK^{-1}mol^{-1}), and the absolute temperature (293K at room temperature), respectively. The voltage dependence of the dissociation equilibrium constant is given by:

$$\frac{k_{-B}(V)}{k_{+B}(V)} = K_B(V) = K_B(0)\exp\left(\frac{\delta zFV}{RT}\right) \tag{6.51}$$

From this relationship it can be seen that a semilogarithmic plot of $\ln K_B(V)$ versus membrane potential will give a straight line with slope of $\delta zF/RT$ and intercept of $\ln K_B(0)$. The inverse of the slope gives the change in membrane voltage required to give an e-fold change in the equilibrium constant. It can be seen that the maximum slope will be obtained when $\delta = 1$. For a blocker with a single charge this will give a maximum slope of 25mV for an e-fold change, while for a divalent ion the maximum slope will be 13mV for an e-fold change. This analysis is illustrated in Figure 6.7 for the block of NMDA receptor channels by Mg^{2+} ions.

Figure 6.7a shows that a plot of log k_{+B} against membrane potential gives a linear relation with the slope corresponding to $\delta = 0.76$, while a plot of log k_{-B} against membrane potential (Figure 6.7b)

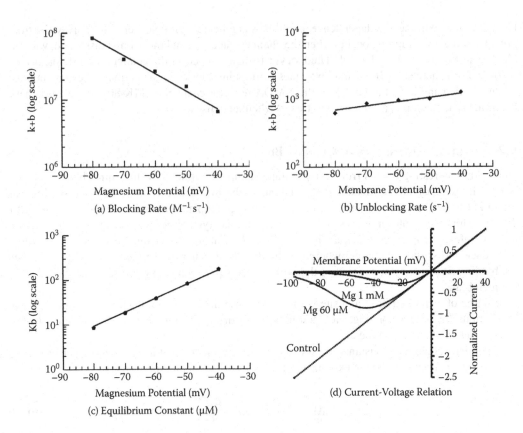

FIGURE 6.7 Analysis of the voltage-dependence of the block of NMDA receptor channels by Mg^{2+}. (a) Channel blocking rate, k_{+B}, estimated from the slope of the lines fitted to the data in Figure 6.6a, is plotted against membrane potential. The solid line shows the fit of Equation (6.49) to the data with $\delta = 0.76$ (reflecting an e-fold increase in blocking rate constant for every 16.6 mV hyperpolarization of the membrane potential) and a blocking rate constant of 2.66×10^7 $M^{-1}s^{-1}$ at –60 mV. (b) Channel unblocking rate, k_{-B}, estimated as the mean of the values at each Mg^{2+} concentration, shows a shallower voltage dependence than that of the channel blocking rate constant. The solid line shows the fit to the data of Equation (6.50) with $\delta = 0.21$ (reflecting an e-fold increase in blocking rate constant for every 61 mV hyperpolarization of the membrane potential) and a blocking rate constant of 2.66×10^7 $M^{-1}s^{-1}$ at –60 mV. (c) Voltage dependence of the equilibrium constant K_B for channel block, calculated from the ratio of k_{-B}/k_{+B}. The solid line shows the fit of the data to Equation (6.51) with $\delta = 0.97$ and illustrates the steep voltage dependence of K_B, which increases e-fold for every 13mV depolarization. (d) Simulation of the current-voltage relationship in the presence of a steeply voltage-dependent channel block. The control current is a linear function of the membrane voltage. However, in the presence of a low concentration (60 μM) or a physiological concentration (1 mM) of Mg^{2+} the current through the channel rectifies steeply at negative potentials reflecting the steep voltage-dependence of the equilibrium constant K_B.

is also linear but not as steeply voltage-dependent with $\delta = 0.21$. How should these results be interpreted? They may either mean that the energy barriers for Mg^{2+} approaching its binding site and dissociating from its binding site back to the extracellular solution are not symmetrical, or that a proportion of Mg^{2+} ions leave their binding site by permeating through the channel to the inside of the cell membrane. The voltage dependence of the equilibrium constant, K_B, shows that the affinity of Mg^{2+} for the channel is steeply voltage-dependent with $\delta = 0.97$, implying that Mg^{2+} ions sense almost 100% of the membrane electric field at their binding site (Ascher and Nowak, 1998).

Given that channel blocking drugs, by definition, act within the permeation path of the channel, it is not unexpected to discover that interaction between the channel blocking drug and the normal permeant ions may affect the behavior of a channel blocker. This is the case for NMDA receptors where occupation of permeant ion binding sites has a significant effect on the observed voltage dependence of Mg^{2+} block. Antonov and Johnson (1999) have demonstrated that taking this effect into account places the Mg^{2+} ion binding site at a much shallower position ($\delta = 0.47$) in the membrane electric field, which is, however, consistent with the predicted position of two asparagine residues near the apex of the M2 loop of the NMDA receptor subunits that have been identified from structural modification of the NMDA receptor as crucial for Mg^{2+} block of the channel (see also Chapter 3).

The steep voltage dependence of channel block underlies the crucial role Mg^{2+} block of NMDA channels plays in giving NMDA receptors the property of *coincidence detectors* in the nervous system. Calcium is able to flow through the channel and influence the mechanisms controlling synaptic strength only when there is coincident depolarization of the neurone to relieve the Mg^{2+} block. This property can, in principle, allow networks of neurones to adapt their behavior according to experience and hence, in effect, allows the nervous system to "learn" from experience. A simulation of the effect of Mg^{2+} block on the steady-state current through NMDA receptor channels is illustrated in Figure 6.7d. It can be seen that the linear relationship between membrane potential and NMDA receptor current becomes steeply voltage-dependent with increasing Mg^{2+} concentration. At physiological levels of Mg^{2+} (1 mM) the current through the channels increases between –80 mV and –20 mV as the Mg^{2+} block is decreased by depolarization. It is important to appreciate that this type of effect will also happen to a greater or lesser extent with any drug that acts to block ion channels and makes predicting the action of channel blocking drugs, particularly on the nervous system, extremely complicated. For example, ketamine, an anesthetic; PCP, a powerful psychoactive drug of abuse; and memantine, used to treat Alzheimer's disease, all act to block the NMDA receptor channel. The main difference between these drugs is their dwell time in the channel. With memantine, this time scale is milliseconds; with ketamine, seconds; and with PCP, tens of seconds (Lipton, 2006).

Figure 6.8 shows a diagrammatic representation of the energy barriers that a channel blocking drug might be supposed to overcome to reach its binding site within the channel. This diagram allows

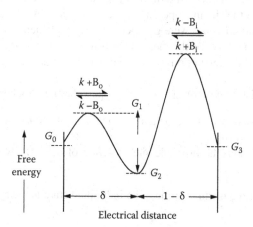

FIGURE 6.8 Diagrammatic representation of a two-energy barrier model. A model that can be used to describe the energy barriers a channel blocking drug might be supposed to overcome to reach its binding site within the channel. The barriers are shown as symmetrical in this case, although they need not necessarily be so. This diagram allows for the possibility that the blocking drug could actually permeate the channel after binding rather than returning to the same side of the membrane it had originally come from. This generalized mechanism can be used to describe channel block from either side of the membrane, ease of access to the binding site being dependent on the height of the energy barriers that the drug has to cross. The free energy G is shown relative to that outside the membrane. The transition rates k_{+Bo}, k_{-Bo}, k_{+Bi}, k_{-Bi} will depend on both the height of the energy barrier and the membrane potential and can be calculated as described by Hille (1992). (Adapted from Figure 5, Chapter 14 of Hille, 1992, *Ionic Channels of Excitable Membranes*, Sinauer, MA.)

for the possibility that the blocking drug could actually permeate the channel after binding rather than returning after dissociation to the same side it had originally come from. This generalized mechanism can be used to describe channel block from either side of the membrane, access to the binding site being dependent on the height of the energy barriers that the drug molecule has to cross. More generally, Figure 6.8 helps to illustrate the idea that the difference between permeation of an ion through the channel and block of the channel may be one of degree and not necessarily a reflection of any fundamental difference in the way a permeant ion or blocker interacts with the channel protein.

6.4 CONCLUDING REMARKS

The material in this chapter has centered on the effects of drugs at receptors in the ligand-gated ion channel class. In particular, the aim has been to emphasize that a quantitative treatment of some simple mechanisms can allow experimentally testable predictions to be made for the effects of a drug and estimates of the affinity of a drug for its binding site/sites on the receptor. Insofar as quantifying the interactions of drugs with their receptors is at the heart of advances in the development of selective drugs and the classification of receptors, this approach is likely to continue to be an essential part of pharmacology. This is particularly so for studies in the central nervous system where a bewildering array of receptor subtypes await the development of subtype-selective drugs in order that the functional and therapeutic significance of this receptor diversity can be determined.

PROBLEMS

PROBLEM 6.1

An experiment in which single AChR ion channel currents were recorded at a membrane potential of −60 mV showed that the duration of individual channel openings followed a single exponential distribution. The mean open time was 5.0 ms. When the experiment was repeated in the presence of an antagonist, drug B, in a concentration of 10μM, it was found that the mean open time was reduced to 2.5 ms, and that the channel openings were interrupted by brief shut periods with a mean duration of 1.0 ms such that openings were grouped into bursts. When the experiment was repeated at a membrane potential of −120 mV the mean open time was 10 ms in the absence of drug B but only 2 ms in its presence; the interruptions of the channel openings had become longer, lasting 2 ms on average at −120 mV.

These results are consistent with drug B being an open channel blocker.

(a) Calculate the microscopic association and dissociation rate constants and equilibrium constant for the action of drug B.
(b) What can you say about the probable site of action of drug B given that the drug has a single positive charge?

Hint: The reciprocal of the mean lifetime of an individual state is the sum of the rates (in s⁻¹) for *leaving* that state.

PROBLEM 6.2

With endplate nicotinic receptors it has been found that, as well as activating the receptor, acetylcholine (ACh) blocks the ion channel. A possible mechanism to describe this situation (assuming for simplicity only a single agonist binding is required to activate the receptor) might therefore be:

$$A + R \underset{k_{-1}}{\overset{k_{+1}}{\rightleftharpoons}} AR \underset{k_{-2}}{\overset{k_{+2}}{\rightleftharpoons}} AR^* + A \underset{k_{-3}}{\overset{k_{+3}}{\rightleftharpoons}} ARA \tag{6.52}$$

$$\text{closed} \qquad \text{closed} \qquad \text{open} \qquad \qquad \text{blocked}$$

TABLE 6.1
Data for Problem 6.2

[ACh]	τ_o	τ_b	p_{open}
300µM	0.2ms	0.04ms	0.5
800µM	0.1ms	0.04ms	0.4

(a) Stating any assumptions you need to make, derive an expression for the equilibrium occupancy of the AR* state (p_{AR*}) in Equation (6.52).
(b) Write down expressions for the mean open time (τ_o) and mean duration of the blocked state (τ_b).

Hint: The mean lifetime of any state is equal to the reciprocal of the sum of the rates for leaving that state.

In experiments designed to test the mechanism in scheme (1), two high concentrations of ACh (300 µM and 800 µM) were tested in single channel recording experiments and the mean open time τ_o, mean closed time τ_b, and the channel open probability (p_{open}) measured. The results were as follows:

(c) Using a plot of $1/\tau_o$ versus [ACh], calculate k_{-2} and k_{+3}. In addition, calculate k_{-3} from the duration of the blockages (τ_b), and hence calculate the equilibrium constant (K_3) for block of the channel by ACh.

In other experiments values of 10^7 M^{-1} s^{-1}, 10^4 s^{-1} and 10^4 s^{-1} were found for k_{+1}, k_{-1} and k_{+2}.

(d) Using the expression you derived in (a), calculate the p_{AR*} you would expect at 300 µM and 800 µM ACh. How does this compare with the experimentally observed p_{open} given in Table 6.1? Suggest reasons why the calculated and observed p_{open} might be different.

PROBLEM 6.3

A simple mechanism for competitive antagonism of a ligand-gated ion channel receptor would be as follows:

$$BR \underset{k_{+B}}{\overset{k_{-B}}{\rightleftharpoons}} B+R+A \underset{k_{-A}}{\overset{k_{+A}}{\rightleftharpoons}} AR \qquad (6.53)$$

(a) Derive an expression for the equilibrium occupancy of state AR given the concentration of antagonist [B] and agonist [A] and their microscopic rate constants for association and dissociation with the receptor.

In an experiment designed to measure k_{-B} and k_{+B} the agonist was applied at a concentration of 100 µM (the equilibrium constant for the agonist is known to be 11 µM). Then, a step change in the antagonist concentration was made from zero to [B] and back to zero again. On application of the antagonist the response was observed to decline ("relax") exponentially toward a steady-state level of block with time constant τ_{on}.

If it is assumed that equilibrium with the agonist is much faster than equilibrium with the antagonist, then the relaxation time constants, τ_{on}, can be shown for scheme 1 to be described by

TABLE 6.2
Data for Problem 6.3

[B]	τ_{on}	% block at equilibrium
7.5µM	0.4s	62%
20µM	0.2s	83%
45uM	0.1s	95%

the equation:

$$\tau_{on} = \frac{1}{p_{free}k_{+B}[B] + k_{-B}} \tag{6.54}$$

where p_{free} is the fraction of receptors in state R before the antagonist is applied.

The antagonist was tested at three concentrations, and the results are shown in Table 6.2:

(b) Calculate the microscopic rate constants k_{+B} and k_{-B} and hence the equilibrium constant K_B. Using these and the equation you derived in part (a), calculate the percent block expected at equilibrium for each of the antagonist concentrations used. How well do these calculated values agree with those observed experimentally?

Suggest possible reasons why the calculated equilibrium block might not agree with that observed experimentally. Describe what a single channel recording of the receptor activity would look like at equilibrium in the presence of the agonist alone and in the presence of agonist plus antagonist.

SOLUTIONS TO PROBLEMS

PROBLEM 6.1

Notice that the question states that the distribution of open times is a single exponential. This tells you that a mechanism containing a single open state of the receptor can describe the data. Using the above hint, the channel closing rate (call this α) is therefore the reciprocal of the mean open time. Thus at −60 mV $\alpha = 1/5$ ms or 200 s^{-1} and at −120 mV $\alpha = 1/10$ ms or 100 s^{-1}. This indicates that the channel closing conformational change is affected by the electric field across the membrane.

In the presence of drug B, the mean duration of the blockages (assuming a single blocked state) will be the reciprocal of the rate for leaving the blocked state (k_{-B} say). Thus at −60 mV $k_{-B} = 1/1.0$ ms or 1000 s^{-1} and at −120 mV $k_{-B} = 1/2.0$ ms or 500 s^{-1}. Apparently the rate of dissociation of drug B from the channel is slowed when the membrane potential is made more negative. For a positively charged drug this is a common finding and suggests the drug is binding within the membrane electric field. However, it could also be that the change in membrane potential has altered the receptor protein conformation and so affected the binding of the drug to the receptor.

To calculate the microscopic association rate for drug B, use the hint above to show that the mean open time in the presence of drug B will be equal to $1/(\alpha + [B]k_{+B})$. Thus the reciprocal of the mean open time in the presence of drug B will be equal to $(\alpha + [B]k_{+B})$ and so $(\alpha + [B]k_{+B}) = 400$ s^{-1} at −60 mV and 500 s^{-1} at −120 mV. α was 200 s^{-1} at −60 mV and 100 s^{-1} at −120 mV so $[B]k_{+B} = 200$ s^{-1} at −60 mV and 400 s^{-1} at −120 mV. Dividing these numbers by the [B] gives $k_{+B} = 2 \times 10^7$ M^{-1}s^{-1} at −60 mV and 4×10^7 M^{-1}s^{-1} at −120 mV.

The equilibrium constant is therefore 50 µM at −60 mV and 12.5 µM at −120 mV.

If the voltage dependence of k_{+B} is described by Equation (6.49), then a plot of $\ln(k_{+B}(V))$ versus membrane potential (V) will be a straight line of slope $-\delta zF/RT$. In this case, the slope of this plot is -11.6 V^{-1} and the reciprocal of this indicates an e-fold increase in k_{+B} for every 0.086V hyperpolarization (86 mV) of the membrane potential. At room temperature (293K) F/RT = 39.6 V^{-1}, so for a drug with a single positive charge, $\delta = 11.6/39.6 = 0.29$, suggesting that when at its binding site the drug has passed through 29% of the membrane electric field (note that this is probably not the same as 29% of the distance across the membrane since the membrane electric field is unlikely to fall linearly across the channel protein).

Notice that in this example the slope of the relationship between membrane potential and $\ln(k_{-B})$ is equal in magnitude, but opposite in sign to that for k_{+B} and $\delta = 0.58$ for the voltage dependence of K_B as expected if the blocker traverses a symmetrical energy barrier (Figure 6.8) when exiting from the channel as when blocking the channel. A voltage dependence for k_{-B} of the same *sign* as for k_{+B} would suggest that unblocking occurred by permeation of the blocker to the other side of the channel. A difference between the magnitudes of δ for k_{+B} and k_{-B} could mean that the energy barrier for access to and exit from the channel is not symmetrical or it could mean that the drug partly permeates the channel and partly exits back to the outside of the membrane.

PROBLEM 6.2

(a) Assume the system is at equilibrium and the Law of Mass Action holds. Use the procedures described in Chapter 1 to derive an expression for p_{AR*} at equilibrium. At equilibrium, the forward and backward rates for each reaction in the mechanism must be equal. The forward and backward rates are defined using the Law of Mass Action.

$$p_R[A]k_{+1} = p_{AR}k_{-1}, \quad p_{AR}k_{+2} = p_{AR*}k_{-2}, \quad p_{AR*}[A]k_{+3} = p_{ARA}k_{-3} \tag{6.55}$$

Each expression is re-arranged to give an expression in p_{AR*}

$$p_{AR} = \frac{k_{-2}}{k_{+2}}p_{AR*}, \quad p_R = \frac{k_{-1}}{k_{+1}[A]}\frac{k_{-2}}{k_{+2}}p_{AR*}, \quad p_{ARA} = \frac{k_{+3}[A]}{k_{-3}}p_{AR*} \tag{6.56}$$

The proportions of the receptor in each state must add up to 1.

$$p_R + p_{AR} + p_{AR*} + p_{ARA} = 1 \tag{6.57}$$

Substituting into this equation and then rearranging the result gives the desired expression.

$$p_{AR*} = \frac{[A]}{\dfrac{k_{-1}k_{-2}}{k_{+1}k_{+2}} + [A]\left(1 + \dfrac{k_{-2}}{k_{+2}} + \dfrac{[A]k_{+3}}{k_{-3}}\right)} \tag{6.58}$$

(b)

$$\tau_o = \frac{1}{k_{-2} + [A]k_{+3}}, \quad \tau_b = \frac{1}{k_{-3}} \tag{6.59}$$

(c) $1/\tau_o = 5000$ s^{-1} when [ACh] = 300 µM and $1/\tau_o = 10000$ s^{-1} when [ACh] = 800 µM.

From the answer to (b) we know that $1/\tau_o = (k_{-2} + [A]k_{+3})$. This has the form of a straight line of slope k_{+3} and intercept k_{-2} when $1/\tau_o$ is plotted against [A]. Thus, k_{+3} = slope = (10,000 – 5000 s^{-1})/(800 – 300 µM) = 10^7 M^{-1}s^{-1}. The intercept = k_{-2} = 2000 s^{-1}. The dissociation rate for the blocker,

$k_{-3} = 1/40$ μs = 25,000 s^{-1}. The equilibrium constant for block of the channel is therefore $K_3 = k_{-3}/k_{+3} =$ 2.5 mM.

(d) Substituting into Equation (6.56) allows the equilibrium occupancy of AR* to be calculated at 300 μM and 800 μM ACh. The results are 0.503 and 0.565, respectively. Therefore, at 300 μM, the calculated p_{AR*} is close to that observed experimentally. However at 800 μM, the calculated p_{AR*} is higher than observed.

Reasons: Possibly desensitization is affecting the p_{open} at higher [A]. In addition, the mechanism used to derive Equation (6.58) may not be correct (as would be the case if a desensitized state must be added to the mechanism).

PROBLEM 6.3

(a) The derivation of an expression for p_{AR} in the presence of the antagonist, B, is achieved using standard procedures. The result is given in Equation (6.60).

$$p_{AR} = \frac{[A]}{[A] + \dfrac{k_{-A}}{k_{+A}}\left(1 + \dfrac{[B]k_{+B}}{k_{-B}}\right)}$$

(6.60)

(b) A plot of the reciprocal of τ_{on} versus [B] will be a straight line of slope $p_{free}k_{+B}$ and y-axis intercept k_{-B}. Using the data in the table the slope is found to be 2×10^5 M^{-1}s^{-1} and intercept 1 s^{-1}. p_{free} is 1-p_{AR} in the absence of antagonist. Thus $p_{free} = K_A/([A]+K_A) = 0.1$. As $p_{free}k_{+B} =$ slope, k_{+B} = slope/$p_{free} = 2 \times 10^6$ M^{-1}s^{-1}. The equilibrium constant $K_B = k_{-B}/k_{+B} = 0.5 \times 10^{-6}$ M. Finally, calculate p_{AR} in the absence of antagonist and then in the presence of each [B] and then use these to calculate the percentage block produced at equilibrium by each antagonist concentration. When [A] = 100 μM, K_A = 11 μM, p_{AR} = 0.9 in the absence of antagonist and with K_B = 0.5 μM and [B] = 7.5 μM, p_{AR} = 0.36. %Block = (0.9 – 0.36)/0.9 × 100 = 60%. When [B] = 20 μM, p_{AR} = 0.191 and %Block = 79%. When [B] = 45 μM, p_{AR} = 0.098 and %Block = 89%.

The calculated values for %Block are close to those observed at low blocker concentrations, but at higher concentrations, the observed block is greater than predicted. Possible reasons for this may lie in the measurement of the onset time constants, in the assumption about the agonist equilibrating much faster than the antagonist, or the mechanism may be wrong perhaps because the receptor has more than one binding site, or binding of the antagonist promotes desensitization of the receptor.

FURTHER READING

TEXTBOOKS WITH RELEVANT MATERIAL

Hille, B. (2001). *Ionic channels of excitable membranes*, 3rd ed. Sinauer, MA. (In-depth chapters on ion channel permeation and block.)

Ogden, D. C. (1994). *Microelectrode techniques: The Plymouth workshop handbook*, 2nd ed. The Company of Biologists Ltd, Cambridge, UK. (Excellent discussion of both methods and principles.)

Sakmann, B., and Neher, E. (1995). *Single channel recording*. 2nd Ed. Plenum Press, NY. (Many good articles that discuss methods and principles.)

ORIGINAL PAPERS

Antonov, S. M., and Johnson, J. W. (1999). Permeant ion regulation of N-methyl-D-aspartate receptor channel block by Mg^{++}. *Proc. Natl. Acad. Sci.* 96, 14571–14576.

Ascher, P., and Nowak, L. (1988). The role of divalent cations in the N-methyl-D-aspartate responses of mouse central neurones in culture. *J. Physiol.* 399, 247–266.

Colquhoun, D. (1986). On the principles of postsynaptic action of neuromuscular blocking agents. In *New neuromuscular blocking agents,* Ed. Kharkevich, D. A. Springer-Verlag. *Handbuch Exp. Pharm.* Volume 79.

Colquhoun, D., Dreyer, F., and Sheridan, R. E. (1979). The actions of tubocurarine at the frog neuromuscular junction. *J. Physiol.* 293, 247–284.

Colquhoun, D., and Hawkes, A. G. (1982). On the stochastic properties of bursts of single ion channel openings and of clusters of bursts. *Phil. Trans. Roy. Soc. Lond.* 300, 1–59.

Colquhoun, D., and Sakmann, B. (1985). Fast events in single-channel currents activated by acetylcholine and its analogues at the frog muscle end-plate. *J. Physiol.* 369, 501–557.

Colquhoun, D., and Ogden, D. C. (1988). Activation of ion channels in the frog end-plate by high concentrations of acetylcholine. *J. Physiol.* 395, 131–159.

del Castillo, J., and Katz, B. (1957). Interaction at endplate receptors between different choline derivatives. *Proc. Roy. Soc Lond.* B. 146, 369–381.

Edmonds, B., Gibb, A. J., and Colquhoun, D. (1995). Mechanisms of activation of muscle nicotinic acetylcholine receptors and the time course of endplate currents. *Ann. Rev. Physiol.* 57, 469–493.

Katz, B., and Thesleff, S. (1957). A study of the "desensitization" produced by acetylcholine at the motor end-plate. *J. Physiol.* 138, 63–80.

Lipton, S. (2006). Paradigm shift in neuroprotection by NMDA receptor blockade: Memantine and beyond. *Nature Reviews Drug Discovery* 5, 160–170.

Neher, E. (1983). The charge carried by single-channel currents of rat cultured muscle cells in the presence of local anaesthetics. *J. Physiol.* 339, 663–678. (Describes deviations from simple channel blocking mechanism.)

Neher, E., and Sakmann, B. (1976). Single-channel currents recorded from membrane of denervated frog muscle fibres. *Nature* 260, 799–802.

Rang, H. P., and Ritter, J. M. (1970). On the mechanism of desensitization at cholinergic receptors. *Molecular Pharmacology* 6, 357–382.

Triggle, D. J. (1980). Desensitization. *Trends in Pharmacological Sciences* 14, 395–398.

Unwin, N. (2005). Refined structure of the nicotinic acetylcholine receptor at 4A resolution. *J Mol Biol.* 346: 967–989.

Wyllie, D. J. A., and Chen, P. E. (2007). Taking the time to study competitive antagonism. *Br. J. Pharmacol.* 150: 541–551.

7 G-Proteins

David A. Brown

CONTENTS

G-proteins are trimeric, signal-transducing, guanine nucleotide-binding proteins. They constitute the first step in transducing the agonist-induced activation of a G-protein coupled receptor (GPCR) (see Chapter 2) to a cellular response.

7.1 THE DISCOVERY OF G-PROTEINS

G-proteins were discovered as a result of some experiments by Martin Rodbell in 1971 on the stimulation of adenylate cyclase by glucagon, in which he found that the addition of guanosine triphosphate (GTP) was necessary to drive the reaction. Using terminology derived from cybernetic information theory, he envisaged a guanine nucleotide regulatory protein, then called an *N* (nucleotide-binding)-*protein*, acting as an intermediary transducer between the *discriminator* (receptor) and *amplifier* (effector; i.e., adenylate cyclase) (Figure 7.1). He subsequently found that adenylate cyclase was activated strongly and irreversibly by a GTP analog, 5′-guanylylimidophosphate [or Gpp(NH)-p]. Because Gpp(NH)-p is resistant to hydrolysis, Rodbell suggested that GTP is "hydrolyzed at the activation site"; that is, the transducer acts as a GTPase. This was subsequently shown directly by Cassell and Selinger in 1976. The presence of a separate GTP-binding protein, distinct from the adenylate cyclase enzyme, was established by Alfred Gilman and colleagues who were able to reconstitute Gpp(NH)-p-stimulated adenylate cyclase activity in membranes from a mutant lymphoma cell line (*cyc–*) that contained adenylate cyclase but lacked the G-protein by adding a separately purified 40-kDa GTP-binding factor.

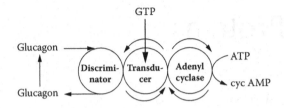

FIGURE 7.1   Martin Rodbell's conception of the role of the G-protein transducer in the activation of adeny-late cyclase by glucagon. (From Birnbaumer, L., *FASEB J.*, 4, 3178, 1990. With permission.)

In 1980, Howlett and Gilman reported that persistent activation of this cyclase-stimulating G-protein (G_s) led to a decrease in the molecular mass of the protein, implying that the G-protein was made up of dissociable subunits. The trimeric nature of G-proteins was then established by Stryer and colleagues. Using the photoreceptor G-protein transducin (G_t), they showed that activation of G_t by Gpp(NH)-p and light led to the dissociation of the trimeric αβγ complex into Gpp(NH)-p-bound $α_t$ and βγ, and that $α_t$ was responsible for phosphodiesterase stimulation. In 1985, α-transducin was cloned by four groups led by Numa, Bourne, Khorana, and Simon; the α subunit of G_s was cloned by Gilman's group in 1986. Rodbell and Gilman were jointly awarded the Nobel Prize in 1994.

7.2   STRUCTURE OF G-PROTEINS

G-proteins are made up of three subunits: an α subunit of molecular mass ~39–45 kDa, a β subunit (~37 kDa), and a smaller γ subunit (~8 kDa). Some 21 different gene products, from 16 genes, encode α subunits, 6 different β subunits (from 5 genes), and 12 different γ subunits (see below). In their native trimeric state, the G-proteins are attached to the inner face of the cell membrane through lipophilic tails on the α and γ subunits (myristoyl and palmitoyl on the α, farnesyl or geranylgera-nyl on the γ) (Figure 7.2). The β and γ subunits are enjoined rather firmly through a coiled–coil

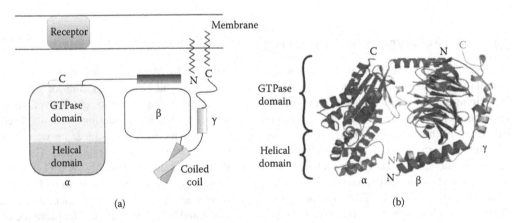

FIGURE 7.2   (a) Diagram to show G-protein α, β, and γ subunits attached to the outer cell membrane. (Adapted from Clapham, D. E., *Nature*, 379, 297, 1996.) (b) Ribbon model of $Gα_{t/i}$-GDP-$β_1γ_1$. (Adapted from Oldham, W. M., and Hamm, H. E., *Q. Rev. Biophys.*, 39, 117, 2006.) **(See color insert following page 116.)**

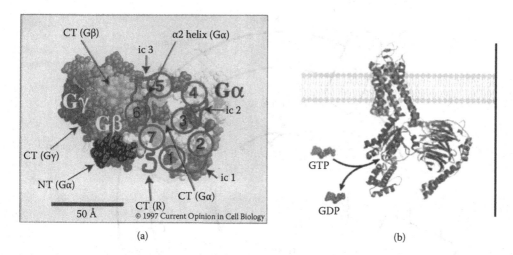

FIGURE 7.3 (a) Superposition of the seven transmembrane helices (numbered 1–7) of a GPCR on the outer surface of a G-protein. (Abbreviations: CT, C-terminus; NT, N-terminus; ic1, ic2, and ic3, first, second, and third intracellular loops of the GPCR.) (From Bourne, H. R., *Curr. Opin. Cell. Biol.*, 9, 134, 1997. With permission.) (b) Representation of the activated receptor–$G\alpha_o\beta\gamma$ complex created by manually docking the G-protein onto an activated receptor model based on the crystal structure of rhodopsin. (Adapted from Oldham, W. M., and Hamm, H. E., *Q. Rev. Biophys.*, 39, 117, 2006.) **(See color insert.)**

interaction to form a βγ-dimer; the β subunit of this dimer is then attached to the α subunit through complementary peptide-binding sites on the two proteins and through interaction of the lipophilic tails.

The α subunit has two other important functional domains in addition to the β-binding domain. First, it interacts with the receptor through a domain that includes the last five amino acids of the C-terminus (Figure 7.3). Second, it bears the guanine nucleotide binding pocket and is responsible for the GTPase activity of the G-protein. On the other hand, both α and βγ subunits can interact with the effector.

Extensive information regarding the three-dimensional structure of a number of G-proteins and their subunits is given in Oldham and Hamm, 2006, in the "Further Reading" section at the end of the chapter.

7.3 G-PROTEIN CYCLE

The cycle of events following receptor activation is summarized in Figure 7.4. The sequence is as follows:

1. In the ground state, the G-protein exists in the trimeric (αβγ) form, with guanosine diphosphate (GDP) bound at the nucleotide-binding site of the α subunit. It is close to (and may be precoupled to) the receptor (see *Note 1* below). On average, there are more G-proteins than receptors, so one might envisage a single receptor surrounded by a ring of nearby G-proteins, providing for multiple sequential receptor–G-protein interactions.

2. The agonist induces a rapid (≤1 msec) conformational change in the receptor, resulting in a realignment and opening up of the transmembrane helices, probably through rotation of helix 6 and separation of helices 3, 6, and 7.

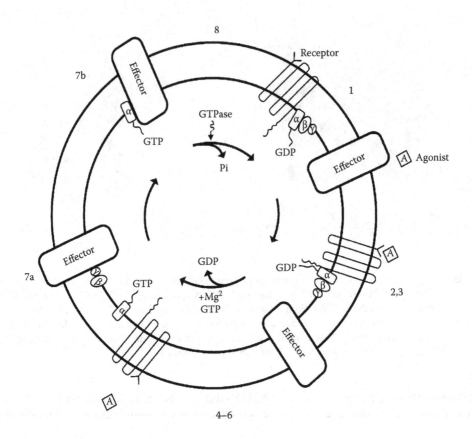

FIGURE 7.4 Diagram of G-protein cycle with activation of the effector by either the β_γ subunit (7a) or the GTP-bound α subunit. (See text for letters.) (Adapted from Neer, E. J. and Clapham, D. E., *Nature*, 333, 129, 1988.)

3. The inner face of the activated receptor binds to the C-terminus of the G-protein α subunit (see Figure 7.3). Inner loop 3 (ic3) between transmembrane helices 5 and 6 of the receptor plays a critical role in this interaction. Note, however, that although the α subunit bears the primary binding site for the receptor, attachment of the $\beta\gamma$-dimer to the α subunit is essential for this interaction to occur. This may require dimerization of the receptor (see *Note 2* below). Activation of the receptor increases its affinity for the G-protein some 50–100-fold; thus, the K_D for transducin binding to rhodospin falls from 64 nM in the dark to <1nM on light-activation.

4. Binding of the receptor induces a rapid conformational change (switch) in the G-protein trimer. This is transmitted to the nucleotide binding site, about 3 nm away, and results in a dissociation of bound GDP.

5. The GDP is replaced at the nucleotide-binding site by guanosine triphosphate (GTP), which is present in a three- to fourfold excess (50–300 μM) in the cytosol.

6. Binding of GTP promotes a disordering of the carboxyl- and amino-termini of the G-protein α subunit. As a result, the GTP-bound α subunit dissociates from the receptor. In addition, the $\beta\gamma$-dimer may dissociate from the α-subunit, releasing free Gα-GTP and free G$\beta\gamma$ (see *Note 3* below). The conformation of G$\beta\gamma$ is not changed on dissociation from the α subunit.

7. Either G$\beta\gamma$ (7a) or Gα-GTP (7b) (or sometimes both) interacts with the effector molecule to activate or inhibit it (see below for examples). This activation is persistent until reversed by Step 8.

8. The terminal (γ) phosphate of GTP is hydrolyzed by the GTPase activity of the G-protein α subunit, leaving GDP bound instead. This reverses the conformational change in Step 5 and allows the α subunit to dissociate from the effector and reassociate with the βγ subunit. The reassociation will also reverse βγ-effector interaction because Gα-GDP effectively competes with the effector for βγ-binding. Though of fairly high affinity (e.g., K_D ~ 50 nM for GIRK [G-protein-activated inwardly rectifying K$^+$ channel] activation) and persistent in the absence of competing Gα-GDP, βγ-effector binding is not irreversible.

The effect of receptor stimulation is thus to catalyze a reaction cycle. This leads to considerable amplification of the initial signal. For example, in the process of visual excitation, the photoisomerization of one rhodopsin molecule leads to the activation of approximately 500 to 1000 transducin (G$_t$) molecules, each of which in turn catalyzes the hydrolysis of many hundreds of cyclic guanosine monophosphate (cGMP) molecules by phosphodiesterase. Amplification in the adenylate cyclase cascade is less but still substantial; each ligand-bound β-adrenoceptor activates approximately 10 to 20 G$_s$ molecules, each of which in turn catalyzes the production of hundreds of cyclic adenosine monophosphate (cAMP) molecules by adenylate cyclase.

The duration of receptor-mediated responses depends, in the first instance, on the rate of the GTPase reaction of the α subunit. In solution, these rates are rather slow (time-constants, 10–60 sec), far too slow to account for the off-rate of many GPCR-induced effects. For example, retinal light responses and cardiac responses to vagal stimulation last less than a second. However, in the intact cell, the GTPase reaction is accelerated 10- to 100-fold by GTPase-activating proteins (GAPs). In some cases, the effector itself acts as a GAP; for example, phospholipase C accelerates the GTPase activity of the G-protein Gα$_q$. However, the principal GAPs are the family of RGS (regulators of G-protein signaling) proteins; these are discussed further below. Normally (but with the exception of cGMP phosphodiesterase), all three components of the system—receptor, G-protein, and effector—are in the plasma membrane and remain there during all of the steps in the cycle.

7.3.1 Notes to the Cycle

1. There is some evidence for a degree of preassociation between some receptors at least and their cognate G-proteins, either by direct interaction or maintained through *scaffolding proteins* (see Gales et al., 2006).
2. There is accumulating evidence that many (if not most) receptors exist as dimers, even if homomeric. This may be necessary for steric reasons to form an appropriate binding to the G-protein trimer. It is envisaged that one monomer attaches to the α-subunit C-terminal and the other to the βγ-subunit (see Oldham and Hamm, 2006).
3. Transducin clearly dissociates into Gα and Gβγ subunits, as depicted in Figure 7.4. However, the α- and βγ-subunits of some other G-proteins appear to remain associated after receptor activation (see Bunemann et al., 2003; Gales et al., 2006).

7.4 PERTURBING THE G-PROTEIN CYCLE

The G-protein cycle can be perturbed in several ways:

1. Reversal of the cycle depends on hydrolysis of the γ-phosphate of GTP. This is prevented if a nonhydrolyzable or slowly hydrolyzable analog of GTP is substituted, for example, Gpp(NH)-p or guanosine 5′-O-(3-thiotriphosphate) (GTPγS), or by adding AlF$_4$, which forms a third "pseudo" phosphate on GDP in Gα-GDP (Figure 7.5). Under these conditions, effector activation becomes virtually irreversible following brief activation of the receptor (see Figure 7.6 for an example). The effect of receptor activation is essentially

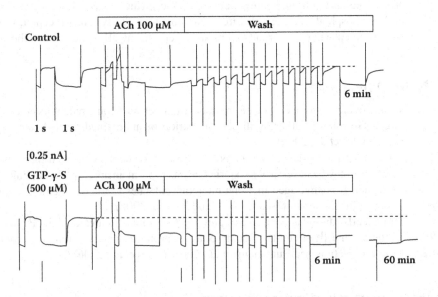

FIGURE 7.5 Some guanosine nucleotides and derivatives. Abbreviations: GDP, guanosine diphosphate; GTP, guanosine triphosphate; GTPγS, guanosine 5′-O-(3-thiotriphosphate); Gpp(NH)-p, 5′-guanylylimido-phosphate; AlF$_4$, aluminum fluoride.

FIGURE 7.6 Irreversible effect of a GTPγS-bound G-protein α subunit. Records show the inhibition of a potassium current in M$_1$ muscarinic acetylcholine-receptor-expressing neuroblastoma hybrid cells by acetyl-choline. The potassium current was recorded as a sustained outward current at a holding potential of −30 mV (dashed line) and was deactivated for 1 sec every 30 sec by hyperpolarizing the cell to −60 mV. In the control cell (upper trace), a brief application of 100 μM acetylcholine (ACh) temporarily inhibited the potassium cur-rent, but this recovered about 6 min after removing acetylcholine from the bathing fluid. However, in another cell patched with an electrode containing 500 μM GTPγS (lower trace), the effect of acetylcholine persisted after washout; indeed, the current continued to decline over the next hour, probably reflecting the slow turn-over of the G-protein cycle in the absence of GPCR activation. Note that this effect of acetylcholine is probably mediated by Gα$_q$. (Adapted from Robbins, J. et al., *J. Physiol.*, 469, 153, 1993.)

PTx
|
∨

α_s — L R Q Y E L L

$\alpha_t, \alpha_{i1,2}$ — L K D $\boxed{C}$ G L F

α_{i3} — L K E $\boxed{C}$ G L Y

$\alpha_{o1,2}$ — L R G $\boxed{C}$ G L Y

α_z — L K Y I G L C

$\alpha_{q,11}$ — L K E Y N L V

α_{12} — L K D I M L Q

α_{13} — L K Q L M L E

α_{14} — L R E F N L V

$\alpha_{15,16}$ — L D E L N L L

FIGURE 7.7   C-terminal residues of G-protein α subunits. The cysteine ADP-ribosylated by Pertussis toxin (PTx) is boxed.

to catalyze the G-protein cycle, accelerating it 100- or 1000-fold. However, even in the absence of receptor activation by a ligand, a slow basal cycling sometimes occurs. This may be due to the fact that a small proportion of receptors exist in the "active" conformation, even in the absence of ligand, as expected from the two-state model of receptors (see Chapter 1). [Rhodopsin is exceptional in this regard, in having a very low (10^{-5}) proportion in the active state in the dark.] As a result, substitution of Gpp(NH)-p or GTPγS for GTP or the addition of AlF$_4$ can itself induce an effector response in the absence of a receptor ligand and, indeed, these techniques were used for this purpose in early experiments on adenylate cyclase; however, onset is much slower than that seen for coaddition of ligand.

2. The cycle may be slowed by adding an excess of GDP or, more commonly, guanosine 5'-O-(2-thiodiphosphate) (GDPβS), a more stable analog. Unlike GTPγS, GDPβS is not bound irreversibly and so only competes with GTP; hence, it is only effective when present in a large (10-fold) excess.

3. In the presence of nicotinamide adonine dinucleotide (NAD$^+$), the G-protein α subunit can be adenosine diphospate (ADP)-ribosylated by two bacterial proteins. *Pertussis* (whooping cough) toxin (PTx) ADP-ribosylates a cysteine residue in the C-terminus of G-proteins of the G$_i$ and G$_o$ group (Figure 7.7; see below). As a result it prevents receptor–G-protein coupling and blocks responses to GPCR activation. *N*-ethyl-maleimide (NEM) alkylates cysteines and has the same effect. *Cholera* toxin (CTx) ADP-ribosylates an arginine in G-proteins of the G$_s$ (adenylate cyclase–stimulating) class, near the catalytic site of the GTPase domain; consequently, it blocks GTPase activity and produces persistent G$_s$/adenylate cyclase activation. Transducin and gustducin (the visual and taste-transducing G-proteins; see below) are ADP-ribosylated by both toxins. This reaction has been very helpful in isolating and purifying G-proteins that can be ADP-ribosylated.

7.5   EXPERIMENTAL EVIDENCE FOR G-PROTEIN COUPLING IN RECEPTOR ACTION

7.5.1   GTP DEPENDENCE

A G-protein-mediated effect has an absolute requirement for GTP. Reference has already been made to the requirement for GTP in reconstituting hormone-stimulated adenylate cyclase activity. A similar requirement can be demonstrated when the effector is an ion channel, such as the cardiac

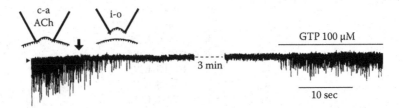

FIGURE 7.8 Requirement for GTP in the activation of inwardly rectifying potassium channels in guinea-pig atrial cell membranes by acetylcholine. The recording started when a pipette containing acetylcholine was attached to an intact atrial cell (c-a). This produced sustained opening of up to three potassium channels (recorded as inward current deflections at −60 mV because the pipette contained 145 mM K+). On excision of the membrane patch in inside-out mode (i-o) into the bathing solution (containing 140 mM [K+]), the activity stopped but was resurrected by adding 100 µM GTP to the solution, bathing the inner face of the membrane patch. (Adapted from Kurachi, Y. et al., *Am. J. Physiol.*, 251, H681, 1986.)

atrial inward-rectifier K+ channel, which is activated following stimulation of the M_2 muscarinic acetylcholine receptor. Thus, in the experiment illustrated in Figure 7.8, the channel recorded with a cell-attached patch pipette from an intact atrial cell is tonically activated when acetylcholine (or adenosine) is present in the patch pipette. This activity is lost when the patch is excised (in inside-out configuration) but is then restored on adding GTP to the solution bathing the inside face of the patch.

Even in the absence of an effector, the linkage of an activated receptor to a G-protein can be detected in a receptor-binding assay by the so-called GTP-shift. The apparent affinity of the agonist (but *not* the antagonist), measured either directly or by displacement of antagonist with agonist, is reduced on adding GTP (or a stable analog, such as GTPγS or even GDP) to the solution (Figure 7.9). This is because a trimeric G-protein, with the guanine nucleotide binding site unoccupied, forms a stable complex with the activated receptor such as to slow the dissociation of agonist. The agonist then has a high affinity for the receptor. The addition of nucleotide breaks this complex to form

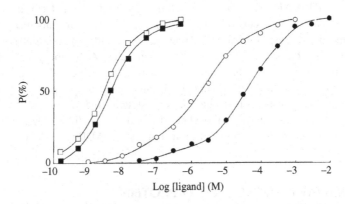

FIGURE 7.9 The GTP shift of agonist binding to a GPCR. Graphs show the binding of carbachol (circles) and atropine (squares) to rat heart homogenates in the absence (open symbols) and presence (closed symbols) of 1 mM GTP. Axes: receptor occupancy (P) and log-molar concentration of ligand. (Adapted from Hulme, E. C. et al., in *Drug Receptors and Their Effectors*, Birdsall, N. J. M., Ed., Macmillan, New York, 1981, p. 23.)

a dissociated GDP-bound trimer or GTP-bound α subunit; the agonist can then dissociate more rapidly from the receptor, conferring low affinity.

7.5.2 Use of GTP Analogs and Toxins

Stable analogs of GTP and GDP can be used to study the role of the G-protein, as indicated above. Thus, stable GTP analogs enhance agonist-induced receptor-mediated effects and slow their reversal, as shown in Figure 7.6. *Pertussis* and *Cholera* toxins can also be used to inhibit or activate certain G-proteins, as indicated.

7.6 MEASUREMENT OF G-PROTEIN ACTIVATION

The most direct way of measuring activation by a receptor is to measure the rate of hydrolysis of GTP in a broken cell or membrane preparation following receptor activation. Unfortunately, this is not always very easy in practice because of the high background rate (reflecting the basal activity of all the G-proteins in the membrane plus other enzymatic reactions), which may mask the response of the particular G-protein activated by the receptor, and because some G-proteins such as G_s have a slow GTPase rate in such preparations. The method works best for members of the G_o/G_i family, which are abundant, high-turnover G-proteins. An alternative and widely used method is to measure the rate of GTPγS binding, which does not depend on GTPase activity, only on the rate of G-protein activation and GDP dissociation.

Methods for measuring fluorescence changes during G-protein activation have also been described. For example, interactions in the cell membrane can be observed using a technique called fluorescence resonance energy transfer (FRET). This involves labeling the receptor and G-protein with two different fluorophores, for example, cyan and yellow jellyfish fluorescent proteins, CFP and YFP. On illumination at ~440 nm, these two emit light at different peak wavelengths (480 and 535 nm, respectively). When the two fluorophores approach to within a few nanometers of each other, energy is transferred from the donor CFP to YFP, so YFP emission is increased and there is a measurable shift in emission wavelength. (See Bunemann et al., 2003, in "Further Reading" for applications of this method.) BRET (bioluminescence resonance energy transfer) is a variant using a naturally luminescent protein such as luciferase or aequorin, which do not need excitation (see Gales et al., 2006, in "Further Reading" for an example of BRET). Though difficult to quantify, these methods have the advantage of good time-resolution, as well as allowing interactions of receptors and G-proteins to be studied in their native environment.

7.7 TYPES OF G-PROTEIN

Traditionally, G-proteins have been classified in terms of the effector coupling of the α subunit. In spite of the facts that (1) this predates information on primary and secondary structure from cloning work, and (2) the $\beta\gamma$ subunits are also involved in effector coupling, this classification is still quite useful.

The first G-protein α subunit to be identified was G_s. The α subunit of G_s (α_s) is responsible for stimulating adenylate cyclase (hence, the s-subscript) and is ADP-ribosylated and activated by CTx. G_s has at least four molecular variants. Some evidence exists that α_s can also enhance the activity of cardiac L-type Ca^{2+} channels, independently of their phosphorylation by cAMP-stimulated protein kinase A. G_{olf} is a cyclase-stimulating homolog in the olfactory epithelium, activated by the large family of olfactory receptors.

G_i is the G-protein responsible for inhibiting adenylate cyclase. The inhibition is mediated by the α subunit. Unlike G_s, G_i is not affected by CTx but instead is ADP-ribosylated (and inhibited) by PTx. Of the three isoforms of G_i (G_{i1-3}), α_{i1} is the most potent inhibitor of cyclase. G_i also activates inward-rectifier (Kir3.1/3.2 and Kir3.1/3.4) K^+ channels (GIRK channels); this activation is mediated by the $G\beta\gamma$ subunits (see below).

G_o was isolated as an "other" PTx-ribosylated G-protein that copurifies with G_i but does not inhibit adenylate cyclase. There are two main isoforms (G_{o1} and G_{o2}), with additional splice variants. G_o is particularly abundant in the nervous system, comprising up to 1% of membrane proteins. Its main function is to reduce the opening probability of those voltage-gated Ca^{2+} channels (N- and P/Q-type) involved in neurotransmitter release. Hence, it is largely responsible for the widespread auto-inhibition of transmitter secretion by presynaptic receptors. This effect is also mediated by $\beta\gamma$-subunits.

G_t (transducin) is the retinal G-protein responsible (through the α subunit) for stimulating phosphodiesterase (PDE) following light activation of rhodopsin. There are two subtypes, in rods and cones, respectively. G_{gust} (gustducin) is a PDE-stimulating homolog in tongue tastebuds involved in bitter-taste reception. Activation of G_{gust} also stimulates phospholipase C (PLC), possibly via the $\beta\gamma$ subunits. G_t and G_{gust} are ADP-ribosylated by both PTx and CTx.

G_q and G_{11} are two closely related and widely distributed G-proteins whose α subunits stimulate PLC. They are not ADP-ribosylated by either PTx or CTx, so they are probably responsible for many instances of PTx-insensitive PLC stimulation. G_{14} and G_{15} are two more distantly related PTx-insensitive G-proteins that can stimulate PLC. G_{12} and G_{13} are other PTx-insensitive G-proteins related to G_q, while G_z is more closely related to G_i; the precise functions of these G-proteins are not yet clear. Though of restricted distribution (to hemopoietic-derived cells), G_{16} is interesting because it lacks receptor specificity and so acts as a universal PLC transducer.

7.8 RECEPTOR–G-PROTEIN COUPLING

The interaction between the receptor and the G-protein is transient and rapidly reversible. This is indicated, for example, by the fact that a single light-activated rhodopsin molecule may activate 500 to 1000 transducin molecules during its 1 to 3 sec lifetime. Hence, the interaction should, in the endpoint, be governed by the normal laws of chemical interaction and expressible in terms of association and dissociation rate constants and binding affinity. The question then arises as to whether the affinity of different receptors for different G-proteins varies. That is, is there specificity in receptor–G-protein coupling, and, if so, what determines this?

Ideally, it might be thought that this question could best be approached by measuring the activation of individual recombinant G-protein trimers (using GTPase reactions, GTPγS binding, or fluorescence methods) by individual recombinant receptors (both in known concentrations) in artificial lipid membranes; however, this is a daunting task. Rubinstein and colleagues have accomplished a near-approach by measuring the GTPase activity of several recombinant α subunits reconstituted with purified β adrenoreceptors and purified bovine G-protein $\beta\gamma$ subunits in phospholipid vesicles. Using a single concentration (10 μM) of isoprenaline, with varying receptor concentrations, they found that the GDP/GTP exchange was stimulated most effectively using α_s, about one-third as effectively using α_{i1} or α_{i3}, one-tenth with α_{i2}, and negligibly with α_o. A more frequent approach is to assess the interaction of recombinant receptors with recombinant or endogenous G-proteins in cell lines, using GTPase measurements or GTPγS binding in membrane fractions or some downstream effector function as endpoints. This has yielded considerable information regarding what might best be termed *preferences* in regard to individual receptor–G-protein interactions and, through the use of point-mutations and chimeras, has been particularly useful in delineating some of the structural features of receptors and G-proteins that determine such preferences. From such work, it is clear that the major determinants are the C-terminal sequence of the α subunit, on the one hand (see Figure 7.3), and the third and second inner loops (i3, i2) of the receptor, on the other hand, although other domains of the α subunit and of the β and γ subunits are also involved in the overall interaction.

Such *reconstitutional* approaches suffer from two problems, however. First, the selectivity of receptor–G-protein coupling in their native cell environment depends not only on the relative affinities of the receptor for different G-proteins, but also on the relative proportions and availability of receptors and G-proteins. Thus, some examples of apparent "promiscuity" in receptor–G-protein coupling can undoubtedly be attributed to receptor overexpression. Second, the response of a G-protein to the receptor can be affected by ancillary factors: for example, the presence of particular RGS proteins (see Section 7.10.1) that may be cell specific. The question then arises as to how the receptor–G-protein coupling selectivity can best be deduced in the normal cell. Several approaches have been used. A simple one is to test whether the response to activating the receptor is prevented by PTx, thus defining the responsive G-protein as a member of the G_i/G_o family. If so, then this may be followed up by trying to "rescue" the response by applying or expressing individual exogenous α subunits in which the ADP-ribosylated cysteine is substituted by some other amino acid such as isoleucine. Another approach is to disrupt coupling to individual G-protein α subunits using antibodies directed against the C-terminal sequences or using competing short-peptide sequences. This will permit discrimination between, say, $G_{i1/2}$ and G_{i3} or G_o, between G_{oA} and G_{oB}, or between $G_{i/o}$ and $G_{q/11}$, but not between G_{i1} and G_{i2} or between G_q and G_{11}, because the C-terminal sequences for these pairs are the same (see Figure 7.7). Greater selectivity may be obtained by deleting individual G-protein subunits using gene knockouts or, more rapidly and less expensively (but less completely), by reducing protein expression with antisense constructs.

Two general points emerge from such work. First, different approaches do not always give concordant results. For example, antisense-depletion suggests that the activation of GIRK channels by the action of noradrenaline on α_2-adrenoceptors in native sympathetic neurons is mediated selectively by G_i-proteins, rather than G_o-proteins, but activation can be equally well rescued in PTx-treated cells by PTx-resistant forms of both α_o and α_i (Figure 7.10). Conversely, inhibition of the N-type Ca^{2+} current in these same cells by noradrenaline can be rescued after PTx treatment by PTx-resistant α_i even though antisense depletion suggests that inhibition is normally mediated by native G_o proteins, rather than G_i proteins. Thus, rescue experiments, like other expression approaches, tend to show what coupling pathways are possible and do not necessarily define what pathway normally operates. Second, and following from this, a rather surprising degree of specificity in receptor–G-protein coupling in native cells has emerged from some of the antisense-depletion studies, extending not only to closely related α subunits but also to associated β and γ subunits. For example, the inhibition of Ca^{2+} currents in GH_3 pituitary tumor cells by somatostatin appears to be preferentially mediated by the combination $\alpha_{o1}\beta_1\gamma_3$, whereas the very similar effect of acetylcholine, via muscarinic M_4 receptors, is most effectively obtunded by antisense depletion of $\alpha_{o1}\beta_3\gamma_4$. One reason for high *in situ* specificity not predictable from reconstitution experiments may be that in the normal cell, receptors and cognate G-proteins are not randomly distributed in the cell membrane but are colocalized in *microdomains*.

On the other hand, some receptors are truly "promiscuous" in that they can activate two or more G-proteins from quite different classes, even in their normal cellular environment. For example, similar concentrations of thyroid-stimulating hormone (TSH; 0.1–100 U/ml) can stimulate the incorporation of ^{32}P-GTP into α_i, α_o, α_{12}, α_{13}, α_s, and $\alpha_{q/11}$ through activation of the thyrotropin receptor in membranes from the human thyroid gland. TRH activation of Ca^{2+} currents in GH_3 cells is obtunded equally by antisense-depletion of α_{i2}, α_{i3}, and $\alpha_{q/11}$ but not of α_o. Some individual genotypic $P2_y$ nucleotide receptors can also couple with equal affinity to PTx-sensitive and PTx-insensitive G-proteins in sympathetic neurons. The degree, or otherwise, of such promiscuity is presumably determined by the structure of the receptor protein itself.

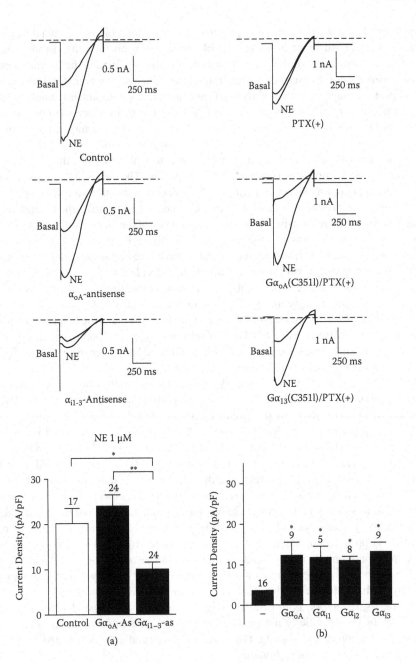

FIGURE 7.10 Contrasting information yielded by antisense depletion and α subunit reconstitution regarding the species of G-protein responsible for adrenergic inhibition of inward rectifier GIRK currents in rat sympathetic neurons. Records show inwardly rectifying GIRK currents generated in cells previously transfected with cDNAs coding for Kir3.1 and Kir.3.2 potassium channels by a voltage ramp from −140 to −40 mV, recorded in the absence (basal) and presence (NE) of 10 μM noradrenaline (norepinephrine). Note that in (a) the coexpression of antisense cDNA directed against $G\alpha_{oA}$ had no effect on the activation of current by noradrenaline, whereas coexpression of an antisense directed against the common coding sequences of $G\alpha_{i1-3}$ reduced the response to noradrenaline by about half (as shown in the bar chart below). In (b), a different approach was used, in which the native α subunit was inactivated with Pertussis toxin (PTx), thereby inhibiting the effect of noradrenaline (top panel), and an attempt was made to rescue the response by cotransfecting cDNAs coding for different α subunits mutated to remove the PTx-responsive cysteine (see Figure 7.7). In this case, the response was rescued to equal extents by all of the expressed α subunits. (Adapted from Fernandez-Fernandez J. M. et al., *Eur. J. Neurosci.*, 2001.)

TABLE 7.1
Some Principal Receptor–G-Protein Coupling Preferences

G-Protein	Receptors
G_s	β-Adrenoceptor; dopamine $D_{1,5}$; histamine H_2; 5-hydroxytryptamine $5HT_{4,6,7}$; glucagon; vasopressin V_2; VIP/PACAP (VPAC$_{1-3}$); prostanoid DP, IP; CRF$_{1,2}$; calcitonin/amylin/CGRP
G_i/G_o	α_2-Adrenoceptor; $M_{2/4}$ muscarinic acetylcholine; dopamine D_{2-4}; 5HT1; opioid δ, μ, κ, OFQ; somatostatin sst$_{1-5}$; GABA$_B$; mGlu$_{2-4}$; cannabinoid CB1,2
G_q/G_{11}	α_1-Adrenoceptor; $M_{1,3,5}$ muscarinic; histamine H_1; 5HT$_2$; mGlu$_{1,5}$; nucleotide P2$_Y$; vasopressin V_1; tachykinin NK$_{1-3}$; bradykinin B$_{1,2}$; neurotensin NTS$_{1,2}$; endothelin ET$_{1,2}$; TRH; cholecystokinin CCK$_2$; prostanoid FP, TP

Abbreviations: VIP, vasoactive intestinal peptide; PACAP, pituitary adenylate cyclase-activating peptide; VPAC, VIP and PACAP receptor; CRF, corticotrophin releasing factor; CGRP, calcitonin gene-related peptide; CB, cannabinoid receptor; TRH, thyrotropin-releasing hormone.

More interestingly, some evidence suggests that the degree of preference that one receptor shows for one or another G-protein may depend on the agonist used. Thus, activation of the *Drosophila* octopamine receptor expressed in Chinese hamster ovary (CHO) cells inhibits adenylate cyclase and raises intracellular Ca^{2+} through activation of two different G-proteins: PTx-sensitive and insensitive, respectively. Tyramine and octopamine have been shown to raise Ca^{2+} with similar potencies, but tyramine was considerably more potent in inhibiting cyclase than octopamine. This is in agreement with previous experiments showing that mutations of the highly conserved aspartate involved in amine agonist binding to nearly all receptors affect G-protein coupling in an agonist-dependent manner. One interpretation of this is that different agonists produce different active states of the receptor, or a different distribution of active states, with different affinities for various G-proteins; however, there is no direct information on whether or not ligand-occupied receptors can form multiple active states. Thus, light-activated rhodopsin goes through multiple conformational states before forming the active-state metarhodopsin-II, but none of the intermediate states has more than ~1/10,000th of the affinity of metarhodopsin-II for transducin.

Notwithstanding the various considerations and caveats regarding receptor–G-protein coupling specificity outlined above, and ignoring variations between coupling to different members of the same class of G-proteins, Table 7.1 may be helpful in providing a broad operational summary of the principal receptor–G-protein coupling preferences. More detailed information is provided in the "Further Reading" section (see Guderman et al., 1996; Wettschurek and Offermanns, 2005).

7.9 G-PROTEIN–EFFECTOR COUPLING

The *effector* in this sense is the direct target protein of the activated G-protein subunit(s). Although initially characterized in terms of effector activation by the GTP-bound α subunit, for example, of adenylate cyclase by α_s, it is now clear that the $\beta\gamma$-subunits also act as independent transducers (see Table 7.2). While allowance has to be made in intact systems for an indirect effect of G$\beta\gamma$ through binding to, and inactivation of, Gα-GTP, a direct interaction of G$\beta\gamma$ with the effector protein has been established for a wide range of effectors, including the β-adrenergic receptor kinase (βARK), adenylate cyclase, phospholipase C-β1,2,3, phosducin, GIRK (Kir3.1 + 3.2/3.4) K^+ channels, and N- and P/Q-type (CaV2.2 and 2.1) Ca^{2+} channels, and several of these complexes have been crystallized (see Oldham and Hamm, 2006). Binding to these effectors appears to be principally via a site

TABLE 7.2
Types of G-Protein

Subscript ($G_{subscript}$)	Toxin Sensitivity		Effectors	
	PTx	CTx	α Subunit	βγ Subunits
s	−	+	Adenylate cyclase ≠	βARK translocation; $I_{Ca(N)}$ ¬
olf	−	+	Adenylate cyclase ≠	—
t	+	+	Phosphodiesterase ≠	Phospholipase A_2 ≠
gust	+	+	Phosphodiesterase ≠	PLC ≠
i	+	−	Adenylate cyclase ¬	GIRK ≠
o	+	−	—	Ca(N, P, Q) ¬
z	−	−	—	Ca(N)¬, GIRK ≠
q	−	−	PLC ≠	PLC ≠
11	−	−	PLC ≠	—
12	−	−	?	—
13	−	−	?	—
14	−	−	PLC ≠	—
15	−	−	PLC ≠	—
16	−	−	PLC ≠	—

Abbreviations: VIP, vasoactive intestinal peptide; PACAP, pituitary adenylate cyclase-activating peptide; VPAC, VIP and PACAP receptor; CRF, corticotrophin releasing factor; CGRP, calcitonin gene-related peptide; CB, cannabinoid receptor; TRH, thyrotropin-releasing hormone.

on the β subunit that overlaps with the site through which βγ binds to the α subunit; hence, the α subunit acts as a competitor with the effector for βγ binding. Complementary binding sites for βγ on the C-terminus of βARK protein, on the I–II linker of the CaV2.2 (α_{1B}) Ca^{2+} channel (overlapping the binding site for the channel β subunit) and on both N- and C-termini of the GIRK channel have been identified. Some effectors are targets for both α and βγ subunits (e.g., PLCβ1–3; some adenylate cyclase isoforms). In these cases, the two subunits have independent and additive effects. Activation of these enzymes by βγ released from PTx-sensitive α subunits may account for the many instances of PTx-sensitive cyclase or PLC responses to receptor activation.

The question then arises as to how, in an unknown system, one can identify which subunit (α or βγ) carries the message. Two main approaches are available for identifying a βγ-mediated response: *replication* (and occlusion) by expressed or applied βγ subunits and *antagonism* by expressed or applied βγ-binding peptides such as a C-terminus peptide from βARK-1 or α-transducin, which, in essence, compete with the target for free βγ subunits. Positive identification of α-mediated effects is more difficult, because Gα antagonists such as PTx or C-terminus antibodies also prevent release of free Gβγ, and the effects resulting from antisense depletion of α subunits might be attributable to excess unbound Gβγ. Replication by GTPase-deficient α subunits in the absence of positive evidence for the involvement of βγ subunits can be useful.

As an example of dual α- and βγ-mediated effects, one might consider the inhibition of N-type Ca^{2+} currents in sympathetic neurons by acetylcholine (Figures 7.11 and 7.12; see also Hille, 1994). Acetylcholine inhibits these currents through two different muscarinic receptors (M_1 and M_4), using two different G-protein pathways.

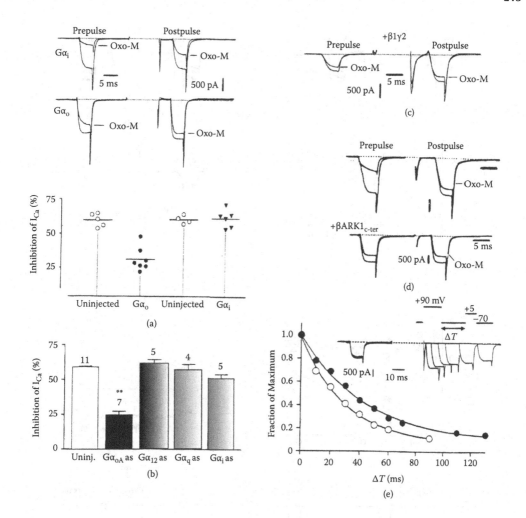

FIGURE 7.11 Experimental approaches to the identification of G-protein subunits responsible for the inhibition of calcium currents in rat sympathetic neurons on stimulating M_4 muscarinic acetylcholine receptors with the muscarinic agonist, oxotremorine-M (Oxo-M). The currents (evoked by 5-msec depolarizing steps to 0 mV from −60 mV) were recorded from dissociated ganglion cells patched with open-tip electrodes containing 20 mM BAPTA; this eliminates the component of inhibition produced by stimulating M_1 receptors. As shown in the upper left traces, Oxo-M produced ~60% inhibition of the current, which was transiently and partly reversed by a 10-msec depolarizing step to +90 mV. Preinjection of an antibody directed against the C-terminus of $G\alpha_o$, but not $G\alpha_{11}/2$, reduced the inhibition (a), suggesting that $G\alpha o$ was the receiving α subunit for this effect. This was confirmed and narrowed down to the $G\alpha_{oA}$ isoform by expressing antisense cDNA constructs to deplete individual α subunits (b). Overexpression of $\beta1\gamma2$ subunits (by cDNA transfection) also inhibited the current and occluded the action of Oxo-M (c), while overexpression of the C-terminal fragment of βARK-1 (which acts as a $\beta\gamma$-binding agent) prevented the voltage-dependent inhibition by Oxo-M (d), implying that inhibition was mediated by $\beta\gamma$ subunits freed from the activated G_{oA}-$\alpha\beta\gamma$ trimer. The freed $\beta\gamma$ subunits interact directly with the calcium channel in a voltage-dependent manner: Depolarization causes the dissociation of the subunits, which then reassociate with an average time-constant of 37 msec on repolarization (e; open circles); overexpression of βARK-1C-ter reduced the effective concentration of free $\beta\gamma$ subunits and lengthened the time-constant for reassociation to 51 msec. Note that noradrenaline, instead of Oxo-M, was used to inhibit the current in (e). (a through d: Adapted from Delmas, P. P. et al., *Eur. J. Neurosci.*, 10, 1654–1666, 1998. (e) Adapted from Delmas, P. P. et al., *J. Physiol.*, 506, 319–329, 1998.)

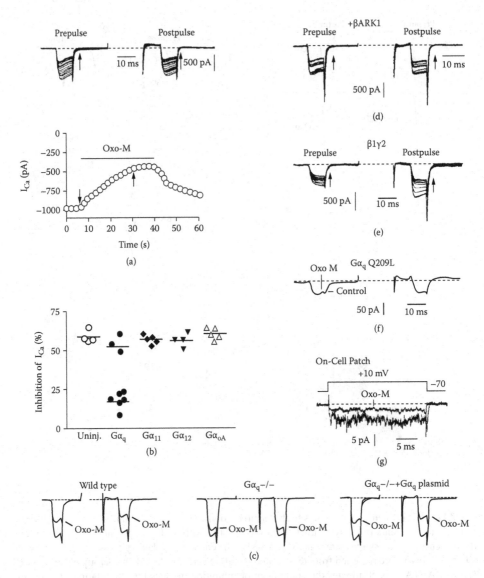

FIGURE 7.12 Experimental approaches to the identification of G-protein subunits responsible for the inhibition of calcium currents in rat sympathetic neurons on stimulating M_1 muscarinic acetylcholine receptors with the muscarinic agonist oxotremorine-M (Oxo-M). In these experiments, the $M_4/G_o/\beta\gamma$-mediated inhibition illustrated in Figure 7.11 has been blocked by prior treatment with *Pertussis* toxin, and the calcium currents were recorded using the perforated-patch variant of the patch-clamp method (which preserves normal cytoplasmic constituents). Under these conditions, oxotremorine-M produces a slowly developing inhibition that is not reversed by strong depolarization (a). This form of inhibition is not affected by expressing antisense to $G\alpha_{oA}$, but instead is selectively reduced by antisense depletion of $G\alpha_q$ (b). In confirmation of this, inhibition is strongly reduced in ganglion cells from transgenic mice deficient in $G\alpha_q$ ($G\alpha_q$ –/–), and inhibition is restored in these cells by expressing free $G\alpha_q$ (c). Unlike M_4-mediated inhibition (Figure 7.11), this form of inhibition is not affected by overexpressing the βARK-1 peptide (d) and persists after overexpressing free $\beta_{1\gamma2}$ subunits (e). Instead, the inhibition is replicated and occluded by overexpressing a GTPase-deficient α subunit of G_q (f), suggesting that it is mediated by the GTP-bound α_q subunit. This probably does not interact directly with the calcium channel but instead generates a signal remote from the channel (see text) so that full inhibition is seen when a cluster of channels is recorded with a cell-attached patch pipette and Oxo-M is added to the bathing solution in contact with the cell membrane outside the patch (g). (a, b, and d through g: Adapted from Delmas, P. P. et al., *Eur. J. Neurosci.*, 10, 1654–1666, 1998. (c) Adapted from Haley, J. et al., *J. Neurosci.*, 20, 3973–3979, 2000.)

Stimulation of M_4 receptors produces a rapid inhibition that is characterized by its voltage dependence. That is, the opening of the channels during a depolarizing voltage step is delayed (so the onset of the current is slowed), and this is temporarily reversed by a strong depolarizing prepulse (Figure 7.11a). Such an effect is prevented by PTx and is mediated by a member of the G_i/G_o family that can be narrowed down specifically to G_{oA}, as it is (1) antagonized by injecting an antibody to the C-terminal domain of $G\alpha_o$ but not to C-terminal $G\alpha_{11/2}$ (Figure 7.11a), and (2) reduced on expressing antisense RNA to $G\alpha_{oA}$ (Figure 7.11b). The final transducer is the $\beta\gamma$-dimer because (1) the effect of M_4 receptor stimulation is replicated and occluded by overexpression of a common $\beta\gamma$ combination ($\beta_1\gamma_2$; Figure 7.11c), and (2), the action of the agonist is prevented by overexpressing the C-terminal peptide domain of βARK-1, which binds and sequesters free $\beta\gamma$ subunits (Figure 7.11d). The small, residual voltage-independent inhibition probably results from an additional effect of the α_{oA}–GTP monomer. The effect of the $\beta\gamma$ subunits on these channels may be interpreted as follows. A "free" $\beta\gamma$ molecule binds directly to the channel protein at one or more sites, including a site on the I–II linker that contains a binding motif (QXXER) that corresponds to a similar motif in the βARK-1 peptide, hence the competition. This binding leads to a retardation in Ca^{2+} channel opening during a voltage step. Strong depolarization causes the temporary dissociation of this bound $\beta\gamma$ molecule and so reverses the inhibition. On repolarization, the dissociated $\beta\gamma$ molecule rebinds and inhibition is restored. Rebinding (reinhibition) follows an exponential time-course, the rate-constant of which is dependent on the concentration of available free $G\beta\gamma$ [$\beta\gamma$], according to the equation $k_{obs} = k_1[\beta\gamma] + k_2$, where k_1 and k_2 are the forward and backward rate constants for the reversible binding of one molecule of $\beta\gamma$ with one channel protein molecule (C): $C + \beta\gamma = C\beta\gamma$. Thus, the rate of reinhibition is accelerated by increasing the concentration of agonist or by applying increasing concentrations of $\beta\gamma$ and is slowed by reducing the amount of available $\beta\gamma$ using βARK-1 peptide (Figure 7.11e). Whereas only one molecule of $G\beta\gamma$ appears to bind to each Ca^{2+} channel molecule, inward rectifier K^+ channels, which are activated by $G\beta\gamma$, are made up of four separate subunits, each of which can bind one molecule of $G\beta\gamma$.

Stimulation of M_1 receptors produces a slower inhibition that is not voltage sensitive and that persists in the presence of PTx (Figure 7.12a). As expected from its resistance to PTx, this is not affected by antisense-depletion of α_{oA} but, instead, is reduced by antisense-depletion of α_q (Figure 7.12b) and is lost in neurons from $G\alpha_q$ knock-out mice (Figure 7.12c). Unlike the voltage-sensitive inhibition produced by stimulating M_4 receptors, it is not mediated by the $\beta\gamma$-subunits because (1) it is not affected by the βARK-1 peptide (Figure 7.12d), and (2) agonist inhibition persists after overexpressing free $\beta_1\gamma_2$ subunits (Figure 7.12e). Instead, the effect of the agonist is replicated and occluded by overexpressing a GTPase-deficient (and therefore permanently active, GTP-bound) form of $G\alpha_q$ (Figure 7.12f). This action of $G\alpha_q$-GTP is unlikely to result from a direct interaction of the α subunit with the Ca^{2+} channel but instead probably results from the $G\alpha_q$-activated PLC-stimulated hydrolysis and consequent membrane depletion of phosphatidylinositol-4,5-bisphosphate (PIP$_2$), which is required to maintain the Ca^{2+} channels in their open state (see Delmas et al., 2005). Since PIP$_2$ is freely mobile in most cell membranes, Ca^{2+} channel activity recorded in a patch pipette attached to the cell membrane can be inhibited by stimulating muscarinic receptors in the cell membrane outside the patch as PIP$_2$ is dragged away from the intrapatch channels down its concentration gradient to the rest of the membrane where PIP$_2$ has been hydrolyzed (Figure 7.12g; also see Section 7.11 below and Figure 7.18).

What is the functional significance of these different modes of Ca^{2+} current inhibition? The $\beta\gamma$-mediated inhibition by acetylcholine, or by other transmitters such as noradrenaline and γ-aminobutyric acid (GABA), and the consequential reduction of Ca^{2+} influx in nerve terminals probably provide an important component of the presynaptic autoinhibitory action of transmitters on their own release in both peripheral and central nervous systems, though other effects beyond the step of Ca^{2+} entry may also contribute to the reduced transmitter release. On the other hand, the more remote α-mediated inhibition appears to be restricted to the somatic membrane. Here, its main effect is to reduce the amount of Ca^{2+} available for opening Ca^{2+}-dependent K^+ channels; this enhances somatic excitability, allowing the neuron to fire longer and more rapid trains of action potentials during continuous or high-frequency excitation.

One problem that arises in connection with $\beta\gamma$-mediated responses is how the specificity of receptor–effector coupling is maintained. Thus, most $\beta\gamma$-mediated effects, on ion channels at least, are inhibited by PTx, implying that they result from activation of G_i or G_o. There are exceptions; for instance, $\beta\gamma$-mediated inhibition of Ca^{2+} currents and activation of GIRK currents in sympathetic neurons can also be induced by vasoactive intestinal peptide (VIP), acting through G_s. However, these are exceptions and, generally speaking, voltage-dependent Ca^{2+} current inhibition or GIRK activation in native cells is restricted to receptors that couple to PTx-sensitive G-proteins such as α_2-adrenoceptors or muscarinic M_2 or M_4 receptors. Adrenoceptors that couple through G_s or $G_{q/11}$ or muscarinic receptors that couple through $G_{q/11}$ do not normally induce these $\beta\gamma$-mediated effects. In contrast, while there are differences in relative affinity between different $\beta\gamma$ combinations, both GIRK channels and Ca^{2+} channels appear to respond to a wide variety of $\beta\gamma$ subunit combinations when directly applied or expressed, including those that normally associate with PTx-insensitive α subunits. Hence, specificity is clearly conferred by the α subunit. How this is translated to specificity of effector response is not yet clear.

7.10 REGULATION OF G-PROTEIN SIGNALING

7.10.1 RGS PROTEINS

RGS proteins are members of a large family of 20 or more loosely related proteins that have in common a 130-amino-acid RGS domain that allows them to bind to G-protein α subunits. (See Vries et al., 2000, and Willars, 2006.) The primary effect of this binding is to accelerate the hydrolysis of GTP by stimulating the GTPase activity of the α-subunit; that is, they act as GAPs. Hence, they accelerate recovery of the effector from activation by $G\alpha_{GTP}$ or by $G\beta\gamma$. They do not affect the rate of GDP–GTP exchange.

One predictable consequence of this is that the steady-state response of the effector to the agonist is also reduced, because the effective dissociation equilibrium constant for G-protein–effector interaction (K_{diss}) is determined by k_{off} / k_{on} x G^* (where G^* is the concentration of activated G-protein). However, they can also reduce binding of $G\alpha_{GTP}$ to the effector, probably by physically blocking the interaction. This may be independent of their GAP activity, as it can be seen when the α subunit is activated by nonhydrolyzable GTPγS. For example, the RGS protein RGS4 inhibits the response of PLC-β1 to GTPγS-activated G_q. This property has sometimes been exploited to assist in the identification of Gq-mediated events, by using RGS2 or 4 as Gq antagonists.

Figure 7.13a shows an example of the effects of an RGS protein on the activation of GIRK channels by stimulating M_2 muscarinic acetylcholine receptors with acetylcholine. This is the K^+ channel in the cardiac pacemaker cells that is opened by acetylcholine released following vagal stimulation and is responsible for the hyperpolarization and slowing of the pacemaker. However, when only GIRK channels and M_2 receptors are reconstituted in oocytes or mammalian noncardiac cells, the channels take several seconds to close down again after removing acetylcholine; whereas, in the heart, the current recovers in less than a second. As shown in Figure 7.13a, the off-rate for GIRK deactivation following acetylcholine removal in the reconstituted system is accelerated more than 10 times by coexpressing RGS4 and now matches the off-rate for the native atrial current.

Figure 7.13a illustrates another common effect of some RGS proteins—namely, that they can also accelerate the rate of G-protein activation. This is not predictable from their primary

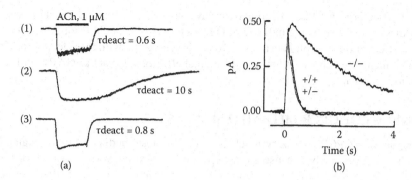

FIGURE 7.13 Role of RGS proteins in accelerating the offset of G-protein-mediated effects. (a) Inwardly rectifying GIRK potassium currents activated by stimulating M_2 muscarinic acetylcholine receptors with acetylcholine (ACh), recorded (1) from a rat atrial myocyte, (2) from a CHO cell cotransfected with the cardiac GIRK channels (Kir3.1 + Kir3.2) plus the M_2 receptor, and (3) from a CHO cell transfected as in (2) but also with RGS protein RGS4. Note that the response in the CHO cell (2) is slower to reach a steady state and much slower to deactivate compared to the atrial cell, but it replicates the response of the atrial cell following transfection of RGS4 (3). (b) Average single-photon responses of retinal rod photoreceptors taken from normal (+/+) mice and from heterozygote (+/−) and homozygote (−/−) RGS9 knock-out mice. The light flash was delivered at time = 0 seconds. (a: Adapted from Doupnik, C. et al., *Proc. Natl. Acad. Sci. USA*, 94, 10461–10466, 1997.) (b: Adapted from Chen C.-K. et al., *Nature*, 403, 557–560, 2000.)

GTPase-activating effect, and indeed appears to be a property of other domains than the RGS-GAP domain within the protein. Instead, it probably results from the ability of many RGS proteins to bind to the effector or the receptor, or both, and thereby to form a link in a G-protein–effector, or receptor–G-protein–effector, complex (see Abramovic-Newerly et al., 2006; Tinker, 2006). This may have the effect of bringing the G-protein and effector in closer proximity, thereby reducing the time required for effector activation.

The large number of RGS proteins have varying degrees of selectivity for different α subunits and varying effects on different effector systems (see Vries et al., 2000). These properties are usually assessed in reconstituted expression systems. However, it is clear that they play an important role in regulating G-protein signaling in native cells, even though experimentally they are more difficult to test. One interesting approach to this question makes use of the fact that coupling of RGS proteins to the α subunit can be disrupted by a point mutation in the α subunit without any other disruption to $G\alpha$ function. By combining such a mutation with another mutation to eliminate PTx sensitivity (see Figure 7.10), it has been established that an endogenous RGS protein is involved in the inhibition of Ca^{2+} currents in sympathetic neurons by noradrenaline-activated G_o, as replacement of the endogenous $G_{o\alpha}$ with the mutated $G_{o\alpha}$ has been shown to reduce the sensitivity to noradrenaline by about 10-fold and to slow the rate of onset and recovery of inhibition. However, even this involves a degree of reconstitution, with the consequent problems addressed earlier. An alternative approach is genetic deletion. Thus, there is a dramatic (greater than 10-fold) slowing of the recovery of the photoresponse of isolated retinal rods in knock-out mice deficient in the retina-specific RGS protein RGS9 (Figure 7.13b).

7.10.2 EFFECTORS AS GTPASE-ACTIVATING PROTEINS

Some enzyme effectors also act as GAPs, accelerating the hydrolysis of GTP and hence promoting the rapid turnoff of the G-protein-activated enzyme itself. For example, the GTPase activity of pure $G\alpha_q$-GTP is very slow (10 to 60 sec) when measured in solution but is increased 50-fold on adding its effector target PLC-β1, to a more physiological half-life of 1 sec. Likewise, addition of phosphodiesterase shortens the half-life of GTP-bound α-transducin from 20 sec to 5 sec. This accelerating effect of the phosphodiesterase effector is synergistic with the effect of the visual RGS protein RGS9 mentioned above. Whether ion-channel effectors also act as GAPs in the absence of RGS proteins is unclear.

7.11   KINETICS OF GPCR-MEDIATED SIGNALS

Effects mediated by GPCRs are very much slower than those mediated by, for example, ligand-gated ion channels, primarily because more steps are involved between activation of the receptor and the final response. For example, even in a simple, three-step, G-protein-mediated effect, such as the opening of atrial GIRK channels following the activation of M_2 muscarinic receptors by acetyl-choline, which follows the scheme:

$$ACh + R \rightarrow R\text{-}ACh + G\alpha\beta\gamma \rightarrow [\alpha_{GTP}] + \beta\gamma + GIRK_{closed} \rightarrow \beta\gamma\text{-}GIRK_{open}$$

the minimum latency to the development of the GIRK current and consequent membrane hyper-polarization, following a pulse-application of acetylcholine, is about 30 msec (Figure 7.14). This contrasts with the <1-msec latency of the opening of nicotinic channels following application of

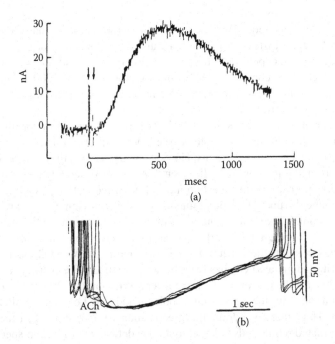

FIGURE 7.14   Time-course of G-protein-mediated activation of GIRK potassium channels in rabbit sino-atrial node cells. (a) Outward current evoked by a 33-msec, 50-nA iontophoretic pulse of acetylcholine (between arrows). (b) Response of the unclamped cell to an iontophoretic pulse of acetylcholine (ACh). (a: Adapted from Trautwein, W. et al., in *Drug Receptors and Their Effectors*, Birdsall, N. J. M., Ed., Macmillan, New York, 1980, pp. 5–22.) (b: Adapted from Noma, A., in *Electrophysiology of Single Cardiac Cells*, Noble, D., and Powell, T., Eds., Academic Press, San Diego, CA, 1987, pp. 223–246.)

acetylcholine to muscle endplate nicotinic receptors. By analogy with the response of rhodopsin to a flash of light, it is likely that the initial binding of acetylcholine to the muscarinic receptor and subsequent conformational change take no more than a millisecond or so; the extra time is required for the diffusion and docking of the activated receptor to the G-protein, the exchange of GTP for GDP, and dissociation of the G-protein, as well as the diffusion and docking of the βγ subunits with the potassium channel. Following its peak, the current then declines over a period of several hundreds of milliseconds; this is determined by the rate of GTP hydrolysis and consequent dissociation of the α subunit from the effector or recapture of the βγ subunit from the effector by the newly formed GDP-bound α subunit. As indicated above, RGS proteins play a major role in accelerating both the onset and offset of muscarinic activation of GIRK channels (see Figure 7.13a above).

The effect of stimulation of cardiac adrenoceptors is even more leisurely because several more steps follow activation of the G_s protein by the β-adrenoceptor. For example, to increase the force of cardiac contraction, we have (1) activation of adenylate cyclase by $G\alpha_s$-GTP, (2) formation of cAMP, (3) activation of protein kinase A by the cAMP, then (4) phosphorylation of the calcium channel protein by the kinase. As a result, it takes about 5 to 6 sec from the time the receptors are activated to the first increase in calcium current amplitude (Figure 7.15a). Most of this time is taken

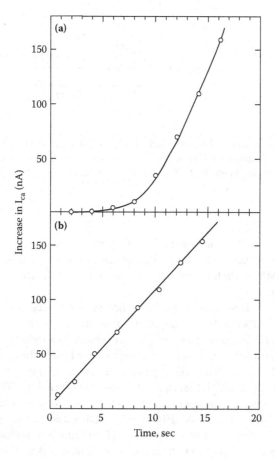

FIGURE 7.15 Time-course of the increases in amplitude of the calcium current recorded from bullfrog atrial trabeculae following (a) rapid application of the β-adrenoceptor agonist isoprenaline (3 μM), and (b) rapid intracellular release of cAMP by flash-photolysis of *o*-nitrobenzyl cAMP. Applications/flashes were made at time zero. (Adapted from Nargeot, J. et al., *Proc. Natl. Acad. Sci. USA*, 80, 2395–2399, 1983.)

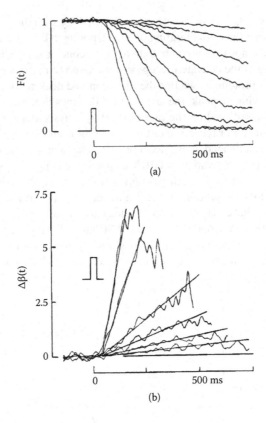

FIGURE 7.16   (a) Photocurrents of salamander rod cells following light flashes giving between 10 and 2000 rhodopsin molecule isomerizations. (b) Calculated increments in phosphodiesterase hydrolytic rate constant. (Adapted from Lamb, T. D., and Pugh, Jr., E. N., *Trends Neurosci.*, 15, 291–299, 1992.)

up with the steps leading to the generation of a sufficient amount of cAMP (adenylate cyclase is a relatively slow-acting enzyme), as the latency is reduced to around 150 msec on applying a concentration jump of cAMP by flash photolysis of an intracellularly accumulated photolabile cAMP precursor (Figure 7.15b).

However, latency alone is not a good guide to the number of steps in the G-protein-mediated cascade; geometry and packing density are also important. Thus, the (almost) equally complex cascade reaction involved in the response of photoreceptors to a light flash (in which rhodopsin activates the G-protein transducin, which in turn activates phosphodiesterase, which reduces the concentration of cGMP and so shuts cGMP-gated cation channels) is very fast, with a minimum latency of around 10 msec at the highest intensity flashes (Figure 7.16). The reason for this is the very high density of receptors, G-proteins, and phosphodiesterase in the rod discs. Also, phosphodiesterase has a much higher (substrate-diffusion-limited) turnover rate than adenylate cyclase. As a rule of thumb, the usual ratio of receptors to G-proteins to ion-channel effectors is probably around 1:10:0.1; because most ion channels seem to have a density of around 1 per square micrometer, this gives about 10 receptors and about 100 G-proteins per square micrometer. In contrast, there are about 2500 transducin molecules and about 167 effector (phosphodiesterase) molecules per square micrometer of rod disc membrane. Conversely, even the direct activation,

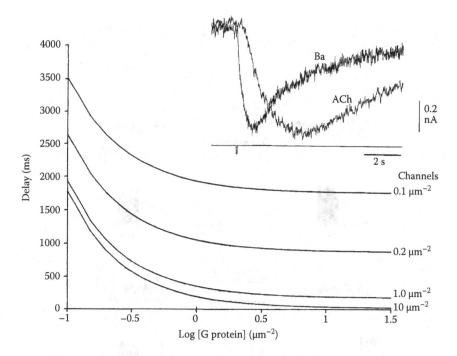

FIGURE 7.17 Calculated latency (delay) between activation of a muscarinic acetylcholine receptor and the closure of a potassium M-channel plotted against the membrane density of G-proteins (in logarithmic units) for different potassium channel densities. It is assumed (for simplicity) that the activated GTP-bound α subunit interacts directly with the potassium channel. Calculations were based on Lamb and Pugh (1992), with the following diffusion coefficients: receptor, 0.7 μm/sec; G$\alpha\beta\gamma$, 1.2 μm/sec; Gα, 1.5 μm/sec; channel, 0.4 μm/sec. Inset: Observed latencies to current inhibition at 35°C in a neuroblastoma hybrid cell expressing M_1 muscarinic acetylcholine receptors following 100-msec pressure application of barium ions (Ba, which directly plugs the channels) and acetylcholine (ACh). The mean latency difference (ACh–Ba) was ~272 msec. At estimated channel and G-protein densities of 1 and 25/μm^2, the direct-hit G-protein–channel interaction would predict a latency of ~180 msec. (Adapted from Robbins, J. et al., *J. Physiol.*, 469, 153–178, 1993; additional unpublished material from J. Robbins.)

or inhibition, of an ion channel might be very slow at low densities of channels and G-proteins (Figure 7.17).

For ion-channel effectors, Figure 7.8 and Figure 7.12 illustrate another way of deciding whether the activated G-protein subunits interact directly with the channel or indirectly through a cascade reaction leading to a cytoplasmic messenger, using the patch-clamp technique shown; the GIRK potassium channels recorded in a cell-attached patch in Figure 7.8 are activated by acetylcholine in the patch pipette but not on adding acetylcholine to the bathing solution outside the patch, implying a local effect of the receptor-activated G-protein on the channel. In contrast, the calcium channels in Figure 7.12 are closed by adding a muscarinic receptor agonist to the extrapatch membrane via the bathing solution, implying that some diffusible messenger system connecting receptors and channels—in this case, the movement of PIP_2 away from the channels as PIP_2 is depleted from the rest of the cell membrane. Another example of such a remote signaling pathway between a muscarinic receptor-activated G-proteins and another type of potassium channel (the M or Kv7.1/7.2 channel), resulting from a similar (channel PIP_2-depletion) mechanism, is illustrated in Figure 7.18.

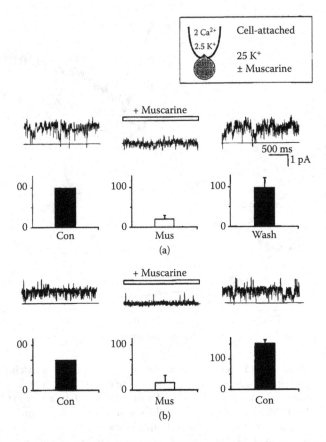

FIGURE 7.18 An example of remote G-protein–effector interaction. Records show M-type potassium channel activity recorded from rat sympathetic neurons in cell-attached patch pipettes held at ~0 mV. Activity is suppressed when the muscarinic acetylcholine receptor agonist muscarine (10 μM) is applied to the cell membrane outside the patch electrode. (The bathing solution contained 25 mM [K⁺] to set the membrane potential at EK (~–30 mV) and prevent depolarization by muscarine.) The fact that muscarine cannot diffuse through the tight seal between the pipette glass and the membrane (and diffusion of an activated G-protein through the membrane to a channel inside the electrode patch would be very slow) implies that some diffusible substance is produced to carry the message from activated receptors and G-proteins outside the patch to the channel inside the patch. The record and bar chart in (b) were obtained using patch pipettes already filled with muscarine solution. In spite of this, channels were active and could still be closed by adding muscarine to the extrapatch membrane. This suggests that channels could not be closed by a local (direct) interaction of the activated G-protein with the channel (also, that not enough receptors were present in the patched membrane to generate a sufficient amount of messenger to close the channels). (Adapted from Selyanko et al., *Proc. Roy. Soc. London* Ser. B, 250, 119–125, 1992.)

This process of receptor-catalyzed PIP$_2$ depletion has been analyzed in some detail in relation to Kv7.1/7.2 inhibition (see Figure 7.19 and Suh et al., 2004). The loss of PIP$_2$ is surprisingly extensive and surprisingly fast (>90% in < 5 seconds); the response of the channel lags behind the fall in PIP$_2$ because of the alinear relation between PIP$_2$ concentration and channel open probability. The inward current produced by acetylcholine in neuroblastoma cells illustrated in the inset to Figure 7.17 probably involves a similar mechanism (closure of Kv7.1/7.2 potassium channels) and shows comparably fast kinetics.

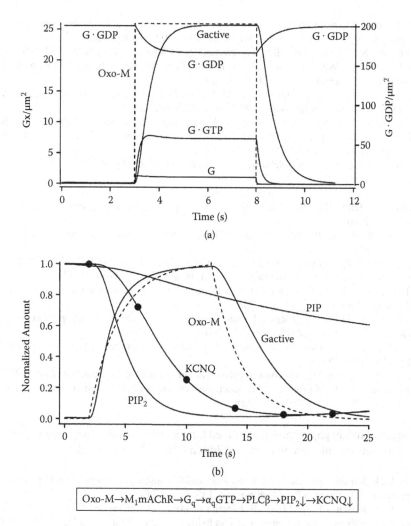

FIGURE 7.19 (a) Calculated time-course of changes in G_q-status following activation of M_1-muscarinic receptors by a stepped-concentration of the muscarinic agonist oxotremorine-M. (b) Calculated changes in downstream effects of G_q activation leading to closure of KCNQ2/3 (Kv7.2/7.3) potassium channels by a rapid bath-application of oxotremorine-M. The pathway is shown below. PLCβ = phospholipase-Cβ; PIP and PIP_2 are phosphatidylinositol-4-phosphate and phosphatidylinositol-4,5-bisphosphate, respectively; KCNQ is the current carried by KCNQ2/3 potassium channels (the channels close as a result of the fall in PIP_2). Points simulate experimental findings. Derived from experiments on human embryonic kidney (HEK) cells express-ing M_1 acetylcholine receptors and KCNQ2+KCNQ3 potassium channel subunits. (Adapted from Suh, B. C. et al., *J Gen Physiol* 123, 663, 2004, *q.v.* for further details.)

FURTHER READING

Abramow-Newerly, M., Roy, A.A., Nunn, C., and Chidiac, P. RGS proteins have a signalling complex: Interactions between RGS proteins and GPCRs, effectors, and auxiliary proteins. *Cellular Signalling* 18: 579–591, 2006.

Birnbaumer, L. Transduction of receptor signal into modulation of effector activity by G-proteins: The first 20 years or so. *FASEB J.*, 4, 3068–3078, 1990.

Bourne, H.R. How receptors talk to trimeric G-proteins. *Curr Opin Cell Biol.* 9, 134–142, 1997.

Bunemann, M., Frank, M., and Lohse, M.J. Gi protein activation in intact cells involves subunit rearrangement rather than dissociation. *Proc Natl Acad Sci USA*. 100, 16077–16082, 2003.

Clapham, D.E., and Neer, E. G-protein βγ subunits. *Annu Rev Pharmacol Toxicol*. 37, 167–203, 1997.

De Waard, M., Hering, J., Weiss, N., and Feltz A. How do G proteins directly control neuronal Ca^{2+} channel function? *Trends Pharmacol Sci*. 26:427–436, 2005.

Delmas, P., Coste, B., Gamper, N., and Shapiro, M.S. Phosphoinositide lipid second messengers: New paradigms for calcium channel modulation. *Neuron*. 47:179–182, 2005.

Galés, C., Van Durm, J.J.J., Schaak, S., Pontier, S., Percherancier, Y., Audet, M., Paris, H., and Bouvier, M. Probing the activation-promoted structural rearrangements in preassembled receptor-G protein complexes. *Nat Struct Mol Biol*. 13:778–786, 2006.

Gudermann, T., Kalkbrenner, F., and Schultz, G. Diversity and selectivity of receptor–G-protein interaction. *Annu Rev Pharmacol Toxicol*. 36, 429–459, 1996.

Lamb, T.D., and Pugh, Jr., E.N. G-protein cascades: Gains and kinetics. *Trends Neurosci*. 15, 291–299, 1992.

Oldham, W.M., and Hamm H.E. Structural basis of function in heterotrimeric G proteins. *Quart Rev Biophys*. 39, 117–166, 2006.

Rodbell, M. The role of hormone receptors and GTP-regulatory proteins in membrane transduction. *Nature*. 284, 17–22, 1974.

Suh, B.C., Horowitz, L.F., Hirdes, W., Mackie, K., and Hille, B. Regulation of KCNQ2/KCNQ3 current by G protein cycling: The kinetics of receptor-mediated signaling by G$_q$. *J Gen Physiol*. 123: 663–683, 2004.

Tinker, A. The selective interactions and functions of regulators of G-protein signalling. *Seminars in Cell & Developmental Biology*. 17: 377–382, 2006.

Vries, L.D., Zheng, B., Fischer, T., Elenko, E., and Farquhar, M. The regulator of G-protein signaling family. *Annu Rev Pharmacol Toxicol*. 40, 235–271, 2000.

Wettschureck, N., and Offermanns, S. Mammalian G proteins and their cell type specific functions. *Physiol Rev*. 85, 1159–1204, 2005.

Wickman, K.D., and Clapham, D.E. G-protein regulation of ion channels. *Curr Opin Neurobiol*. 5, 278–285, 1995.

Willars, G.B. Mammalian RGS proteins: Multifunctional regulators of cellular signalling. *Seminars in Cell & Developmental Biology*. 17: 363–369, 2006.

The following two recent papers provide detailed kinetic information concerning the events linking activation of M1-muscarinic receptors and inhibition of Kv7.2/7.3 channels:

Falkenburger, B.H., Jensen, J.B., and Hille, B. Kinetics of M1-muscarinic receptor and G-protein signaling to phospholipase C in living cells. *J Gen Physiol*. 135: 81–97, 2010.

Falkenburger, B.H., Jensen, J.B., and Hille, B. Kinetics of PIP2 metabolism and KCNQ2/3 channel regulation studied with a voltage-sensitive phosphatase in living cells. *J Gen Physiol*. 135: 99–114, 2010.

8 Signal Transduction through Protein Tyrosine Kinases

IJsbrand Kramer and Elisabeth Genot

CONTENTS

8.1 PHOSPHORYLATION AS A SWITCH IN CELLULAR FUNCTIONING

Phosphorylation of protein was discovered in the era of *allosteric regulation.* Regulation of enzyme activity could be explained by the concentration of substrates, the presence of cofactors, and the concentration of the end product (allosteric effectors). One of the pathways thus analyzed was the glycolysis pathway. The first step in this pathway is the conversion of glycogen to glucose-1-phosphate that is mediated by an enzyme called glycogen phosphorylase. Enzyme activity was found to be regulated through allosteric interactions by adenosine 5'-monophosphate (stimulatory) and glucose-6-phosphate (inhibitory). Glycogen phosphorylase could be isolated in two forms: an active form, designated with an *a*, and a less active form, designated with a *b*. In 1956 Krebs and Fischer discovered that phosphorylase *b* could incorporate one organic phosphate molecule on a serine residue, a process that accompanies an increase in its activity. Through the incorporation of a phosphate, phosphorylase *b* obtained the characteristics of phosphorylase *a*, being less sensitive to the inhibitory action of glucose-6-phosphate and more sensitive to the stimulatory action of adenosin 5'-monophospate. Thus, apart from allosteric regulation, a covalent modification such as phosphorylation could also affect enzyme activity. The phosphorylation is catalyzed by a protein kinase, phosphorylase kinase. Later it was discovered that a phosphorylase phosphatase catalyzed dephosphorylation, and this brings the enzyme back into the phosphorylase *b* state. By 1970 it was clear that almost all enzymes were regulated by phosphorylation/dephosphorylation, and investigators began to question why it was necessary to have two broad systems for controlling enzyme activity: allosteric regulation and phosphorylation. Moreover, in the case of phosphorylase and another enzyme, glycogen synthase, it was clear that allosteric and covalent regulation probably worked through similar conformational changes. A basic difference between these two modes of action became apparent when it was found that hormone receptors, through the release of intracellular second messengers, in turn, controlled the phosphorylase kinase activity. While allosteric control generally reflects intracellular conditions, phosphorylation occurs in response to extracelluar signals. Phosphorylation allows the organism to control metabolism in individual cells. Phosphorylation and dephosphorylation reactions, as will be seen in the following paragraphs, are always part of a cascade of reactions. Cascade systems allow for an enormous amplification as well as fine modulation of an original signal. While the field of serine/threonine protein kinases exploded, a new type of protein kinase entered the arena in 1978 with the discovery that the Rous sarcoma virus contained a protein kinase, named v-src, which phosphorylated protein on a tyrosine residue. It was then discovered that growth factor receptors contain tyrosine protein kinases and a new field of research rapidly developed.

8.2   GROWTH FACTORS, INTERLEUKINS, INTERFERONS, AND CYTOKINES

Research on tyrosine kinase-containing receptors was initiated in the area of cell biology. Factors that could support growth of cells in culture were isolated and named after (1) the cells they were isolated from, (2) the cells they stimulated, or (3) the principle action they performed, for example, platelet-derived growth factor, epidermal growth factor or transforming growth factor. In the area of immunology, factors were studied that directed maturation and proliferation of white blood cells. The factors discovered were named interleukins or colony stimulating factors. In virology, factors were studied that interfered with viral infection: interferons. And in cancer research, factors were studied that could influence the growth of solid tumors: for example tumor necrosis factor. Each area of research believed that the factors functioned by and large only in the category in which they came to light. It was also believed that each factor had a set of additional actions that were related to each other in some obvious way. With progress, it became apparent that growth factors also acted on cells of the immune system and had totally unrelated actions. Moreover, it was shown that the context in which the cells were studied (presence of other factors, presence of other cells, attached or in suspension, type of substrate) also determined the outcome of the cellular response. A good example is transforming growth factor-β, a factor initially shown to enhance cell transformation, hence its name. Later is was found that it also acted as a very potent chemotactic factor for neutrophils and that it played a vital role in the differentiation of hematopoietic cells. It has been proposed that a common name for these factors should be *cytokines*. The definition for a cytokine is a soluble (glyco)protein, nonimmunoglobulin in nature, released by living cells of the host, which acts nonenzymatically in picomolar to nanomolar concentrations to regulate host cell function. Of course there is always an exception to the rule; lysophosphatidic acid also has growth-promoting properties and acts via a specific receptor. This information is not directly relevant for understanding the action of tyrosine protein kinases, but it illustrates that various areas of research are coming together introducing new insights in cell functioning. It also illustrates that tyrosine phosphorylation is not limited to growth-inducing cytokines. Tyrosine phosphorylation has been shown to regulate cell–cell and cell–matrix interactions through integrin receptors and focal adhesion sites. It is also involved in stimulation of the respiratory burst in neutrophils. Occupation of the B cell IgM and high-affinity IgE receptor as well as occupation of the T cell and interleukin-2 receptor results in tyrosine phosphorylation. Last, it is also involved in selection of transmitter responses induced by neuronal contact.

Only a fraction of what is known about the role of tyrosine protein kinases in cellular functioning will be dealt with in this chapter, but it should nevertheless reveal some principles that allow the reader to better understand current literature on the subject. The chapter is divided into two broad sections: one dealing with receptors that contain tyrosine protein kinases (PTKs) as an integral part of the molecule (receptor PTK, or RTK) and one dealing with receptors that associate with cytosolic tyrosine protein kinases (nonreceptor PTK, or NRTK) Because studies with genetically accessible organisms such as *Drosophila* and *Caenorhabditis elegans* have made important contributions to the discovery of signal transduction pathways, we will illustrate some of the analogies between the various species in an appendix to this chapter. Knowledge of these will also facilitate your understanding of the signal-transduction nomenclature.

8.3   COLOR ILLUSTRATIONS

To gain a better insight into the molecular mechanism of signaling through tyrosine protein kinases, color illustrations are helpful. We have therefore prepared color versions of all figures in this chapter, and these are freely available in JPEG format, on a special Web site dedicated to the teaching of signal transduction. You will find them in the "Receptor Pharmacology" section at: http://www.cellbiol.net/ste/book.php.

8.4   RECEPTORS THAT CONTAIN TYROSINE PROTEIN KINASES

8.4.1   Dimerization and Transphosphorylation of Receptors Cause Their Activation

This section of the chapter focuses on the signal transduction pathway initiated by binding of growth factors to their receptors. We will restrict the subject to a number of principles that generally apply for tyrosine kinase containing receptors, with the epidermal growth factor (EGF), platelet-derived growth factor (PDGF), insulin, and nerve growth factor (NGF) receptor as examples. EGF and PDGF are true growth factors, inducing proliferation of epithelial cells and fibroblasts. Insulin has growth-promoting capacities, but we know it best for its role in stimulating glycogen synthesis. The main role of NGF is to ensure survial of neurons and/or neurite outgrowth, not proliferation.

As discussed in Chapter 4, "Molecular Structure of Receptor Tyrosine Kinases," tyrosine kinase–containing receptors come in several different forms, unified by the presence of a single membrane-spanning domain and an intracellular tyrosine protein kinase catalytic domain (receptor PTK). The extracellular chains vary considerably as illustrated in Figure 4.1. Many growth factor receptors contain immunoglobulin domains (Ig-domains) that play a role in ligand binding, and they are therefore part of the Ig-superfamily. Others bind ligand through a leucine-rich repeat. A general feature is that ligand binding results in dimerization of the receptors, and this can be achieved in a

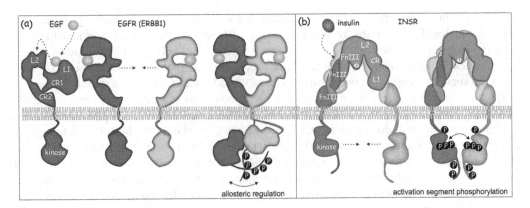

FIGURE 8.1 Receptor dimerization and phosphorylation. (a) On occupation by its ligand, the EGF receptor takes on an extended conformation through which one receptor recognizes the other. Receptor dimerization brings together the tyrosine protein kinase domains that form an asymmetric dimer, leading to a conformational change that renders the kinases catalytically competent. This is followed by phophosphorylation in trans (one kinase phosphorylates the other) of the C-terminal segments of the receptor. The dimerized, phosphorylated molecule constitutes the active receptor, able to attract adaptors and effectors and able to phosphorylate other substrates. (b) The insulin receptor is already dimerized and yet requires ligand to reveal its tyrosine kinase activity. Here it is postulated that receptor occupation causes the correct orientation of the two kinase domains so that they can phosphorylate each others' activation segment. This leads to their activation and is followed by phosphorylation of other receptor residues and then phosphorylate of other substrates. The phosphotyrosines act to recruit adaptors and effectors.

number of ways (Figure 8.1a). The activation signal is, of course, more complicated than this. For activation of all the receptor functions, not only must the receptor molecules be brought together as dimers, but the intracellular protein kinase domains must also be oriented correctly in relation to each other. This is nicely illustrated by the insulin receptor, which shows very little activity without binding of insulin despite its default dimerized state (Figure 8.1b). Although the mechanism remains to be clarified, it is clear that receptor activation constitutes a change in the relative position of the intracellular kinase domains. This change then allows for mutual activation. Activation of the intracellular kinase domain occurs, with the exception of the EGF receptor, through phosphorylation in *trans* (one kinase phosphorylates the other) of one or more tyrosine residue in the activation segment. This induces a conformational change that affects both the coordination of adenosine triphosphate (ATP) and improves access of substrate to the catalytic cleft (for more detail see Figure 4.3). The phosphorylated dimer constitutes the active receptor. It possesses an array of phosphotyrosines that enable it to bind proteins, to form *receptor signaling complexes* (Figure 8.2 and Figure 8.3). Additionally, the dimerized and phosphorylated receptor has the potential of phosphorylating other substrates (its targets).

8.4.2 SRC HOMOLOGY AND PTB DOMAINS AND THE FORMATION OF RECEPTOR SIGNALING COMPLEXES

Having established the formation of receptor signaling complexes, it was important to establish how these proteins interact with the tyrosine phosphorylated receptor. Sequence analysis of proteins that bind has shown that many, but not all of them, contain domains also present in the cytoplasmic tyrosine protein kinase sarcoma (Src), hence named Src homology domain-2 (SH2) domains. Others contain domains that were previously identified as phosphotyrosine-binding domains, phosphotyrosine binding (PTB). Both PTB and SH2 domains recognize the phosphotyrosine in a context of two surrounding amino acids (upstream or downstream) (Figure 8.2). Conclusive evidence for a role

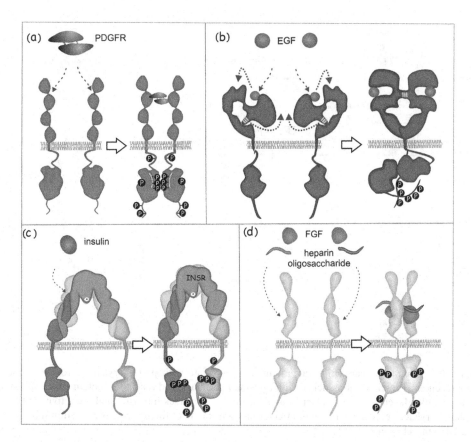

FIGURE 8.2 Recruitment of SH2- and PTB-containing proteins to activated tyrosine kinase receptors. (a) Receptor signaling complex formation through the binding of SH2- and PTB-containing proteins with the EGF receptor (adaptor proteins Grb2 and Shc, respectively). (b) Molecular detail of an SH2-binding sequence interacting with a peptide of the EGF receptor. The phosphotyrosine and asparagine bury themselves into the SH2 domain and constitute the key determinants of the interaction between the receptor and Grb2. The loss of phosphate weakens the interaction and causes separation of the two proteins. (c) Recruitment of Grb2/Sos results in activation of the GTPase Ras. Sos is a guanine exchange factor which facilitates the exchange of GDP for GTP. Ras is active in its GTP-bound state. Hydrolysis brings Ras back in its inactive GDP-bound state. **(See color insert following page 116.)**

of SH2 domains in transmitting the signals due to receptor PTKs came from the finding that deletion of the SH2 domains, in proteins that were found to bind to the activated receptors, abolished the interaction and the cellular response. Further evidence came from the finding that only the γ-isoforms of phospholipase-C (PLC) are directly activated by these receptors.

Significantly, PLCγ, but not the β and δ isoforms, possesses SH2 domains. In conclusion, the assembly of signaling complexes depends on the recruitment by tyrosine phosphorylated receptors of proteins having an SH2 or PTB domain. There are many proteins containing SH2 domains that associate with receptor PTKs in the formation of signaling complexes, and a selection of these is illustrated in Figure 8.3. Some of these proteins themselves become phosphorylated as a result of this association, though it is not clear whether this is always necessary for their activation. In the case of PLCγ, phosphorylation is certainly necessary.

Of the variety of adaptors and enzymes that interact with EGF receptors, some appear to bind more tightly than others, exhibiting sensitivity to the amino acid residues in the immediate vicinity of the phosphotyrosines. Thus, a particular receptor might transmit its signal through a panel of its

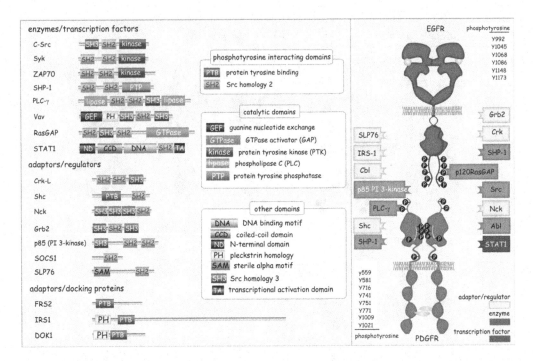

FIGURE 8.3 Domain organization of proteins that associate with phosphorylated tyrosine kinase-containing receptors. Proteins that associate with tyrosine-phosphorylated receptors contain either SH2 or PTB domains. Unlike the enzymes, the adaptors and docking proteins lack intrinsic catalytic activity but serve to link phosphorylated receptors with other effector proteins. Some of the proteins presented in this figure are discussed in this chapter.

favorite SH2- or PTP-containing proteins. This is illustrated in Figure 8.4, where the carboxy terminal segments of the different EGF receptors (erythroblastosis oncogene B-2 [ERBB1], -2, -3, and -4) bind to a range of adaptors and effectors. Many are shared between them, but some are specific for the receptor variant. It remains unclear, however, whether two or more intracellular proteins can bind to a single receptor molecule simultaneously.

8.4.3 BRANCHING OF THE SIGNALING PATHWAY

A number of signal transduction pathways branch out from the receptor signaling complex. Three such branches are described in the next paragraphs (Figure 8.5).

8.4.3.1 The Ras Signaling Pathway

8.4.3.1.1 Ras and Cell Transformation

Infection of rats with murine leukemia viruses can provoke the formation of a sarcoma. A major advance was the discovery that the Harvey murine sarcoma virus encodes a persistently activated form of the H-ras gene, a monomeric guanosine triphosphate (GTP)-binding protein or GTPase, in which valine is substituted for glycine at position-12. GTP-binding proteins act as monostable switches. They are *on* in the GTP-bound state and *off* in the guanosine diphosphate (GDP)-bound

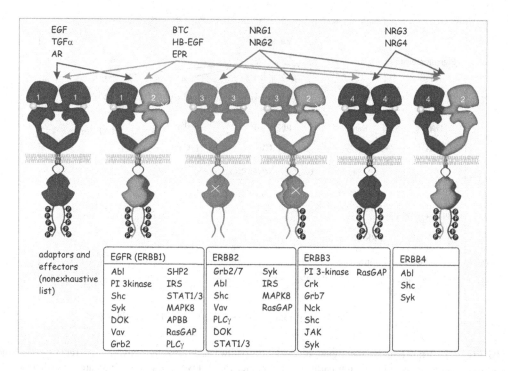

FIGURE 8.4 ERBB receptor family, their ligands and some of their adaptors and effectors. EGF receptors, ERBB1 to 4, form different receptor combinations when bound to ligand. The different receptor dimers, in turn, recruit different sets of effectors and adaptors. Note that ERBB2 does not bind ligand; it naturally occurs in an extended confirmation but cannot form homodimers (ERBB2/ERBB2). It is the favorite partner of ligand-bound EGFR (ERBB1) and of ERBB3. Note also that ERBB3 lacks kinase activity. However, it can nevertheless act as an "active receptor" by recruiting adaptors and effectors after being phosphorylated by ERBB2.

state. Binding of GTP occurs through the dissociation of GDP (exchange reaction), and GTP is subsequently lost through hydrolysis (GTPase reaction). The state of activation is kinetically regulated, positively by the initial rate of GDP dissociation, and subsequent association of GTP, and then negatively by the rate at which the GTP is hydrolyzed. The valine to glycine substitution prevents hydrolysis of GTP, resulting in a constitutive active Ras (also referred to as a gain of function mutation). Expression of this mutant in quiescent rodent fibroblasts resulted in altered cell morphology, stimulation of DNA synthesis, and cell proliferation. When overexpressed, normal H-c-Ras also induces oncogenic transformation, as does microinjection of the mutant protein. Conversely, injection of neutralizing antibodies to inhibit normal Ras function reverses cell transformation. Lastly, stimulation of quiescent cells with serum, or with purified growth factors, causes the activation of Ras, through promotion of the exchange of GDP for GTP. It became apparent that Ras is an important component in the signaling pathways regulating cell proliferation, but how this would fit into the known pathways emanating from growth factor receptors remained unclear for a considerable time.

8.4.3.1.2 Regulation of Ras in Vertebrates

The activated growth factor receptor binds Grb2, an adaptor protein, through its SH2 domain, and this action recruits the guanine nucleotide exchanger hSos to the plasma membrane, bringing it in

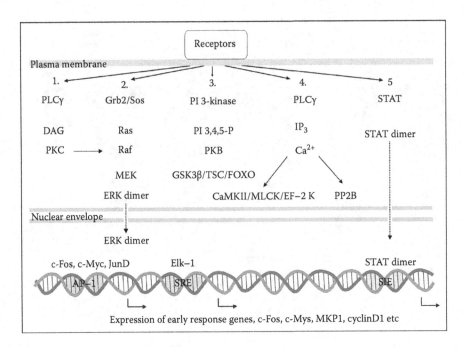

FIGURE 8.5 Branching of the signal transduction pathways. Following activation of receptor tyrosine kinases, several signal transduction pathways can be activated. Five of these are indicated. Further details feature in the text and following figures.

the vicinity of Ras. The activated hSos now exchanges GDP for GTP and brings Ras in its activated state, ready to signal into the cell through interaction with its effector molecules.

The Ras-GTPase activating protein p120[GAP] also contains two SH2 domains (Figure 8.3). It too binds to phosphotyrosines on activated receptors, and it is a component of the signaling complex that assembles on activated PDGF receptors. It is unclear what role the association of GAP plays in signal transduction. For instance, cells that express a mutant of the PDGF receptor that fails to bind GAP manifest normal activation of Ras.

8.4.3.1.3   Other Ras Activators and Effectors

Guanine nucleotide exchange factors other than hSos have also been found to activate Ras, and other effectors have been found too (see Table 8.1). These may interact with unique sequences in the effector-loop. The question remains, how many different effectors can attach to activated Ras and what determines the level of their priority?

TABLE 8.1
Some of the Many Influences of, by, and for Ras

Activators (Guanine Nucleotide Exchanger)	Inhibitors (GTPase)	Effectors
hSos	GAP	Raf
CrkL	neurofibromin	PI 3-kinase
rasGRP		RalGDS
Ras GRF2		
SmgGDS		

8.4.3.1.4   From Ras to ERK and the Activation of Transcription

The events following the activation of Ras ultimately lead to the activation of extracellular signal-regulated kinase (ERK1) and ERK2, members of a large family of protein kinases referred to as mitogen-activated protein (MAP) kinases followed by activation of expression of immediate early response genes. Activation of ERK1 and -2 requires two intermediate steps, and both of these involve a phosphorylation (Figure 8.6). The immediate activator of ERK1 and -2 is MEK1 (MAP kinase-ERK kinase-1, also known as MAP2K or MAP-kinase-kinase), a most unusual enzyme that phosphorylates ERK1 and -2 on both a threonine and a tyrosine residue. These are in the activation segment sequence LTEYVATRWY (residues T183 and Y185, see insert of Figure 8.6). Phosphorylation at these sites renders the protein kinase catalytically competent. To date, ERK1 and -2 (and ERK5) appear to be the unique substrate for phosphorylation by MEK, indicating a particularly high level of specificity (see also Figure 8.9). Moving further upstream, the first kinase downstream of Ras is C-Raf (also known as MAP3K or MAP-kinase-kinase-kinase). This was initially identified as an oncogene product causing fibrosarcoma in the rat. The subsequent finding that activated Ras recruits C-Raf to the membrane and in consequence brings about kinase activation links MAP kinase with the Ras pathway. Ras-mediated activation of C-Raf requires the Ras-binding domain (RBD) and a cysteine rich domain (CRD). How C-Raf is activated is still not fully understood; we return to this subject in Section 8.4.3.1.7, "Activation of the Ras-ERK Pathway Requires Removal of the 14-3-3 Restraint."

8.4.3.1.5   Beyond ERK: Activation of Gene Expression and of Yet Other Protein Kinases

The activated MAP kinase dimerizes and through an as yet unrecognized mechanism translocates to the nucleus there to phosphorylate transcription factors. In the case of stimulation by EGF and PDGF, the activation of MAP kinase is an absolute requirement for cell proliferation. In the case of NGF, its stimulation plays a role in neurite outgrowth and survival. The early response genes become activated within an hour of receptor stimulation. Their activation is transient, and it can occur under conditions in which protein synthesis is inhibited. Activation of the EGF, PDGF, or NGF receptor results in the rapid induction of the transcription factor c-Fos, one of the first cytokine-inducible transcription factors to be discovered. It occupies a central position in the regulation of gene expression. Other early response genes include c-myc, junB and c-jun. The promoter region of the c-fos gene contains a serum-response element (SRE), a DNA domain that binds the transcription factors p67[SRF] (serum-response factor) and Elk-1. Phosphorylation of Elk-1 at residue ser-383 and ser-389 by ERK2 increases the formation of a complex of both transcription factors with the DNA to promote transcription of the c-fos gene (Figure 8.6). ERK1 or -2 also phosphorylates the c-Fos protein, and this prolongs its half-life. C-Fos binds c-Jun, and together they bind the AP-1 sequence.

Apart from transcription factors, other protein kinases are also important substrates of ERK1 and -2. These are the members of the ribosomal sb kinase (RSK) and mitogen and stress-activated kinase (MSK) family of kinases. Both families phosphorylate numerous substrates and these are listed in Table 8.2.

8.4.3.1.6   Fine-Tuning the Ras-ERK Pathway

Activation of the Ras-ERK pathway appears to be a rather complicated procedure. Numerous barriers have been put into place to prevent accidental growth-promoting signals. Moreover, studies in yeast have demonstrated that the different components of the kinase cascade are bound to a scaffold protein. In mammalian cells this role is taken by the kinase suppressor of Ras-1 (KSR1) protein, which binds C-Raf, MEK1, and ERK2. This organization has a number of important consequences. First, it means that the signal trickles down in a one-to-one stoichiometry and excludes amplification. C-Raf phosphorylates and activates one MEK1, and this phosphorylates and activates one ERK2. Second, it makes the system very sensitive to relative expression levels of the different components. Third, it introduces new levels of regulation of the activity of the kinase cascade.

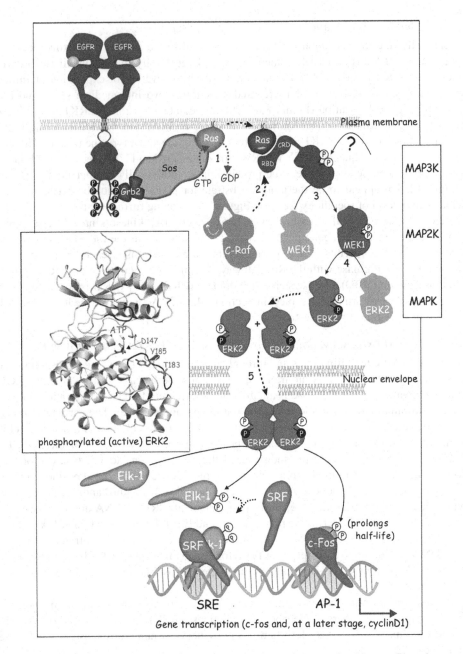

FIGURE 8.6 Regulation of the Ras-ERK pathway by receptor protein tyrosine kinases. The adaptor protein Grb2, in association with the guanine exchange factor Sos, attaches to the tyrosine-phosphorylated receptor through its SH2 domains. This brings the Grb2/hSos complex into the vicinity of the membrane where it catalyzes guanine nucleotide exchange on Ras. The activated Ras associates with the serine/threonine protein kinase C-Raf. Its localization at the membrane results in activation and subsequent phosphorylation of the dual specificity kinase MEK1 (at S217 and S221), which in turn phosphorylates ERK2 on a threonine residue (T183) and on a tyrosine (Y185) residue. Dimerization allows ERK2 to enter the nucleus (by an as of yet unknown mechanism). The insert shows a ribbon presentation of the kinase domain of ERK2 with its two phosphorylated residues (pT183 and pY185). Inside the nucleus ERK2 phosphorylates Elk-1, which then associates with SRF to form an active transcription factor complex. This binds to DNA at the serum response element (SRE). ERK2 also phosphorylates and stabilizes c-Fos, which, in complex with c-Jun, binds to DNA at the AP-1 sequence. Both SRE and AP-1 induce a strong expression of c-Fos as well as genes involved in the onset of cell proliferation (e.g., cyclin D).

TABLE 8.2
Substrates of the MAP Kinases

Substrates of the MAPkinases			
	ERK 1 & 2	**p38α, β, γ, δ**	**JNK1, 2, 3**
Membrane	CD120a, Syk, calnexin		
Transcriptional regulation (nucleus)	SRC-1, Pax6, NF-AT, Elk-1, MEF2, c-Fos, c-Myc, STAT3, JunD, Ets-2	ATF1/2, MEF2a, Sap-1, Elk-1, NFκB, Ets-1, p53	c-jun, JunD, ATF-2, NF-Acc1, HSF-1, STAT3, p53
Actin cytoskeleton and focal adhesion	Neurofilament, paxillin, vinexin	Tau	
Signaling	MEK, Lin-1, RSK, MSK, MNK, TSC2	PLA2, MNSK, MSK, MK2	Shc

Substrates of the MAPkinase-Activated Kinases (MK)				
	RSK1–4	**MSK1 & 2**	**MNK 1 &2**	**MK2 & 3**	**MK5**
Transcription	TIF-1, ER81, ERα, Mi, CBP, CREB, c-Fos, c-Jun, Nur77, SRF, ATF-4	Histone H3, HMG14, CREB, ATF1, p65, ER81, STAT3	ERβ	CREB, SRF, ER81, E47	
RNA stability, translation		4E-BP1	eIF-4E	hnRNP, TTP, PABP1, HuR, eEFkinase	
Cell cycle	P27kip, Myt1, Bub1				
Cell survival	Bad, LKB1, GSK3β, IkBα, C/EBPβ	Bad			
Signaling	Sos, TSC2	PKB			
Miscellaneous				glycogen synthase, 14-3-3ζ, 5-LO	

8.4.3.1.7   Activation of the Ras-ERK Pathway Requires Removal of the 14-3-3 Restraint

Both C-Raf and the MEK1/ERK1 signaling cassette are restrained in their activity by the scaffold protein 14-3-3. It holds C-Raf locked in a folded state, which prevents both its access to RasGTP and its activation by upstream protein kinases, and it sequesters the signaling cassette in the cytoplasm (Figure 8.7a). The scaffold protein 14-3-3 attaches to phosphoserine residues. The serine/threonine protein kinase Cdc25C-associated kinase-1 (C-TAK1) plays an important role in keeping two serine residues (S297 and S392) phosphorylated on KSR1 (Figure 8.7a; Figure 8.8b). Growth factors signal the assembly of an active protein phosphotase-2A (PP2A) complex by providing the missing regulatory subunit B (Figure 8.7b). As a result of PP2A activity, C-Raf opens up and binds to RasGTP and the plasma membrane with its Ras binding domain (RBD) and cystein-rich-binding domain (CRD), respectively. The signaling cassette is also liberated and translocates to the plasma membrane, where it binds to RasGTP. However, it still cannot associate with C-Raf. Its access is prevented by impedes mitogenic signal propagation (IMP), and this protein has first to be destroyed in order to allow C-Raf to reach the signaling cassette.

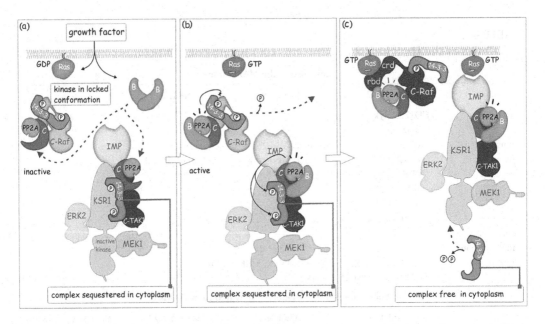

FIGURE 8.7 Central role of the serine/threonine phosphatase PP2A in the formation of a productive Ras-MAP kinase signaling cassette. The serine/threonine phosphatase PP2A plays two important roles in the onset of the Ras-ERK pathway. Both effect the relief of inhibitory constraints imposed by the phosphoserine-binding scaffold protein 14-3-3. (a) C-Raf and the MEK/ERK-signaling cassette are blocked through their association with the scaffold protein 14-3-3. With respect to the signaling cassette, this attachment is made possible through phosphorylation of KSR1 on serine residues by the kinase C-TAK1. Growth factor signaling causes the release of a regulatory subunit of PP2A (PP2A-B) which binds the catalytic domain, leading to its activation. (b) Activated PP2A dephosphorylates C-Raf on S259, causing detachment of 14-3-3 from the C-terminus. This allows C-Raf to associate with RasGTP. PP2A also dephosphorylates two residues in KSR1 (S297 and S392). (c) Dephosphorylation of KSR1 causes detachment of 14-3-3 and translocation of the signaling cassette to the membrane, there to bind to RasGTP.

8.4.3.1.8 Docking of the MEK/ERK Kinase Signaling Cassette Requires Destruction of IMP

IMP is a latent ubiquitin E3-ligase. Binding to RasGTP reveals its catalytic activity and this causes auto-ubiquitylation (Figure 8.8a). Poly-ubiquitylated IMP is recognized by the 26S proteasome and degraded. Removal of this constraint allows KSR1 to associate with C-Raf. Once C-Raf has attached to the signaling cassette, it is fully activated through phosphorylation by an as yet unknown protein kinase. C-Raf then phosphorylates MEK1, followed by phosphorylation of ERK2.

8.4.3.1.9 A Family of MAP Kinase-Related Proteins

Following the cloning of ERK1 and 2, it became apparent that they are members of a substantial family, the MAP kinases. Based on sequence analysis and the composition of their activation segments, they may be classified into five groups, each operating in different signal transduction pathways (Figure 8.9).

- *ERK*—ERK1 and ERK2 are the *prototypic* or *classical* MAP kinases, operating mainly in mitogen-activated signal transduction pathways.
- *JNK (c-Jun N-terminal kinase)*—JNK and SAPK (stress-activated protein kinase) are kinases that phosphorylate c-Jun and are activated in response to "stress." They emerged

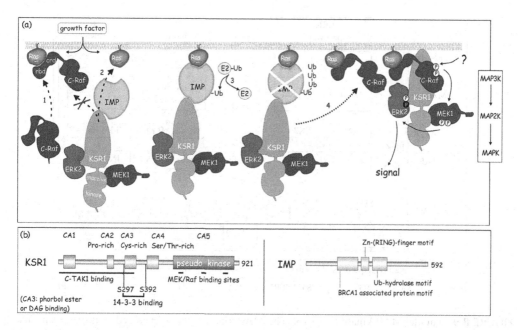

FIGURE 8.8 Dual effector interaction of RasGTP that leads to effective signaling to ERK. (a) In order to activate the ERK pathway, Ras has not only to recruit C-Raf (1), but also to remove IMP, the inhibitor that prevents formation of the Raf-MEK-ERK signaling cassette. RasGTP binds IMP (2), and this initiates a series of ubiquitylations that mark the protein for destruction by the proteasome (3). MEK1 and ERK2, linked to the scaffold protein KSR1, are now able to join C-Raf, enabling the signal to pass from one kinase to another. (b) KSR1 has a number of conserved domains: CA2, proline-rich domain; CA3, cysteine-rich domain that resembles the PMA/DAG binding site (C1 domain) of PKC; CA4, Ser/Thr-rich domain; and CA5, a kinase domain that resembles that of Raf but lacks an essential lysine and is therefore inactive. The domain architecture of IMP reveals a Zn-(RING)-finger, a motif known to be involved in the ubiquitylation of protein. IMP qualifies as an E3-ligase and binds E2-ubiquitin. The E3-ligase activity is activated by binding to RasGTP, and this results in the autoubiquitylation of IMP, followed by its destruction.

in experiments in which rat livers were challenged by injection of cycloheximide.* Other activating factors include growth factor deprivation, UV irradiation, or treatment with inflammatory cytokines (IL1β, TNF). The JNKs include JNK1, 2, and 3.

- *p38 kinase*—p38/HOG came to light in genetic deletion studies in yeast (*S. cerevisiae*) as a protein kinase involved in the generation of glycerol in response to osmotic stress. HOG1 induces expression of glycerol-3-phosphate dehydrogenase, related to glycerol synthesis. In mammalian cells, it is also activated in response to stress stimuli. p38/HOG is now generally referred to as p38 kinase, of which there are four variants: p38α, β, δ, and γ.
- *ERK3 and ERK4*—These are distinguished from other ERKs by the absence of a tyrosine in the activation segment. Thus they possess only a single phosphorylation site at a serine in the motif SEG. Little is known about their upstream regulators and substrates. ERK3 has two gene variants: ERK3α and 3β.
- *ERK5*—Originally called Big MAP kinase or BMK1, ERK5 is activated by mitogens, but its unique C-terminal domain gives rise to a protein twice the size of ERK1 or ERK2. This has transcriptional activity, either on its own, binding direct to DNA, or through its

---

* Cycloheximide, a product of the bacterium *Streptomyces griseus*, is an inhibitor of protein biosynthesis in eukaryotic organisms. It interferes with the activity of peptidyl transferase activity, thus blocking translational elongation.

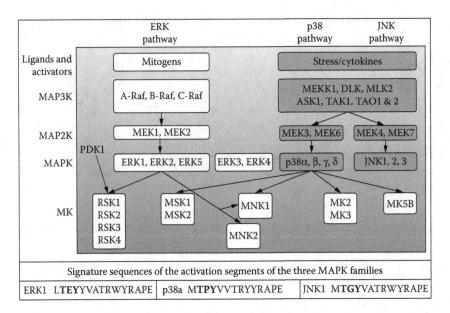

FIGURE 8.9 Parallel MAP kinase pathways. The MAP kinases can be classified in three groups, based on the identity of the intermediate residue in their dual phosphorylation motifs (TEY, TGY, or TPY) in the activation segment. This classification also defines three distinct signal transduction pathways indicated as the ERK, the P38, and the JNK kinase pathway, each having unique upstream activators. The ERK pathway is said to act in response to mitogens, whereas the p38 and JNK pathways are reserved for the response to stress and inflammatory cytokines.

association with other transcription factors (for instance the AP-1 complex). It operates in a similar pathway as ERK1/2 and has many substrates in common. It has a unique role in cardiovascular development and neural differentiation

8.4.3.1.10   Switch in Receptor Signaling: Activation of ERK by 7TM Receptors

G-protein linked receptors are substrates for protein kinase A (PKA) and protein kinase C (PKC) and for receptor specific kinases, which preferentially target occupied (and therefore activated) receptors. These receptor-specific kinases (GRKs), such as the β-adrenergic receptor kinase GRK2, are only called into action under conditions of more robust stimulation. The β-receptor phosphorylated by GRK2 recruits β-arrestin2, a scaffold protein, so blocking the transmission of signals through the heterotrimeric G$_s$ protein (Figure 8.10). Upon binding, β-arrestin2 interacts with the adaptor protein-2 (AP-2), and this causes endocytosis of the G-protein linked receptor. Importantly, the bound β-arrestin2 offers an alternative means to activate the Ras-ERK pathway through interaction with the SH3 domain of the Src tyrosine kinase. This initiates a signaling pathway that activates ERK1/2. The steps following the recruitment of Src are not yet clear. It is possible that it initiates a series of events resulting in the phosphorylation of the adaptor Shc-1, which in turn binds to the Grb2/Soscomplex. Finally, β-arrestins also act as scaffolds for other MAP kinases, binding Jun N-terminal kinase 3 (JNK3), apoptosis signaling kinase-1 (Ask1), and MAP kinase-kinase-4 (MKK4).

Other seven transmembrane (7-TM) receptors may employ different pathways to reach Ras. For instance, the lysophosphatidic acid receptor, LPA, also activates ERK, but in this case dominant negative Src is without effect. Here the signal appears to involve PI 3-kinase, an unidentified tyrosine kinase, a docking protein, and finally Grb2/Sos.

8.4.3.2   The PI 3-Kinase/PKB Signaling Pathway

In this section we focus on insulin-mediated activation of the PI 3-kinase/PKB signal transduction pathway. This pathway is of course stimulated by a variety of receptor tyrosine protein kinases,

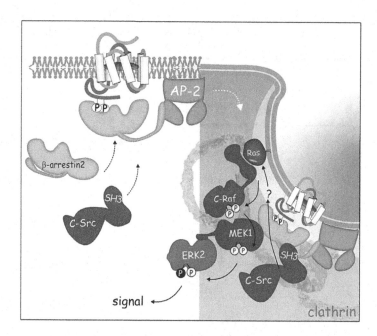

FIGURE 8.10 Phosphorylation of the β-adrenergic receptor by GRK2 activates the Ras-ERK pathway. Phosphorylation of the β-adrenergic receptor by GRK2 allows recruitment of the adaptor β-arrestin2 and terminates communication with the G protein. It also activates the Ras-ERK pathway by recruitment of Src (via its SH3-domain) and MEK1/ERK2. β-arrestin2 also directs the receptor to clathrin-coated pits, there to be removed from the cell surface by endocytosis and degraded in the lysosomal pathway.

among which are the EGF and PDGF receptors. It is also activated by adhesion molecules of the integrin family. The PI 3-kinase/PKB pathway regulates a number of cellular processes: glycogenesis, regulation of cell size, migration, survival, and proliferation. In this section we shall focus on its role in the regulation of protein synthesis. Later in the chapter we will return to its role in protection against apoptosis (programmed cell death).

8.4.3.2.1 PI 3-Kinase

The PI 3-kinases comprise a family of enzymes subdivided in three classes. They have distinct substrates and various forms of regulation. They all have four homologous regions, the kinase domain being most conserved. Uniquely, the class I enzymes activate protein kinase B and will therefore be discussed in this chapter. This class of phospholipid kinases phosphorylate PI, PI-4-P and PI-4,5-P2 (the preferred substrate) at the 3-position of the inositol ring (Figure 8.11a,b). These enzymes comprise two subunits, a regulatory (p55 or p85) and a catalytic subunit (p110), each existing in various forms (Figure 8.11c).

The multidomain structure of the regulatory subunit, in particular p85α, suggests that it should be able to interact with a number of signaling proteins. The SH2 domains enable them to bind to phosphotyrosine residues (on a variety of proteins such as insulin receptor substrate-1 (IRS1), PDGFR, EGFR, Grb2-associated binder-1 (Gab-1), or linker of activated T cells (LAT), and the SH3 domains allow interaction with proline-rich sequences, present for instance in the adaptor molecule Shc, the GTPase-activating protein Cdc42GAP, or the regulator of T-lymphocyte receptor (TCR) signaling, Cositas B-lineage lymphoma oncogene (Cbl). In addition, the p85 subunit contains a B-lymphocyte receptor (BCR)/GTPase activator protein (GAP) homology domain that interacts with members of the Rho family of GTPases, Rac, and Cdc42, providing yet further opportunities for regulation.

There are four isoforms of the catalytic p110 subunit. All contain a kinase domain and a Ras interaction site. In addition the α, β, and δ isoforms (type 1A PI 3-kinases) possess an interaction site for the p85 subunit (Figure 8.11c).

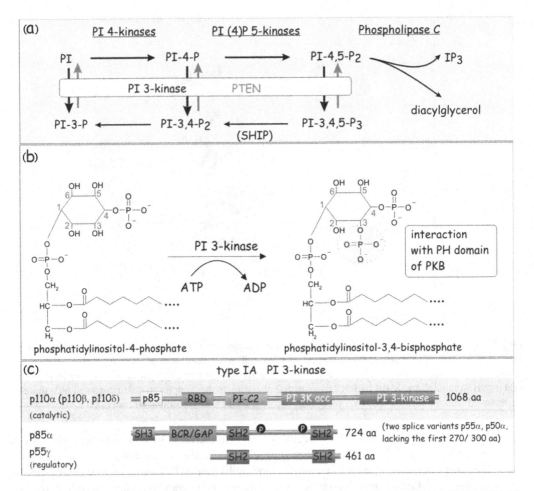

FIGURE 8.11 Phosphoinositide 3-kinases and the generation of 3-phosphorylated lipids. (a) The PI 3-ki-nases phosphorylate the 3 OH-position in the inositol ring of the phosphatidylinositol lipids. The 3-OH phos-phorylated inositol lipids are not substrates for PLC. The phosphatases PTEN and SHIP reverse the reaction. (b) Composition of inositol lipids before and after phosphorylation by PI 3-kinase. The PH domain of PKB interacts preferentially with the PI-3,4-P2 product. (c) Domain architecture of the type 1A PI 3-kinase family. The catalytic subunits (α, β, and δ) all possess a p85- and Ras-binding site. They also have a PI-C2 domain with which they interact with phospholipids. The PI 3K accessory domain serves as a spine on which the other domains are fastened. Of the regulatory subunits, p85a is particularly versatile, its SH3 domain interacts with proline-rich sequences, its BCR/GAP domain interacts with monomeric GTPases of the Rho family (Cdc42 and Rac), whereas its SH2 domain interacts with phosphotyrosines.

8.4.3.2.2 *Phosphatidyl Inositol Phosphatases*

The phosphorylation of inositol can be counteracted by two lipid phosphatases: SH2-containing inositol phosphatase, SHIP, and phosphatase and tensin-homologue deleted from chromosome 10, PTEN. SHIP dephosphorylates at the 5-position of inositol and was discovered as a protein that associates with the adaptor protein Shc in hemopoietic cells. SHIP plays a major role in modu-lating the signaling of hemopoietic cell surface receptors. Its absence, through targeted disrup-tion in mice, is associated with increased numbers of granulocyte-macrophage progenitors and with excessive infiltration of tissues by these cells. PTEN was discovered as a tumor suppressor because inactivating mutations were detected in glioblastomas, melanomas, and breast, prostate, and endometrial carcinomas. Its sequence reveals the characteristics of a dual specificity protein phosphatase but its favorite substrate is phosphoinositides. It dephosphorylates at the 3-position of

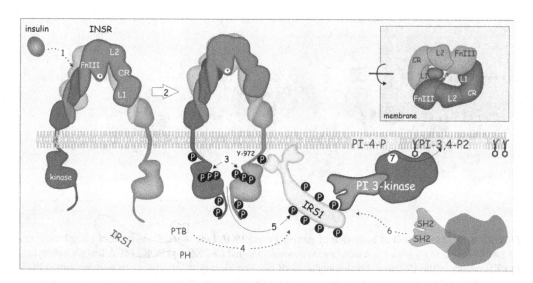

FIGURE 8.12 Activation of PI 3-kinase by the insulin receptor. Insulin binding to the insulin receptor dimer (1) induces a conformational change (2) (as of yet to be determined how) that causes trans-phosphorylation of the activation segments at three tyrosine residues (3). Further phosphorylation follows both upstream and downstream of the catalytic domain. The IRS-1 (insulin receptor substrate-1) binds phosphotyrosine-972 (also numbered Y960, situated in the NPEY motif) with its PTB domain (phosphotyrosine binding domain) (4). Phosphorylation of a number of tyrosine residues follows (5), which then serves as a docking site for the SH2-domains of the p85 regulatory subunit of PI 3-kinase (6), leading to the generation of phosphatidylinositol-3,4,5-trisphosphate.

the inositol ring, counteracting the phosphorylation by PI 3-kinase (Figure 8.11a). Ectopic expression in PTEN-deficient tumor cells results in arrest of the cell cycle in the G1 phase eventually followed by apoptosis. It also reduces cell migration, a finding that may explain why the loss of the gene product is frequently associated with late-stage metastatic tumors.

8.4.3.2.3 Activation of PI 3-Kinase

The tyrosine phosphorylated insulin receptor binds a large docking protein, IRS1, with numerous tyrosine phosphorylation sites. After phosphorylation, IRS1 recruits the 85 kDa regulatory subunit of PI 3-kinase (p85$^{\text{PI 3-kinase}}$). This is attached to a p110 catalytic subunit (p110$^{\text{PI 3-kinase}}$). IRS1-mediated recruitment of p85 has two consequences: It brings the catalytic subunit to its substrate localized in the membrane, and it modifies p85 such that an auto-inhibitory constraint is removed from the catalytic subunit.

The EGF and PDGF receptors directly bind the p85-adaptor subunit of PI 3-kinase through the interaction of their phosphorylated tyrosine residues with the SH2 domain of the adaptor. This recruitment is most likely enforced by a simultaneous binding of activated Ras to the p110-catalytic domain of the lipid kinase. In the case of NGF the situation is different. Activation of the NGF receptor (TrkA) causes the phosphorylation of a docking protein at a number of tyrosine residues. This docking protein, named Grb-2-associated binder-1 (Gab-1) resembles one of the main substrates of the insulin receptors, IRS-1, a protein with a similar function. The SH-2 domain of the p85-adaptor protein now binds to Gab-1. Binding of PI 3-kinase to the activated receptor or docking protein recruits it to the membrane and brings it into contact with the phospholipids (its substrate); this constitutes its activation. The catalytic subunit (p110) can also be activated by direct binding to Ras, independent of p85. Importantly, the subsequent generation of PI 3,4,5-P3 results in activation of a serine/threonine protein kinase-B, PKB.

8.4.3.2.4 Protein Kinase B and Activation through PI 3,4-P3

PKB, or Akt, was discovered as the product of an oncogene of the acutely transforming retrovirus AKT8, causing T-cell lymphomas in mice. It encodes a fusion product of a cellular serine/threonine protein kinase and the viral structural protein Gag. This kinase is similar to both PKCε (73% identity

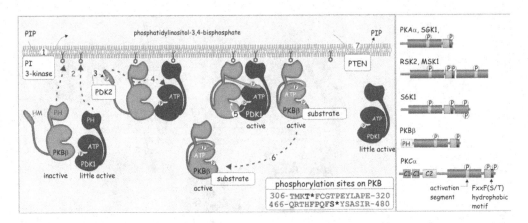

FIGURE 8.13 Mechanism of activation of protein kinase PKB. Left panel. Generation of phosphatidylinositol 3,4-bisphosphate (1) serves as a membrane recruitment signal for PKB and PDK1 (2). A first phosphorylation of PKB occurs in the C-terminal hydrophobic motif (3). The identity of the kinase, tentatively named PDK2, remains elusive. Possible candidates are the complex mTOR/Rictor and PKB itself (low level of autophosphorylation). Close apposition of PKD1 causes binding of the phosphorylated hydrophobic motif to the αC-helix of PDK1 (4). The kinase now fully competent and phosphorylates the activation segment of PKB. Full kinase activity is achieved (5). Detachment of activated PKB from the membrane may occur after dephosphorylation of PI-3,4-phosphate by PTEN (or SHIP) (6). The sequences in the lower right-hand corner box shows the position of the phosphorylated threonine (T*) and serine(S*) residues (the hydrophobic motif is FPQFS). Right panel. Domain architecture of AGC kinases whose activity is controlled by two phosphorylation sites, one in a hydrophobic motif, which is sometimes part of a bigger autoregulatory C-terminal domain, and one in the activation segment. For these protein kinases, PDK1 acts as the "master switch" by phosphorylating the activation segment.

to the catalytic domain) and protein kinase A (68%). It differs from other protein kinases since it contains a PH domain, which allows it to bind to polyphosphoinositide head groups (and also G-protein βγ subunits). To date there are three subtypes, α, β, and γ, all of which show a broad tissue distribution. It was found that PI 3-kinase, through the production of PI-3,4-P2, is the activator of PKB. The mechanism of this activation has turned out a multistep process with the phosphatidylinositol-3,4-P2 playing an important role: bringing together PKB and PDK1 (3-phosphoinositide dependent protein kinase-1), through binding of their PH-domains (Figure 8.13, left panel). In order to understand the next section dealing with activation of PKB, it should be appreciated that PKB belongs to a family of protein kinases (AGC kinase) that requires two phosphorylations in order to become catalytically competent (Figure 8.13, right panel). One phosphorylation occurs in the C-terminal hydrophobic motif (FxxF(S/T)) and the other in the activation segment. PDK1 also requires two modifications, one in the C-terminal lobe and one in the activation segment, but it is different from PKB in two respects. First, it phosphorylates its own activation segment; and secondly, rather than being phosphorylated, it uses the interaction with substrate to obtain the second modification (rearrangement of the αC-helix in the C-lobe). PDK1 is therefore referred to as a constitutively active protein kinase; it only requires the right substrate in order to express its activity.

The sequence of events is as follows. Both PKB and PDK1 attach to phosphatidylinositol-3,4-P2 with their PH domains. PKB is first phosphorylated in its hydrophobic motif by an as yet unknown protein kinase, tentatively named PDK2. The phosphorylated C-terminal binds to the C-lobe of PDK1, which now becomes fully active and phosphorylates the activation segment of PKB. When the two kinases separate, the hydrophobic motif of PKB embraces its own C-lobe, leading to a fully competent protein kinase. Substrate is phosphorylated at the membrane, as long as PI-3,4-P2 is produced, or in the cytoplasm, when PTEN or SHIP have removed the 3-phosphorylated inositol.

The viral oncogene product, v-Akt, has a lipid anchor (myristoyl group), which means that the protein kinase is already located at the membrane, and this may facilitate its activation or alter the range of substrates, both of which may play a role in the transformation process.

8.4.3.2.5 The Role of PI 3-Kinase in Activation of Protein Synthesis

Insulin controls glycogen synthesis but also has a growth factor action. It acts to increase protein synthesis by a mechanism that involves the PI 3-kinase pathway acting through a number of intermediates on two downstream effector proteins: the eukaryotic translation initiator factor-4E (eIF-4E) and the ribosomal p70 S6-kinase-1 (S6K1).

eIF-4E is the limiting initiation factor in most cells, playing a principal role in the determination of global translation rates. It is regulated by phosphorylation, for instance through the ERK pathway (phosphorylation of eIF-4E by MNK kinase) (see Table 8.2), but more importantly by binding to the translational repressor protein, 4E-BP. eIF-4E binds to the 7-methylguanine (m7G) cap at the 5'-end of mRNA. It protects the mRNA from degradation by exo-nucleases and enables the recruitment of other translation initiation factors. These, together with the 40S ribosomal subunit, form a translation initiation complex that enables the search for the start (AUG) codon on the mRNA (Figure 8.14). The movement is facilitated by a helicase (protein complex eIF4A/eIF4B) that breaks the intramolecular base-pairing. Recognition of the AUG codon requires the presence of tRNA^{Met} that contains the anticodon 3'-UAC-5'. This comes into the ribosomal preinitiation complex bound to eIF-2γ.GTP. As the AUG-codon is recognized, GTP is hydrolyzed; and the ribosomal 60S particle, carrying the peptidyl transferase activity, joins the initiation complex in order to start the elongation phase of protein synthesis. Binding of 4E-BP to eIF-4E prevents all this.

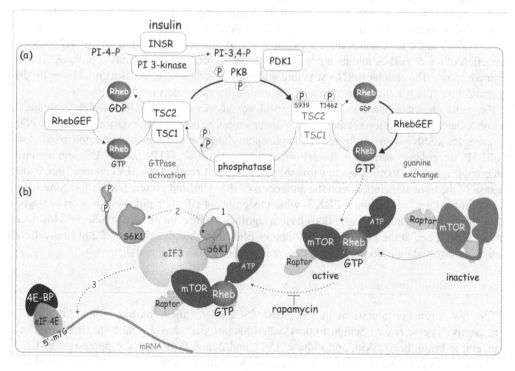

FIGURE 8.14 Regulation of mTOR by PKB-mediated phosphorylation of TSC2. (a) One of the substrates of PKB is the protein TSC2. This, in complex with TSC1, acts as a GTPase activing protein (GAP) of the monomeric GTPase Rheb. TSC1/TSC2 keeps Rheb in its inactive state and this holds protein synthesis in check. Insulin augments the rate of protein synthesis by activation of Rheb. This occurs through phosphorylation and inactivation of TSC2 by PKB. Rheb gradually accumulates in its GTP bound state (by an as yet unidentified guanine exchange factor) and interacts with the protein kinase mTOR, complexed to Raptor (and GαL, which is not shown). (b) Binding of Rheb to mTOR/Raptor somehow unveils its kinase activity and causes the complex to associate with eIF3. The first action of mTOR/Raptor is to phosphorylate S6K1 (1), in its C-terminal segment, which causes its detachment from eIF-3 (2). This enables the initiation factor to join the mRNA (3) and to start to assemble other initiation factors that eventually form the protein translation initiation complex.

The S6K1 acts to phosphorylate the rbS6 protein, a component of the 40S ribosomal subunit. rbS6 is phosphorylated in response to numerous growth factors and to glucagon. Cells lacking rbS6 are smaller in size, but how rbS6 and its phosphorylation regulates cell size remains an enigma. Cellular localization of RbS6 is not restricted to the 40S ribosomal particle; thus it may control cell size independently of regulation of protein synthesis at the ribosomal level. S6K1 also phosphorylates the regulatory domain of eIF-4A (helicase). In the next section we will describe how activation of PKB affects the above-mentioned proteins. We will first introduce two new signaling components that act immediately downstream of PKB: the monomeric GTPase Rheb, Ras homologue-enriched brain, and its GTPase activating protein complex tuberous sclerosis complex 1 (TSC1)/TSC2.

TSC1 and TSC2 are downstream components of the PI 3-kinase pathway, discovered as loss-of-function mutants in patients suffering from tuberous sclerosis, a syndrome of benign tumors. The complex of TSC1/TSC2 harbors GTPase-activating activity that holds the GTPase Rheb in its GDP-bound inactive state. Phosphorylation of TSC2 by PKB inhibits the GTPase-activating activity and this allows Rheb to accumulate in its GTP loaded state. Rheb-GTP interacts with and activates the protein kinase mTOR (Figure 8.14).

Initially recognized as the target of the immunosuppressant rapamycin (a component structurally related to FK506), when complexed with yet another protein Raptor, mTOR binds to eIF-3 and coordinates the assembly of the initiation complex through a series of ordered phosphorylation events. First, mTOR/Raptor phosphorylates S6K1 in its hydrophobic motif (Thr-389), which then dissociates from eIF-3. Loss of S6K1 allows eIF-3 to join the mRNA and brings mTOR/Raptor near its next substrate 4E-BP. This is phosphorylated at multiple sites, provoking its detachment, and allows the association of eIF-4G to the initiation complex (Figure 8.15a,b). Importantly, binding of eIF-4G causes the interaction of the 5'-mRNA initiation complex with the 3'-mRNA poly A binding proteins (BAPBs) (Figure 8.15a,c). The circular mRNA structure thus created is thought to act as a critical step for driving translation. It may represent a mechanism to ensure that only intact mRNA is translated.

The partly phosphorylated and liberated S6K1 next associates with PDK1, which subsequently phosphorylates the activation segment (in a manner similar to the phosphorylation of PKB by PDK1 (Figure 8.15b). S6K1 is now fully active and phosphorylates the S6 ribosomal protein (rpS6) as well as eIF-4B, a regulatory subunit of the eIF-4A helicase. As eIF-2γ.GTP and tRNA^Met join the initiation complex, it starts to progress towards the 3' end until it reaches the AUG codon. Here it stops because of the tight association with the anticodon of tRNA^Met, and protein translation commences.

Insulin-mediated activation of ERK is without significant effect on glucose transport or the activation of glycogen synthesis, but it does have a significant effect on protein synthesis. This occurs through RSK1, one of the kinases downstream of ERK that phosphorylates TSC2 at sites different from those targeted by PKB, and it also causes inhibition of the GAP activity.

The loss-of-function mutations in TSC1 and TSC2 (also called "harmatin" and "tuburin," respectively) give rise to benign tumors called hamartomas, having the form of nodules or tubers, in brain, heart, skin, and kidney. TSC1 and 2 qualify as tumor suppressors. PTEN, which acts in the same signal transduction pathway, is also a tumor suppressor, but loss of its function is linked to Cowden disease in which patients have a predisposition to malignancies such as prostate cancer, glioblostoma, endometrial tumors, and small-cell lung carcinoma.

Rapamycin is a triene macrolide antibiotic obtained from the soil microorganism, *Streptomyces hygroscopius*, found in Rapa Nui (Easter Island). It binds to a cellular receptor protein FKBP12, and together they form a complex with mTOR and Raptor (mTORC1). This prevents interaction with substrates. Such inhibitory complex formation does not occur when mTOR is associated with Rictor (mTORC2). Raptor: **R**egulatory **a**ssociated **p**rotein of m**TOR** (rapamycin sensitive). Rictor: **R**apamycin **i**nsensitive **c**ompanion of m**TOR**.

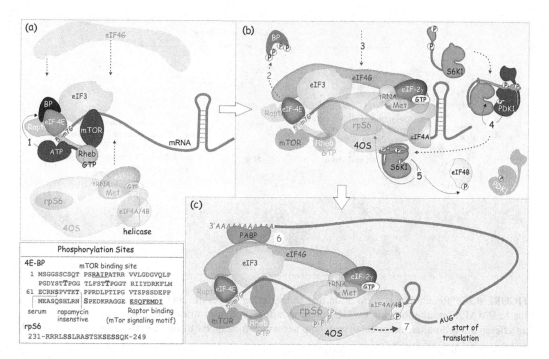

FIGURE 8.15 A series of ordered phosphorylation events facilitate the assembly of the translation initiation complex on the mRNA. (a) Activation and association of mTOR with the initiation complex causes the phosphorylation of 4E-BP (indicated as "BP") (1). Phosphorylated 4E-BP detaches from eIF-4E. (b) The dissociation of 4E-BP (2) permits the association of a big initiation factor eIF-4G that interacts with eIF-4E, eIF-3 and eIF-4A (3). Partly phosphorylated S6K1 is now fully activated by PDK1 through phosphorylation of its activation segment (4). S6K1 phosphorylates the ribosomal S6 protein (rbS6) and phosphorylates eIF-4B, a regulatory component of the RNA helicase that next joins the subunit eIF-4A (5). (c) The conditions are now favorable for binding of PABP (poly-A binding protein) which is attached to the 3'-poly A tail of the mRNA (6). The initiation complex now moves toward the start AUG codon (7) where it will be joined with the 60S ribosomal particle. **(See color insert following page 116.)**

8.4.3.2.6 *Control of Translation and Transcription*

Both the Ras/ERK and PI 3-kinase/PKB pathways have profound effects on the pattern of expression of individual proteins, independent of their effects on gene transcription. This has been demonstrated in mouse glial-progenitor cells after ectopic expression of constitutively activated forms of K-Ras or PKBβ. Here, poly-ribosome complexes engaged in the translation of mRNA that encode proteins involved in the regulation of growth, transcription, and cell–cell interactions are enriched. How the mRNAs are selected remains to be determined. Thus it seems that protein translation, in addition to gene transcription, is also an important target of transforming proteins (Figure 8.16).

In order to boost protein synthesis further, mTOR/Raptor also controls the nuclear transcription of the different forms of RNA required for ribosome biogenesis and formation of the translation machinery. It stimulates RNA polymerase-I, leading to the transcription of ribosomal RNA; RNA polymerase-II, leading to the transcription of mRNA coding for ribosomal proteins (about 82 in total); and RNA polymerase-III, which transcribes the 32 different transfer RNAs.

8.4.3.2.7 *Activation of PKB and the Regulation of Cyclin D Expression*

Another substrate of PKB is glycogen synthase kinase3β (GSK3β), whose phosphorylation causes its inactivation. As its name indicates, this protein kinase was originally discovered as a regulator

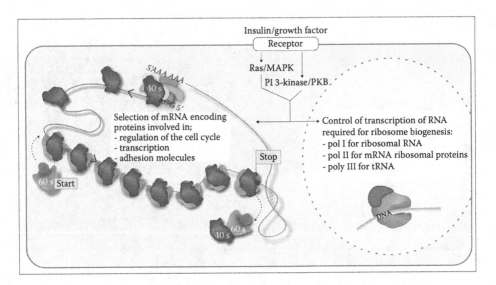

FIGURE 8.16 Regulation of translation and transcription by insulin and growth factor receptors. Both the Ras/MAPK and the PI 3-kinase/PKB pathway affect protein synthesis and gene transcription. This is an effective way to alter the cellular proteome necessary to respond to the signals of insulin and growth factors.

of glycogen synthase. GSK3β also plays an important role in the destruction of protein mediated via the ubiquitination pathway. When cylinD1 is phosphorylated by GSK3β it becomes ubiquitylated, a process that involved the addition of a number of small ubiquitin peptides in sequence, which serves as recognition signal for the proteosome. Phosphorylation and inhibition of GSK3β by PKB therefore prevents destruction of cyclinD1.

In addition, activation of PKB also enhances transcription of the cyclinD1 gene, although the signal transduction pathway causing this effect has not yet been revealed. The combination of an increased expression and a reduced destruction causes accumulation in the cell of the cyclinD1 protein. CyclinD1, associated with its catalytic subunit, cyclin-dependent kinase 4 or 6 (CDK4 or 6), is the driving force of the cell cycle during the G1 phase. It therefore is one of the most important cyclins in regulating cellular proliferation.

8.4.3.3 Direct Phosphorylation of STAT Transcription Factors

The simplest way by which a plasma membrane receptor can alter gene expression is through the direct phosphorylation of a transcription factor. The activation of transcription by interferons is an example. Transcription factors known as STATs are targets of interferon receptors, and they also mediate EGF and PDGF signaling. STAT1a (p91) and STAT1b (p84) possess SH2 domains, enabling them to associate with the phosphotyrosines of an activated receptor (Figure 8.17). Following binding, they themselves are phosphorylated on tyrosine residues, causing them to form a STAT dimer that can translocate to the nucleus. Here it promotes transcription of early response genes such as c-fos. The STAT dimer formed after phosphorylation by the PDGF receptor was originally described as Sis-inducible factor (SIF), because it was observed in cells exposed to the viral oncogene product v-Sis. This is closely related to PDGF and activates the same signal transduction pathway.

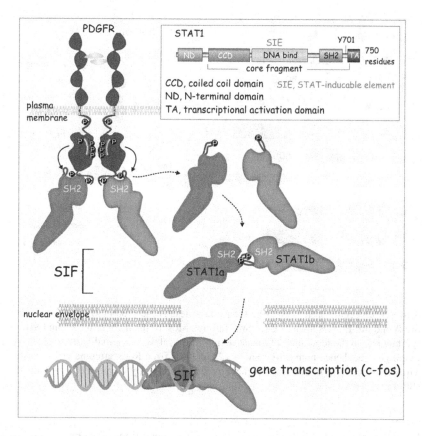

FIGURE 8.17 Direct phosphorylation of STAT transcription factors. Through their SH2 domains, STAT1a and STAT1b bind to the tyrosine-phosphorylated receptor and become phosphorylated. They then form a dimer, (called a Sis-inducible factor, SIF) which translocates to the nucleus, where it binds to a Sis-inducible element (SIE) within the fos promoter.

8.5 RECEPTORS THAT ASSOCIATE WITH TYROSINE PROTEIN KINASES

8.5.1 FAMILY OF NONRECEPTOR TYROSINE PROTEIN KINASES

This section deals with an important family of receptors that have no intrinsic catalytic activity but nevertheless induce responses similar to those of the receptor tyrosine kinases. The question of how they signal was resolved with the finding that many of these receptors recruit catalytic subunits from within the cell in the form of one or more NPTKs. These can be divided into 10 families (Figure 8.18). These proteins exist within the cytosol as soluble components, or they may be membrane-associated through farnesylation (C15 isoprenoid) or palmitoylation (C16) of the C-terminal region (Src, Fyn, Lyn, or Yes) or through the presence of a PH domain (Tec family members). A large number of vertebrate genes encode for NPTKs (a minimum of 33). Recruitment of NPTKs and the consequent tyrosine phosphorylations are usually the first steps in the assembly of a substantial signaling complex consisting of a dozen or more proteins that bind and interact with each other.

Examples of the class of receptors that recruit NPTKs include those that mediate immune responses:

- *T-lymphocyte receptor (TCR)*—Involved in detection of processed antigens, presented in the context of the major histocompatibility complex (MHC). Subsequently it regulates the clonal expansion.

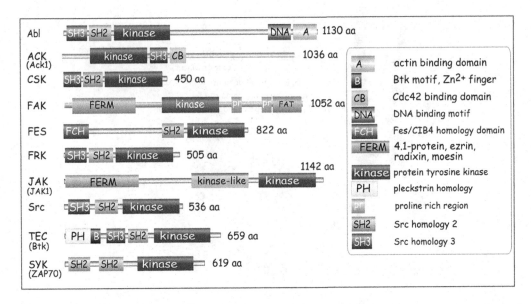

FIGURE 8.18 Nonreceptor protein tyrosine kinase families. These protein kinases are subdivided into 10 families (Src-A and Src-B are shown as one "Src" family). Most of them contain SH2 and SH3 domains that play an important role in the regulation of kinase activity. Several were originally discovered as transforming genes of a viral genome, hence names like Src or Abl, derived from Rous sarcoma virus or Abelson murine leukemia virus. The acronym in between brackets indicates the family member of which the domain architecture is illustrated.

- *B-lymphocyte receptor (BCR)*—Involved in the detection of nonprocessed antigens. Important for the elaboration of antigen-specific immunoglobulins necessary for the defense against infection by microorganisms.
- *Interleukin-2 receptor (IL-2R)*—The cytokine IL-2, secreted by a subset of T-helper cells, enhances the proliferation of activated T- and B-cells and increases the cytolytic activity of natural killer (NK) cells and the secretion of IgG.
- *High-affinity receptor for IgE (IgE-R) present on mast cells and blood-borne basophils*— This plays an important role in hypersensitivity and in the initiation of acute inflammatory responses.
- *Erythropoietin receptors*—The cytokine erythropoietin (Epo) plays an important role in the final stage of maturation of erythroid cells into mature red blood cells. For this reason it has been used by athletes to boost their performance in endurance sports such as cycling. The erythropoietin receptor is present on a number of cell types in addition to erythroid progenitor cells, suggesting that erythropoietin may have effects on other tissues, still to be discerned (see also Figures 4.14 and 4.15 in Chapter 4).
- *Prolactin receptors*—Involved in the regulation of lactation. In addition, prolactin has been implicated in modulation of immune responses. For instance, it regulates the level of NK-mediated cytotoxicity. It has also gained attention as a potential male contraceptive.

8.5.2 Mode of Activation of Nonreceptor Protein Tyrosine Kinases

The nonreceptor PTKs are a large group of signaling proteins that have diverse roles in the control of cell proliferation, differentiation, and death. Some are widely expressed; others are restricted to particular tissues. Their early classification was dominated by the discovery of pp60[src], to the extent that the major group of tyrosine kinases was simply known as the Src family.

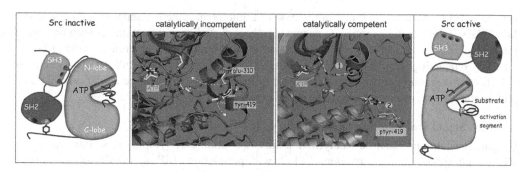

FIGURE 8.19 Regulation of Src kinase activity. Phosphorylation of the C-carboxy terminal tyrosine of Src causes binding of its own SH2 domain. This event places the SH3 domain adjacent to the N-terminal lobe of the kinase domain, which affects the coordination of ATP through a change in the position glutamate-310 in the C-helix. Detachment of the SH2 domain, through dephosphorhylation of the carboxy terminal tyrosine (or through binding of the SH2 domain to tyrosine phosphates of other proteins) removes this restraint (1). Subsequent phosphorylation of tyrosine-419 in the activation segment liberates the entry path for substrate (2); the protein kinase is now catalytically competent.

The Src family kinases share a similar structure. A unique domain at the N-terminus is followed by an SH3 domain and an SH2 domain (prototypes of the domains that are widely expressed). The SH2 domain is then attached by a linking region to a kinase domain and finally a C-terminal tail (see Figure 8.19). Many of these kinases function by becoming associated with macromolecular signaling complexes assembled at membrane sites. Regardless of their location, most Src family kinases are generally inactive. They are commonly held in this state by a crucial phosphorylated tyrosine (Y527 in the C-terminus of c-Src) that engages N-terminal SH2 domain. Furthermore, a sequence in the linker takes on a structure that resembles a proline-rich region, so that it binds to the SH3 domain. These interactions cause the molecule to adopt a compact structure. The bending of the carboxy tail causes a rotation of the smaller lobe of the kinase domain, which distorts the active site. Activation therefore requires removal of the C-terminal phosphate. This is made possible because the sequence of amino acids immediately adjacent to the phosphotyrosine in the C-terminal is not optimal for tight binding to the SH2 domain. SH2 domains bind phosphotyrosines most effectively when they reside in a pYEEI motif. The sequence in the Src C-terminus lacks the isoleucine at pY+3 and is not so tightly bound. This gives the opportunity for access by a phosphatase. Having lost the carboxy tail phosphate, the activation loop at the edge of the catalytic site can then become autophosphorylated, greatly increasing the catalytic activity. Activation of Src family kinases therefore requires first a dephosphorylation and then a phosphorylation.

8.5.3 T CELL RECEPTOR SIGNALING

8.5.3.1 Activation of T Lymphocytes, Interaction between T Cell Receptor and Major Histocompatibility Complex

T lymphocytes have a central role in cell-mediated immunity. When activated, they proliferate and differentiate to become either cytotoxic natural killer (NK) or helper T-helper (Th) T cells. Cytotoxic T cells kill specific targets, most commonly virus-infected cells, while helper T cells assist other cells of the immune system, like B lymphocytes, to induce the production of antibodies, and macrophages, to augment the release of inflammatory cytokines that enables an effective host defense. T lymphocytes are activated through interaction with cells that present antigen in the context of a major histocompatibility complex (MHC). The cell–cell interaction occurs in the following manner. The selective event is the recognition of an antigen placed in the groove of the MHC by the T cell receptor (TCR). In the case of an intracellular or viral antigen, protein fragments (antigens) are presented by MHC class I, and in the case of a microbial infection antigens are presented by MHC class II. Before the lymphocyte becomes fully activated, the interaction between the antigen presenting cell and the T lymphocyte has to be enforced by a number of other interactions, like CD4 (or CD8) interacting with MHC and B7 with CD28 (among others). The full response comprises induction of expression of IL-2 and its receptor followed by autocrine stimulation resulting in cell proliferation, an event also referred to as clonal expansion.

8.5.3.2 Signal Transduction Downstream of the T Cell Receptor

In spite of having no intrinsic catalytic domains, activation of T lymphocytes commences with tyrosine phosphorylations, activation of PLCγ with production of IP$_3$ and DAG, and elevation of cytosolic free Ca^{2+}. Thus, the consequences of receptor Ligation are not dissimilar from those induced by the receptors for EGF or PDGF. An early candidate explaining the induction of tyrosine kinase activity emerged with the discovery of the nonreceptor protein tyrosine kinase Lck (p56^{lck}), a T cell–specific member of the Src family. Lymphocyte-specific kinase (Lck) is associ-ated with the cytosolic tail of CD4 (in helper T cells) or CD8 (in cytotoxic T cells) (Figure 8.20). As mentioned, the extracellular domains of these molecules bind to the MHC protein, and this not only strengthens the rather weak interaction established between the TCR and the antigen, but it also brings CD4 (or CD8) into the vicinity of the TCR complex, leading Lck to its targets on the ζ–chains. However, as with other Src family kinases, Lck is inactive until specific residues have been dephosphorylated. This is accomplished by yet another transmembrane protein, CD45,

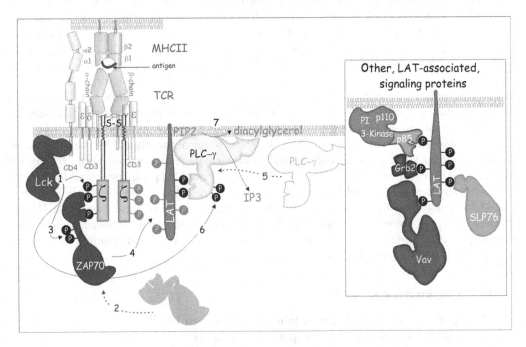

FIGURE 8.20 Signaling complex formation at the TCR complex. The TCR bound to antigen/MHC activates Lck that phosphorylates the two CD3 ζ-chains in the ITAM motif (1). The phosphotyrosine residues form a docking site for the SH2 domains of ZAP70 (2), another cytosolic PTK. ZAP70 is phosphorylated by Lck in the linker region between the SH2 domains and the catalytic domain (3). Phosphorylated and activated ZAP70, in turn, phosphorylates several (maximally nine) tyrosine residues on the transmembrane adaptor protein LAT (4). Various proteins attach onto LAT. These include PLC-γ (5), which upon attachment gets phosphorylated and activated by Lck (6). Other proteins are the guanine exchange factor Vav, the adaptor proteins Grb2 and SLP76, and the p85 regulatory subunit p85 of PI 3-kinase. All of these play important roles in the activation of the IL-2 gene. Production of diacylglycerol and IP3 (7) by PLCγ is an important starting point for the two signaling pathways described in more detail in this section.

that possesses protein tyrosine phosphatase activity. Loss of CD45 makes T-cell unresponsive to antigen signaling.

Activation of Lck results in the phosphorylation of the ζ-chains of the TCR. The target tyrosines are confined to amino acid sequences referred to as ITAM motifs (immunoreceptor tyrosine-based activation motifs). ITAMs are also present in the δ, γ, and ε chains of CD3 and are targets of another Src family kinase, Fyn (p59^{fyn}), associated with the ε chain. Fyn is also activated by dephosphorylation. Both Fyn and Lck are needed for efficient TCR signaling. Phosphorylation of ITAMs provides docking sites for SH2 domain-bearing molecules, and the immediate result is the recruitment of yet another nonreceptor protein tyrosine kinase ZAP-70 (ζ-chain-associated protein-tyrosine kinase of 70 kDa). Once bound, this in turn becomes phosphorylated and thereby activated, causing phosphorylation of multiple substrates. As with growth factor receptors, the sequence of events follows a pattern in which phosphotyrosines bind SH2-domain-containing (or PTB-) proteins that may themselves be PTKs, which can phosphorylate other proteins in succession. At each stage there is the opportunity for branching, through a range of effectors. By successive recruitment, an extensive signaling complex is assembled that includes multiple effector enzymes (Figure 8.20, insert). An important branch-point is offered by the integral membrane protein LAT (linker for activation of T-cells) that presents no less than nine substrate tyrosine residues. When phosphorylated, these recruit a broad range of signaling molecules, all through interaction with SH2-domains. These include the adaptor proteins Grb2 and SLP76 (SH2 domain-containing leukocyte protein of 76 kDa, an adaptor protein), the enzymes PLCγ and PI 3-kinase (through its p85 regulatory subunit), and the guanine nucleotide exchange factors Dbl and Vav.

The formation of a signaling complex around the TCR and the branching pathways that emanate from it resemble the mechanisms used by the growth factors. However, the destinations of these pathways are not all clear. We will elaborate on the PLCγ pathway (DAG, IP3, and elevation of intracellular free Ca^{2+}), which leads to the activation of the phosphatase calcineurin, which activates the transcription factor NFAT (nuclear factor of activated T cells) and leads to activation of PKCθ (theta) and ultimately activation of the transcription factor NFκB (Figure 8.21).

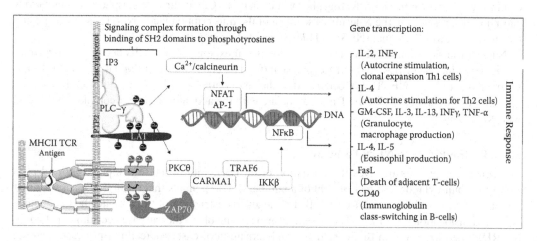

FIGURE 8.21 Two signaling pathways downstream of PLC-γ. Activation of PLC-γ results in the production of diacylglycerol and IP3. These second messengers activate two signaling pathways. One involves IP3-mediated release of Ca2+ from intracellular stores and result in the activation of the serine/threonine phosphatase calcineurin. This leads to activation of NFAT. The other involves the diacylglycerol-mediated activation of PKCθ, which phosphorylates the adaptor protein CARMA1. The unfolded protein acts as a docking site for the assembly of a TRAF6-ubiquitin ligase complex that results in the activation of IKKβ and subsequent nuclear translocation of NFκB. The genes whose transcription is regulated by NFAT and NFκB are involved in the regulation of the immune response. Expression of IL-2 is particulary important for the clonal expansion of the activated T cells (Th1 subtype).

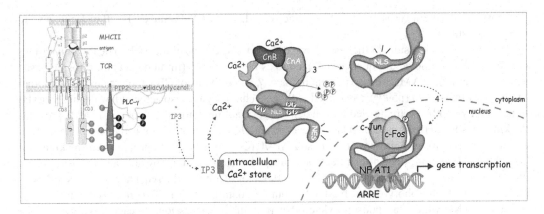

FIGURE 8.22 Calcineurin-mediated activation of NFAT1. Activation of PLCγ results in the liberation of IP3 into the cytosol. This binds to its receptor and causes release of Ca2+ from intracellular stores. Ca^{2+} binds to calmodulin (CaM) and calcineurin B (CnB), leading to the activation of the serine/threonine phosphatase PP2B. The phosphatase dephosphorylates numerous phosphoserine residues in the N-terminal segment of the transcription factor NFAT1, and this causes exposure of the nuclear localization signal (NLS) together with a masking of the nuclear export signal (NES). NFAT enters the nucleus and associates with c-Jun and c-Fos (AP-1 complex) to drive gene expression.

8.5.3.3   The PLCγ1 to NFAT Pathway

Phosphorylated LAT recruits PLCγ1 to the TCR/CD3 complex. This recruitment is facilitated by the concerted action of other proteins such as Vav1, SLP-76, Itk, and c-Cbl (not shown in the illustrations). In the complex, PLCγ1 is activated through phosphorylation by Lck (in the linker region between SH2 and SH3 at Y753 and Y759) (Figure 8.22). The consequent production of diacylglycerol, inositol-1,4,5-trisphosphate (IP_3) and elevation of Ca^{2+} leads to the activation of the serine/threonine phosphatase calcineurin (classified as PP2B or PPP3). This phosphatase is associated with two Ca^{2+} sensors, calmodulin and calcineurin B, each affecting phosphatase activity. Calcineurin dephosphorylates numerous phosphoserine residues in the N-terminal segment of the transcription factor NFAT, thereby exposing the nuclear localization signal (NLS) and hiding the nuclear export signal (NES).

Nuclear translocation of NFAT is essential for clonal expansion of T cells because of its pivotal role in the induction of IL-2 and INFγ expression (for Th1 cells) and IL-4 (for Th2 cells). Full transcriptional activity of NFAT only occurs after phosphorylation by ERK1 or -2 or p38. In order to drive full expression of IL-2, NFAT must associate with the activator protein-1 complex (AP-1) and with NFκB (see below).

8.5.3.4   The PLCγ1 to NFκB Pathway

In essence this process involves the formation of an E3 ubiquitin-ligase complex followed by a K63-type ubiquitylation and recruitment of a number of components that result in the activation of inhibitor of NFκB-kinase (IKK)-α and -β. This leads to destruction of the inhibitor IκB and hence nuclear translocation of NFκB. The assembly process involves the caspase recruitment domain (CARD), first discovered in the recruitment and activation of caspases (cellular proteases leading to apoptosis). All depends on the activation of PKC-θ (PKC-theta) by diacylglycerol in the lipid raft supporting the TCR-CD3 complex.

Activated PKCθ phosphorylates a rather big membrane-bound adaptor protein CARD-containing MAGUK protein-1 (CARMA1). This causes the protein to unfold, resulting in the attachment of the adaptor protein Cbl-10, through a CARD–CARD domain interaction. Cbl-10 is associated with the adaptor protein Malt1, which in turn binds to the TNF receptor-associated factor 6 (TRAF6) E3-ubiquitin ligase complex (comprising TRAF6, ubiquitin-conjugating enzyme 13 [Ubc13], and Mms2) (Figure 8.23). K63-type ubiquitylation of TRAF6 ensues, and this causes the recruitment of

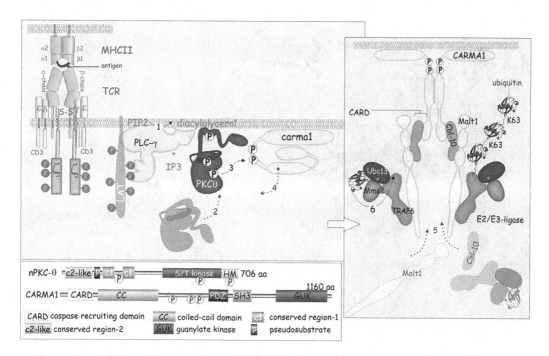

FIGURE 8.23 PLC-γ-mediated activation of PKCθ (theta) causes activation of the TRAF6 E3-ubiquitin ligase complex. The production of diacylglycerol by PLC-γ causes membrane attachment, followed by multiple phosphorylations and activation of PKCθ, a member of the nPKC subfamily, which lacks a functional C2-domain and therefore does not require Ca^{2+} for its activation. PKCθ phosphorylates the adaptor protein CARMA1 resulting in its unfolding. The CARD domain of CARMA1 recruits another adaptor, Cbl-10, via its CARD domain. This brings Malt1, TRAF6 (E3-ligase) and Ubc13/Mms2 (E2-conjugating enzyme) into the complex. As a result, TRAF6 is polyubiquitylated. The K63-type ubiquitin chain acts as a docking site for the NEMO/IKKα/IKKβ as well as the TAB1, -2/TAK1 protein kinase complex (not shown).

NFκB essential modulator (NEMO)/IKKα/IKKβ, as well as TAK1-binding (TAB1), -2, -3/TAK1 (Figure 8.24). K63-type ubiquitylation is not primarily involved in labeling proteins for destruction by the proteasome. The chain of ubiquitins act as docking peptides to which certain proteins can bind. One such protein is NEMO; it recognizes and binds the K63-linked ubiquitins. NEMO in turn is attached to IKK-α and -β, two serine/threonine protein kinases. The other is TAB2, and it is bound to the serine/threonine protein kinase TAK1 and its regulatory subunit TAB1. This is yet another example of how cells exploit posttranslational modifications to recruit proteins that form signaling complexes. The assembly of these protein kinase complexes allows phosphorylation and activation of IKK-β by TAK1. Activated IKK-β in turn phosphorylates IκB, and this makes the inhibitor susceptible to ubiquitylation (this type concerns a K48-type ubiquitination) by the SCF E3-ubiquitin ligase complex. Ubiquitylated IκB is destroyed by the S26 proteasome. The liberated NFκB now exposes its nuclear localization signal and translocates to the nucleus, where it participates in the induction of expression of interleukins together with the transcription factors NFAT and AP-1.

As already mentioned, full T cell activation requires a second, costimulatory signal, derived through the engagement of a separate receptor. For some helper T cells, this must be provided by CD28 on the lymphocyte that binds to the B7 molecule on an antigen-presenting cell. The signaling pathway activated by CD28 involves PI 3-kinase and *mammalian target of rapamycin* (mTOR), and it plays a crucial role in the expression of cyclin E necessary for T cell proliferation. In fact, prolonged occupation of both TCR and CD28 reduces the requirement of the autocrine IL-2 signal. The involvement of mTOR in the costimulatory signal explains why rapamycin, an inhibitor of mTOR (see Figure 8.14), acts as a potent inhibitor of T cell function (immunosuppressant).

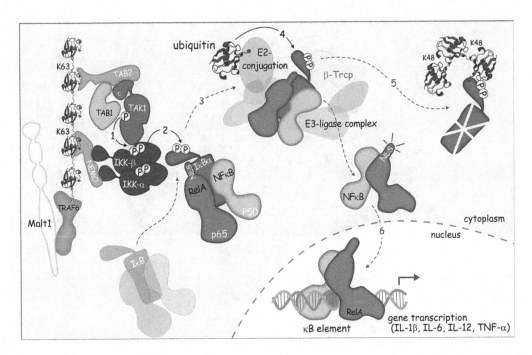

FIGURE 8.24 IKK-β-mediated activation of the RelA/NFκB complex. Phosphorylated/activated IKK-β phosphorylates IκB on two serine residues in its N-terminal domain, allowing its recognition by the SCF/bTrcp ubiquitin-ligase complex. Following ubiquitylation (K48-type), IκB is marked for destruction by the S26 proteasome, thus liberating RelA (p65) and NFκB1 (p50) and exposing their nuclear localization signal (NLS). They enter the nucleus, there to bind DNA at the kB-element, driving expression of inflammatory cytokines.

8.5.4 INTEGRINS, TYROSINE KINASES, AND CELL SURVIVAL

8.5.4.1 The Formation of an Integrin Signaling Complex

Integrins are adhesion molecules that can bind both components of the extracellular matrix, such as fibronectin, laminin, or collagen, and cellular adhesion molecules of the immunoglobulin superfamily, such as intercellular adhesion moleculer (ICAM) and vascular cellular adhesion molecule (VCAM). They often cluster in focal adhesion complexes at discrete sites on the cell surface. At these sites signaling complexes are formed, as well as extensive contacts with the actin cytoskeleton (stress fibers) or with intermediate filaments (in the case of hemi-desmosomes). The focal adhesion complex forms the site of attachment for the tyrosine kinase FAK (focal adhesion kinase) (Figure 8.25a). Although the focal adhesion targeting domain (FAT) has been described, it is unclear which structural component of the adhesion complex acts as the docking site for FAK: Both paxillin and talin having been suggested. Attachment, resulting in autophosphorylation and activation, enables FAK to act as a docking site for the tyrosine kinase Src (but also other members of the Src family of kinases such as Fyn and Yes). Src phosphorylates further tyrosine residues converting FAK into an SH2-domain docking protein. Besides binding SH2 domains, FAK also possesses two proline-rich regions, one of which interacts with the SH3 domains of CAS (Crk-associated substrate of tyrosine kinases). CAS, with its many tyrosine phosphorylation sites, acts as a docking protein attracting numerous SH2-containing effectors and adaptors (a role similar to IRS-1/2 for the insulin receptor or LAT in the case of TCR signaling). A lack of CAS prevents integrin-mediated FAK signaling.

The importance of FAK is underlined by the finding that cells expressing a constitutively active form of this tyrosine kinase survive in suspension, even though they are effectively "homeless." Here, FAK is active regardless of the failure to make contact with an extracellular matrix.

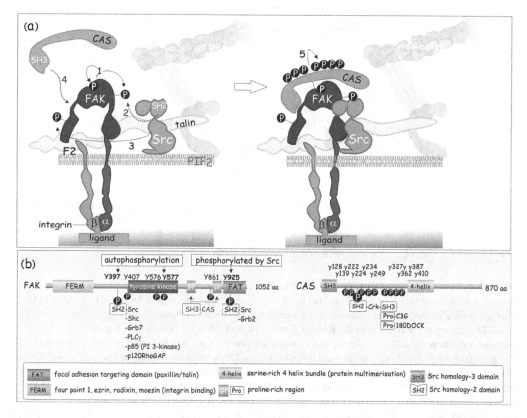

FIGURE 8.25 A two-step process to create an integrin signaling complex. (a) Once the structural components of the focal adhesion site have been put into place, the tyrosine focal adhesion kinase FAK associates with the FERM-F2 domain of talin. This causes its autophosphorylation on residue Tyr397 and on residue Y577 in the activation segment. (1) The phosphotyrosine at residue 397 acts as a docking site for the SH2 domain of Src. (2) Src binding causes a second phosphorylation of FAK, on residue Tyr925 (in the FAT domain). (3) Src and FAK next phosphorylate the FAK-associated docking protein CAS on multiple tyrosine residues. (4) An integrin-signaling complex is formed and this acts in a manner similar to growth factor–receptor signaling complexes, that is, attachment of adaptors and effectors and tyrosine phosphorylation of substrate. (b) Phosphorylated FAK and CAS act as docking protein to which several adaptors and effectors can bind. A signaling complex forms in a way similar to those surrounding the activated tyrosine kinase receptors.

The CAS protein family: CAS (Crk-associated substrate) (P56945) and EFS (embryonal Fyn-associated substrate (O43282)) are SH3-containing docking proteins with multiple tyrosine phosphorylation sites that interact with SH2 domains of Crk (adaptor) and Nck and Abl (tyrosine protein kinases). In humans, CAS was identified as a protein whose overexpression confers resistance to antiestrogen treatment (tamoxifen) of breast cancer (BCAR1). CAS is an important mediator of Src-mediated cell transformation. CAS phosphorylation correlates with inhibition of expression of Fhl1, a transcription factor. Loss of Fhl1 is a marker of anchorage-independent cell growth.

8.5.4.2 Focal Adhesion Kinase–Mediated Activation of Protein Kinase-B

Among the proteins that attach to tyrosine phosphorylated FAK is the p85-regulatory subunit of PI 3-kinase (bound to the catalytic domain p110) (Figure 8.26). This leads to the generation of 3-phosphorylated inositol lipids and the subsequent activation of PKB. It effects a number of phosphorylations which, if inhibited, prevent rescue from apoptosis. PKB promotes rescue by at least four

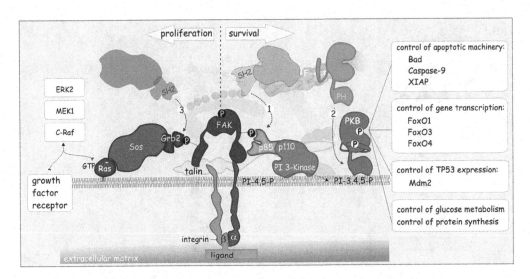

FIGURE 8.26 Adhesion-mediated survival. The focal adhesion site promotes cell proliferation signals through activation of Ras. The Src phosphorylated Tyr925 acts as a binding site for the SH2 domain of Grb2. This interaction recruits the Ras guanine exchange factor Sos to the membrane, leading to activation of Ras. Ras-GTP initiates the activation of the Raf-ERK pathway, necessary for initiation of the cell cycle. The focal adhesion site promotes cell survival signals through activation of serine/threonine protein kinase-B (PKB). The phosphorylated Tyr397 residue of focal adhesion kinase (FAK) provides a binding site for the SH2 domain of the regulatory subunit (p85) of the lipid kinase phosphatidyl inositol 3-kinase (PI-3 kinase). Subsequent production of PI-3,4,5-P3 provides a binding site for the PH domain of PKB (and PDK1). After its activation through phosphorylation of a serine (in hydrophobic motif) and a threonine (in activation segment) residue, PKB phosphorylates a large number of proteins that directly or indirectly deal with cell death (see text for further details).

different mechanisms (Figure 8.26). The first is by direct phosphorylation of components of the apoptotic machinery, like Bad, Caspase-9, or XIAP. Phosphorylation of Caspase-9 prevents its proteolytic activation while phosphorylation of Bad shifts its location from the mitochondrial membranes to the cytosol due to sequestration by 14-3-3 proteins. Since the phosphorylation site of human caspase-9 is not conserved in mouse and rat, it seems unlikely that this is a major control mechanism. Secondly, PKB acts to control transcription of a number of genes that regulate apoptosis by phosphorylating the three members of the FoxO subfamily of Forkhead transcription factors (FoxO1, FoxO3 and FoxO4, previously known as FKHR, FKHRL1, and AFX), causing cytosol retention, again by 14-3-3 proteins (phosphoserine binding scaffold protein). In this way, they are prevented from activating genes critical for induction of factors that promote cell death such as the Fas ligand, TRAIL (TNF-related apoptosis inducing ligand), TRADD (TNF receptor-1-associated death domain), and the pro-apoptotic protein Bim (Blc-2 interacting mediator of cell death). That this constitutes an essential survival mechanism is indicated by the finding that overexpression of FoxO3 triggers a program of cell death in the interleukin-3 dependent hematopoietic cell line Ba/F3. The death process is identical to the one observed after withdrawal of the BalF3 cells, for vital cytokine interleukin-3.

Another substrate of PKB is Mdm2 (mouse double minute-2, so called because the gene that codes the protein has been amplified on minute chromosomes present in cancer cells). Mdm2 is a component of an E3-ubiquitin ligase complex that ubiquitylates the tumor suppressor protein p53 (TP53). Poly-ubiquitylation of TP53 causes its destruction by the proteasome. Mdm2-assisted destruction of p53 occurs in cells that have undergone DNA damage ("genotoxic stress") but that aspire to prevent the TP53-mediated induction of apoptosis. PKB phosphorylation of Mdm2 causes its nuclear localization and renders TP53 ubiquitylation more efficient. As with Caspase-9, this mechanism of protection by PKB is operational in human cells, although the phosphorylation sites are not conserved throughout mammalian species.

PKB also protects against apoptosis by intervening in carbohydrate metabolism. When cells are starved of growth factors, nutrient uptake is severely reduced and they become quiescent. This may reach such a point that they fail to maintain their size, and this inevitably results in a loss of viability. The apoptotic process that ensues is due to the enhanced permeability of the mitochondrial outer membrane to cytochrome c. In cells starved of glucose, this is signaled by detachment of hexokinase from the mitochondrial outer membrane. Beyond its widely recognized role in phosphorylating glucose, hexokinase may also be involved in the linkage between the mitochondrial outer membrane pores and the inner membrane adenine nucleotide transporter, thus ensuring pore integrity selective transport (by an as yet unknown mechanism). Sustained activation of PKB prevents apoptosis of cells even in the absence of growth factors by maintaining the cell surface expression of the glucose transporter GLUT4. As a consequence, the activity and the mitochondrial association of hexokinase are maintained and leakage of cytochrome c is prevented.

The above-described processes are thought to represent the underlying mechanism of attachment-dependent cellular growth and survival. Without contact, epithelial cells die through the controlled process of cell death, apoptosis. In the case of cell detachment, the situation provoking programmed cell death has been called *anoikis*, meaning homelessness. The intrinsic drive of detached cells to self-destruct may protect the organism against dysplastic growth (meaning wrongly formed), preventing stray cells from colonizing inappropriate locations. The importance of FAK in all this is underlined by the finding that cells expressing a constitutively active form survive in suspension even though they are "homeless." Here, the protein kinase is active regardless of the failure to make contact with an extracellular matrix. Rescue from apoptosis also occurs when cells express constitutively activated oncogenic forms of Ras or Src, and thus activate PI-3 kinase and the MAP kinase pathway.

8.5.5   INTEGRINS, TYROSINE KINASE, AND CELL PROLIFERATION

8.5.5.1   FAK Signaling Reinforces the Ras-ERK Pathway

The formation of focal adhesion sites also is an essential requirement for the proliferation of tissue cells, driven by growth factors. If, for instance, EGF or PDGF are added to suspended fibroblasts, the activation of the MAP kinase pathway is merely transient and the cells fail to proliferate (and in the long run die through apoptosis). Proliferation only proceeds under the influence of two independent stimuli, one due to a growth factor, the other from adhesion molecules. With most integrins, the phosphorylated FAK binds the adaptor protein Grb2/Sos complex, causing activation of the Ras-ERK pathway (Figure 8.27). With some ($\alpha1\beta1$, $\alpha5\beta1$, and $\alpha V\beta3$), activation of ERK requires the palmitoylated kinase Fyn that links to the integrin α-subunit. Fyn is activated and binds, via its SH3 domain, to Shc. Shc is then phosphorylated, and this leads to recruitment of the Grb2/Sos complex.

An alternative route for the stimulation of ERK is through phosphorylation of CAS by Src/FAK (Figure 8.27b). Tyrosine phosphorylated CAS preferentially binds the SH2/SH3 adaptor protein Crk, which is either linked to the Rab1 guanine exchange factor C3G or to the Rac1 exchange factor 180DOCK (180 kDa downstream of Crk). This results in activation of both Rab1 and Rac1, leading to activation of B-Raf, resulting in prolonged activation of ERK, and leading to activation of JNK-1. The sustained signal ensures progression from G_0 to G_1 and entry into the cell cycle.

8.5.5.2   FAK-Mediated Activation Growth Factor Receptors

Growth factor receptors play a role in the activation of integrins, but the reverse is also true. A good example is the interaction between the integrin $\alpha V\beta3$ and the epidermal growth factor receptor (EGFR). Adherence to extracellular matrix causes phosphorylation of four tyrosine residues on the EGFR in a manner dependent on the adaptor protein p130[Cas] and the kinase Src. The number of receptors activated, and the number of tyrosines phosphorylated, is less than that induced by EGF,

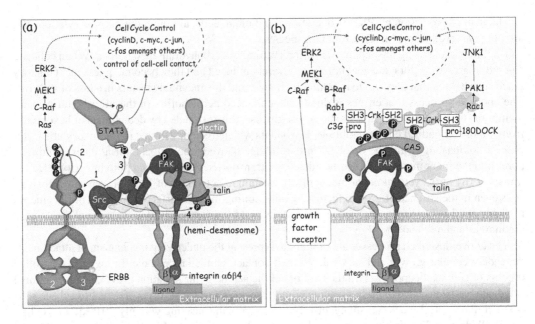

FIGURE 8.27 Adhesion-mediated cell cycle control. (a) In epithelial cells, intergrin α6β4, attached to the extracellular matrix, forms a special adhesion complex named hemi-desmosome. These complexes are linked to intermediate filaments via plectin (a protein that resembles plakoglobin). ERBB2/3 receptors are recruited into these complexes leading to phosphorylation of ERBB2 onTyr869 by Src bound to FAK (1). This phosphorylation promotes the catalytic activity of the tyrosine kinase domain of ERBB2 and enhances growth factor receptor signaling output. (Note that ERBB3 is kinase dead and cannot phosphorylate ERBB2). Src also phosphorylates STAT3, and this signal is enforced by a second phosphorylation on serine through ERK2 (3). Both phosphorylations enhance its transcriptional activity. In the case of breast tumor cells, this pathway promotes cellular invasion. Finally, the α4-integrin subunit is also a target of Src and this may affect its interaction with plectin (4). (b) Two examples of FAK signaling via the intermediate of CAS. The phosphotyrosines of CAS bind the SH2 domain of Crk. The proline-rich region (pro) of the guanine exchange factors C3G and 180DOCK bind the SH3 domain of Crk. Their recruitment to the focal adhesion complex causes the activation of Rabl and Racl. Rabl signals to B-Raf, which then phosphorylates MEK1, thus enforcing the growth factor receptor–stimulated Ras-ERK pathway, whereas Racl stimuates PAK1, which signals to JNK1. Both ERK and JNK stimulate expression of genes that initiate progression into the G1 phase of the cell cycle (cyclinD, c-myc, etc.).

and there is a failure to achieve a full cell proliferation response. Addition of EGF phosphorylates a fifth tyrosine residue on the EGFR, and so we understand that the full response to low levels of EGF requires the additional integrin-mediated phosphorylation of the receptor. The importance of the interplay between integrins and growth factor receptor is further highlighted by the finding that integrin α6β4 (forming adhesion structures called hemi-desmosomes) amplifies transformation of breast cancer cells overexpressing the ERBB2 receptor. This amplification occurs through Src-mediated phosphorylation of ERBB2 on tyr869 (Figure 8.27a). This tyrosine is normally not phosphorylated by the EGFR itself (see also Figure 8.3). Src also phosphorylates the transcription factor STAT3, and this event relates to enhanced invasiveness of the epithelial cells. This change of phenotype may be due to a STAT3-mediated loss of adherens junctions (cadherin/β-catenin).

Numbering of amino acids occurs in two different fashions. They either include the signal peptide of the protein or they do not. The data presented in Protein Data Bank (PDB) are often lacking the signal peptide, whereas Swiss Prot/TrEMBL includes it. Thus tyrosine 845 of the human EGFR (ERBB1) corresponds to tyrosine 869 because the signal peptide is 24 amino acids.

8.6   TERMINATION OF GROWTH FACTOR SIGNAL TRANSDUCTION PATHWAYS

The ability to terminate signals initiated by growth factors is crucial. There are numerous ways in which they may be attenuated, and these can operate at different stages. Here we limit the discussion to events affecting the growth factor receptor itself and the adaptors and effectors that bind to it.

A first mechanism of negative feedback is the removal of cell surface receptors through endocytosis. In the case of EGF, endocytosis following the application of low concentrations of the ligand actually induces a burst of signaling before suppressing it. This is due to a contribution from the internalized receptor, which still interacts with adaptors and effectors. Signaling effectively terminates when the receptors reach the late endosome and are degraded by acid hydrolases. Tyrosine-phosphorylated receptors are preferentially endocytosed and directed by vesicular transport to the late endosomal compartment, through the action of Grb2 and Cbl (an E3-ubiquitin ligase) (Figure 8.28). Both bind to receptors through their (atypical) SH2 domains and both play a role

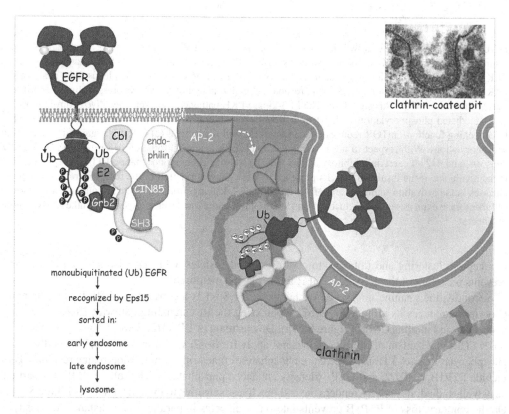

FIGURE 8.28   Removal of the EGFR from the cell surface and sorting into the lysosome pathway. Activated EGF receptors are recognized by Cbl, which either binds directly through a phosphotyrosine-binding motif or by interaction with the SH3 domain of Grb2. Cbl causes monoubiquitylation of the EGFR, and this acts as a sorting signal directing the receptor into the lysosomal pathway for degradation. The receptor-Cbl complex is recognized by CIN85 and endophilin, which couple the receptor to a complex of proteins that includes the key endocytic adaptor AP-2. The complex then recruits clathrin monomers. As a result, active EGFRs accumulate in clathrin-coated membrane pits, which then pinch off from the plasma membrane as endocytic vesicles. Within the intracellular network of vesicular transport pathways, the receptors are sorted into a pathway that takes them via the early and late endosomes towards the lysosome. They are thus destroyed.

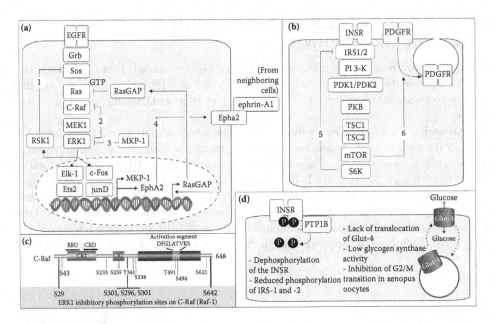

FIGURE 8.29 Attenuating growth factor signaling. (a) The Ras-ERK1 pathway has a number of feedback controls. The activated ERK1 or its downstream kinase RSK1 negatively feed back on Sos (1) and on C-Raf (2). ERK1 also induces expression of the dual specificity phosphatase MKP-1 (3), which leads to its deactivation. ERK1 also induces expression of the Epha2 receptor, which, if neighboring cells express its ligand ephrin-A1, causes attenuation of the Ras signal. (b) The PI 3-kinase/PKB pathway also exerts negative control, in part by S6K1-mediated phosphorylation of IRS1 and IRS2 (serine/threonine phosphorylations that block the SH2/PTB docking function). mTOR reduces expression of the PDGF receptor. (c) C-Raf is regulated by numerous phosphorylations. With respect to negative regulation by ERK1, phosphorylation of serine residues 29, 289, 296, 301, and 642 all exert an inhibitory action. (d) The tyrosine protein phosphatase PTP1B plays a key role in the regulation of the insulin signal. Its presence reduces phosphorylation of the receptor (removal of phosphatases in the activation segment) and of the IRS-1 and -2 docking proteins. The consequences are a lack of cell membrane expression of the glucose transporter Glut-4 and a low level of glycogen synthesis (symptoms of diabetes).

in receptor clustering and uptake into clathrin-coated vesicles. Cbl may also act as a marker that prevents recycling of the activated EGFR to the plasma membrane.

Secondly, the guanine nucleotide exchange factor Sos1 is a substrate of ERK1/2 and its phosphorylation reduces its affinity for Grb2, suppressing the Ras signaling pathway. ERK1 also phosphorylates and inhibits C-Raf (Figure 8.29a). Downstream of ERK1/2, RSK can also phosphorylate Sos1. (This mechanism of inhibition does not apply for Sos2, which lacks several serine/threonine phosphorylation sites.) Thirdly, there are phosphatases that strip the phosphotyrosine residues. They include PTP1B, SHP1/2, and DEP1 (density enhanced phosphatase). The role of PTP1B is particularly well studied; its activity renders the cell much less sensitive to insulin signaling (Figure 8.29d). On the contrary, loss of PTP1B prevents late-onset diabetes in parallel to a resistance to obesity in rats. This particular aspect of PTP1B is widely studied in order to define inhibitors that may treat both pathological states. Among the genes induced by ERK1 are the dual specificity phosphatase MKP-1, which dephosphorylates members of the MAP kinase family, and the Epha2 receptor. Expression of the Epha2 receptor creates a negative feedback loop when neighboring cells express its ligand ephrin-A1. Activation of Epha2 causes an elevated expression of RasGAP, thus attenuating the Ras signal (Figure 8.29a). Finally, mTOR and S6K1 also block growth factor signaling by phosphorylating the docking protein IRS1 or -2, and thereby inhibiting its docking function, and by reducing the expression levels of the PDGF receptor (Figure 8.29b).

THE CBL FAMILY PROTEINS

Cbl was discovered as an oncogenic protein v-Cbl, carried by the Cas NS-1 retrovirus, which causes B cell lymphomas in mice. The protein acts as an E3-ubiquitin ligase, and it plays a role in downregulating PTK-induced signaling pathways. It works by transfering ubiquitins at various sites to activated kinases. In the case of the EGF receptor and the TCR, this has the effect of directing the receptor to late endosomes, so preventing recycling to the outer membrane. Cbl also downregulates other effectors such as tyrosine phosphorylated Vav (RhoGEF), tyrosine phosphorylated STAT5, or the FcεRI in mast cells. The oncogenic form, v-Cbl, may act as an inhibitor of endogenous Cbl activity, hence preventing downregulation of a number of tyrosine protein kinase pathways. Finally, Cbl members also act as adaptors for numerous proteins such as PI-3 kinase, c-Src, tubulin, or yet another adaptor protein SLAP.

8.7 APPENDIX

8.7.1 Homologous Pathways in *Drosophila*, *C. Elegans*, and Mammals

This section is meant to explain how genetic studies with *Drosophila* and *C. elegans* have contributed to the discovery of the Ras signal transduction pathway operative in mammalian cells.

8.7.2 Photoreceptor Development in the Fruit Fly

The compound eyes of insects are formed of a hexagonal array of small units, ommatidia, (in the case of the fruit fly, approximately 800 "small eyes"). Each is composed of eight photoreceptor cells (R1–R8) and 12 accessory cells. On the basis of their morphology, order of development, axon projection pattern, and spectral sensitivity, the photoreceptor cells can be classified in three functional classes, R8, the first to appear, followed by R1–R6, and then R7. The photosensitive pigment resides in a microvillus stack of membranes, the rhabdomere. The larger rhabdomeres of cells R1–R6 are arranged as a trapezoid surrounding the rhabdomeres of cells R7 and R8, the R8 rhabdomere being located below R7 (Figure 8.30). The development of R7 requires the products of two genes, *sevenless* (*sev*) and *bride-of-sevenless* (*boss*). The phenotypes generated by loss-of-function mutations in either of these genes are identical, R7 failing to initiate neuronal development. These mutations are readily detected in a behavioral test. Given a choice between a green and a UV light, normal (WT) flies will move rapidly toward the UV source. Failure to develop cell R7, the last of the photoreceptor cells to be added to the ommatidial cluster, correlates with the lack of this fast phototactic response, and the flies move toward the green light.

While the *sev* product is required only in the R7 precursor, boss function must be expressed in the developing R8. Cloning revealed the boss product as a 100kD glycoprotein having seven transmembrane spans and related to the metabotropic receptors. Although ultimately expressed on all of the photoreceptor cells, at the time that R7 is being specified it is only present on the oldest, R8. The product of the *sev* gene is a receptor protein tyrosine kinase (member of the insulin receptor family). Evidence for direct interaction between the products of these two genes came with the demonstration that cultured cells expressing the *Boss* product tend to form aggregates with cells expressing *Sev*. It is now understood that the binding of Boss (the ligand) to Sev (the receptor tyrosine kinase) leads to the activation of kinase activity and that this ultimately determines the fate of R7 as a neuronal cell. Since a reduction in the gene dosage of the fly *ras1* impairs signaling by Sev, and persistent activation of *Ras1* obviates the need for the *boss* and *sev* gene products, it follows that the activation of *Ras1* is an early consequence of *Sev* activity.

Further genetic screens of flies expressing constitutively activated Sev led to the identification of two intermediate components of this pathway as *Drk* (*downstream of receptor kinase*) and *Sos*

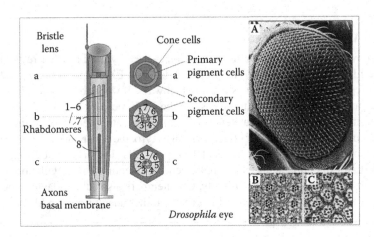

FIGURE 8.30 The sevenless mutation in fly eyes. The events leading to the development of cell R7 in eyes of *Drosophila* have provided a key to understanding the pathway downstream of receptor PTKs. Genes acting downstream of the sevenless receptor were revealed by screening for mutations that affect the development of cell R7. The eye of the fly (A) is built up of ommatidia, groups of eight photoreceptor cells each covered by a single lens. The drawing illustrates the basic anatomy of a single ommatidial unit in longitudinal section. Sections cut at a, b, and c are shown in transverse section on the right. Since two of the cells, R7 and R8, do not extend the full length of the ommatidial unit, the transverse sections b-b and c-c only reveal seven, not all eight, cells. The scanning electron microscope image shows the geometrical arrangement of ommatidia, units of eight photoreceptor cells. The thin sections B and C are both representative of cuts through section b-b in the drawing. Note that in B, taken from a wild type fly, seven cells are evident, while in C, taken from a fly having the sevenless mutation, there are only six. For further information, visit: http://flybase.bio.indiana.edu/.

(*son of sevenless*, see column 1 of Figure 8.31). The Sos protein shows substantial homology with the yeast CDC25 gene product, a guanine nucleotide exchange catalyst for RAS. While reduction in the gene dosages of *drk* and *sos* impairs the signal from constitutively activated Sev, there is no effect on signaling from constitutively activated Ras. Thus, in the pathway of activation, this places the functions of the *drk* and *sos* products into positions intermediate between Sev and Ras. The *drk* gene codes for a small protein consisting exclusively of Src homology domains, two SH3 flanking a single SH2 domain. Having no catalytic activity of its own, Drk acts as an adaptor. It binds to the tyrosine-phosphorylated receptor and links it to the proline-rich domains of Sos.

8.7.3 VULVAL CELL DEVELOPMENT IN NEMATODE WORMS

In the nematode *C. elegans*, a similar pathway of activation involving autophosphorylation of a tyrosine kinase receptor leads to activation of the GTPase Let-60, a homolog of Ras (column 2 of Figure 8.31). This determines the development of vulval cells (Figure 8.32). Again, these proteins were first identified from genetic analysis of lethal mutations (let, lethal mutants), morphological changes in vulval development (sem, sex muscle mutants), or alterations in cell lineage (lin, lineage mutants). They constitute the components of a signal transduction pathway based on Lin-3 (a product of the anchor cell), Let-23 (a tyrosine kinase receptor of the p5.p cell), and Sem-5 that associates with a (Sos-like) guanine nucleotide exchange protein. This brings about nucleotide exchange on Let-3 (Figure 8.32). Lin-3 and Let-23 are, respectively, members of the neuregulin (ligand) and ERBB (receptor) family.

In both nematode and fly, the Ras protein acts as a switch that determines cell fate. In *C. elegans*, the activation of Ras determines the formation of vulval as opposed to hypodermal (skin) cells. In *Drosophila* photoreceptors, the activation of Ras determines the development of R7 as a neuronal as opposed to a cone cell. In both cases, Ras proteins operate downstream of receptor tyrosine kinases that are activated by cell–cell interactions.

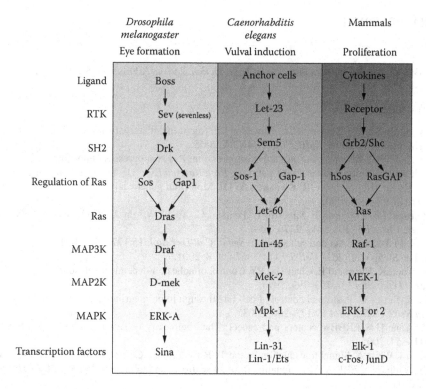

FIGURE 8.31 Comparison of signaling pathways activated by a receptor protein tyrosine kinase in species from different phyla. The striking homologies that exist between the proteins operating downstream of RTK in distant phyla have enabled the elucidation of the EGF receptor pathway.

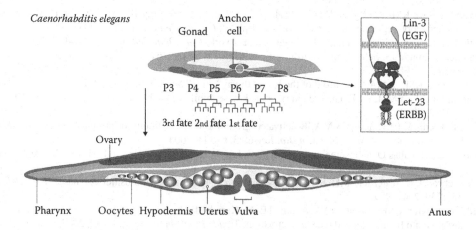

FIGURE 8.32 Vulval development in *Caenorhabditis elegans*. Because it is a relatively simple structure, formed from just a few cells, the vulva is well suited for the genetic analysis of cell differentiation during embryological development. It is the product of just three cell lineages, the descendents of cells p5.p, p6.p, and p7.p. Development is initiated by a signal from the anchor cell that lies adjacent to p6.p. The ligand, lin-3 (a homolog of EGF), produced by the anchor cell binds its receptor, Let-23, (homologous to the EGF-R) on the surface of cell p6.p. Cell p6.p in turn releases signals to its neighbors, p5.p and p7.p. This initiates a sequence of events involving the MAP kinase pathway that determines the fate of these cells as components of vulval tissue. For more information consult: http://www.wormbook.org/.

FURTHER READING

BOOKS

Gomperts BD, Kramer IM, Tatham PER. *Signal Transduction,* 2nd ed. AP/Elsevier, San Diego, 2010.

REVIEW ARTICLES

Braiman A, Barda-Saad M, Sommers CL, Samelson LE. Recruitment and activation of PLCγ1 in T cells: A new insight into old domains, *EMBO J* 25:774–784, 2006.

Cantley LC, Neel BG. New insights into tumor suppression: PTEN suppresses tumor formation by restraining the phosphoinositide 3-kinase/AKT pathway. *Proc Nat Acad Sci* (USA) 96:4240–4245, 1999.

Cheadle JP, Reeve MP, Sampson JR, Kwiatkowski DJ. Molecular genetic advances in tuberous sclerosis. *Hum Genet* 107:97–114, 2000.

Chen Z, Gibson TB, Robinson F, Silvestro L, Pearson G, Xu B, Wright A, Vanderbilt C, Cobb MH. MAP kinases. *Chem Rev* 101:2449–2476, 2001.

Downward J. PI 3-kinase, Akt and cell survival. *Semin Cell Dev Biol.* 15:177–182, 2004.

Elion EA. The Ste5p scaffold. *J Cell Sci* 114:3967–3978, 2001.

Frisch SM, Vuori K, Ruoslahti E, Chan-Hui PY. Control of adhesion-dependent cell survival by focal adhesion kinase. *J Cell Biol* 134:793–799, 1996.

Giancotti FG, Tarone G. Positional control of cell fate through joint integrin/receptor protein kinase signaling. *Annu Rev Cell Dev Biol* 19:173–206, 2003.

Hynes NE, Lane HA. ERBB receptors and cancer: The complexity of targeted inhibitors. *Nat Rev Cancer* 5:341–354, 2005.

Kane LP, Lin J, Weiss A. Signal transduction by the TCR for antigen. *Curr Opin Immunol* 12:242–249, 2000.

Kolch W. Coordinating ERK/MAPK signaling through scaffolds and inhibitors. *Nat Rev Mol Cell Biol* 6:827–837, 2005.

Krebs EG, Fischer EH. The phosphorylase *b* to *a* converting enzyme of rabbit skeletal muscle. *Biochim Biophys Acta* 20:150–157, 1956.

Kyriakis JM, Avruch J. Mammalian mitogen-activated protein kinase signal transduction pathways activated by stress and inflammation. *Physiol Rev* 81:807–869, 2001.

Luttrell LM, Lefkowitz, RJ. The role of beta-arrestins in the termination and transduction of protein-coupled receptor signals. *J Cell Sci* 115:455–465, 2002.

Macrae M, Neve RM, Rodriguez-Viciana P, Haqq C, Yeh J, Chen C, Gray JW, McCormick F. A conditional feedback loop regulates Ras activity through EphA2. *Cancer Cell* 8:111–118, 2005.

Martin DE, Hall MN. The expanding TOR signaling network. *Curr Opin Cell Biol* 17:158–166, 2005.

Miranti CK, Brugge JS. Sensing the environment: A historical perspective on integrin signal transduction. *Nat Cell Biol* 4:E83–90, 2002.

Morrison DK. KSR: a MAPK scaffold of the Ras pathway? *J Cell Sci* 114:1609–1612, 2001.

Robinson DR, Wu YM, Lin SF. The protein tyrosine kinase family of the human genome. *Oncogene* 19:5548–5557, 2000.

Roux PP, Blenis J. ERK and p38 MAPK-activated protein kinases: A family of protein kinases with diverse biological functions. *Microbiol Mol Biol Rev* 68:320–344, 2004.

Ruvinsky O, Meyuhas O. Ribosomal protein S6 phosphorylation: from protein synthesis to cell size. *Trends in Biochem Sci* 31:342–348, 2006.

Vanhaesebroeck B, Waterfield MD. Signaling by distinct classes of phosphoinositide 3-kinases. *Exp. Cell Res.* 253:239–254, 1999.

Ward CW, Lawrence MC, Streltsov VA, Adams TE, McKern NM. The insulin and EGF receptor structures: new insights into ligand-induced receptor activation. *Trends Biochem Sci* 32:129–137, 2007.

Weston CR, Davis RJ. The JNK signal transduction pathway. *Curr Opin Cell Biol* 19:142–149, 2007.

ARTICLES

Collett MS, Erikson RL. Protein kinase activity associated with the avian sarcoma virus Src gene product. *Proc Natl Acad Sci (USA)* 75:2021–2024, 1978.

Dijkers PF, Birkenkamp KU, Lam EW, Thomas NS, Lammers JW, Koenderman L, Coffer PJ. FKHR-L1 can act as a critical effector of cell death induced by cytokine withdrawal: Protein kinase B-enhanced cell survival through maintenance of mitochondrial integrity. *J Cell Biol* 156:531–542, 2002.

Ferguson KM, Berger MB, Mendrola JM, Cho HS, Leahy DK, Lemmon MA. EGF activates its receptor by removing interactions that autoinhibit ectodomain dimerization. *Mol Cell* 11:507–517, 2003.

Elchebly M, Payette P, Michaliszyn E, Cromlish W, Collins S, Loy AL, Normandin D, Cheng A, Himms-Hagen J, Ramachandran C, Gresser MJ, Tremblay ML, Kennedy BP. Increased insulin sensitivity and obesity resistance in mice lacking the protein tyrosine phosphatase-1B gene. *Science* 283:1544–1548, 1999.

Harvey JJ. An unidentified virus which causes the rapid production of tumours in mice. *Nature* 204:1104–1105, 1964.

Holz MK, Ballif BA, Gygi SP, Blenis J. mTOR and S6K1 mediate assembly of the translation preinitiation complex through dynamic protein interchange and ordered phosphorylation events. *Cell* 123:569–580, 2005.

Hunter T, Sefton BM. Transforming gene product of Rous sarcoma virus phosphorylates tyrosine. *Proc Natl Acad Sci USA.* 77:1311–1315, 1980.

Sun L, Deng L, Ea CK, Xia ZP, Chen ZJ. The TRAF6 ubiquitin ligase and TAK1 kinase mediate IKK activation by BCL10 and MALT1 in T lymphocytes. *Mol Cell* 14: 289–301, 2004.

Ushiro H, Cohen S. Identification of phosphotyrosine as a product of epidermal growth factor-activated protein kinase in A-431 cell membranes. *J Biol Chem* 255:8363–8365, 1980.

Zhang X, Gureasko J, Shen K, Cole PA, Kuriyan J. An allosteric mechanism for activation of the kinase domain of epidermal growth factor receptor. *Cell* 125:1137–1149, 2006.

Section V

Receptors as Pharmaceutical Targets

9 Receptors as Pharmaceutical Targets

*James W. Black**

CONTENTS

9.1 HORMONE RECEPTORS

The objective of pharmaceutical research is to discover and develop new substances that can be characterized by their selectivity and specificity. *Selectivity* describes the particular effects on physiological or pathological states that the substance can produce. These descriptions, such as hypnotic, hypoglycemic, hypotensive, and antiinflammatory, may be wholly empirical; however, this does not impede their therapeutic utility. Thus, the clinical utility of drugs such as morphine and digitalis was established long before we had biochemical explanations for their actions. *Specificity*, on the other hand, refers to the biochemical hypotheses that claim to explain the selectivity of a substance. Thus, activation of enkephalin receptors is proposed as the mechanism by which morphine acts, and inhibition of Na^+-/K^+-dependent adenosine triphosphatase (ATPase) has been claimed to specify the activity of digitalis. All kinds of biochemical events have been used to specify drug actions. Interactions with enzymes, ion channels, and membrane transporters have been widely used to explain drug actions. However,

---

* During production of the third edition of this book Sir James Black died on March 22, 2010. James Black was a pioneer in the application of careful quantitative pharmacology to the development of new therapeutic agents. He developed the first of the β-blocking drugs, propranolol, to relieve angina pectoris which subsequently became for many years a mainstay in the treatment of high blood pressure. His approach was to take the structure of the natural hormone and then in collaboration with medicinal chemists, make chemical analogues that would be effective antagonists with selective affinity for the receptor of interest, while lacking the agonist efficacy of the natural hormone. He used a similar approach to develop histamine H_2 antagonists for the treatment of stomach and duodenal ulcers. He shared the 1988 Nobel Prize for Physiology or Medicine with George H. Hitchings and Gertrude Elion. β-blockers and H_2-receptor antagonists have benefited millions of patients and often saved lives. By his example, Black made a massive contribution to establishing the importance of receptor pharmacology in drug discovery.

Professor Black graduated in medicine from St. Andrews University in 1946 and, after academic posts at the University of Glasgow, joined ICI as a pharmacologist (1958–1964) where he worked on the development of β-blockers. After working with Smith, Kline and French, where he developed the H_2 antagonists, he became Professor of Pharmacology at University College London (1973–1977), before joining Wellcome as the Director of Therapeutic Research (1978–1984). Since 1984, he was a professor of Analytical Pharmacology at King's College London.

pharmacological receptors are probably the favorite site of drug action used in explanatory models of their selective activity.

Receptor is a much-used term in biology: sensory receptors, telereceptors, mechanoreceptors, baroreceptors, chemoreceptors, T cell receptors, and so on. Plainly, *receptor* requires an adjective or prefix to be informative. As used here, a receptor is the site of action of hormones, neurotransmitters, modulators of various kinds, and autocoids. As yet, no class name has been agreed upon for the receptors associated with these agents; however, all of these agents fulfill the role of intercellular messengers. As this was the concept behind Bayliss and Starling's invention of the term *hormone*, it is convenient to think that a class of molecules (e.g., hormone receptors) has common features in the same way that a class of enzymes has common features. Thus, enzymes induce chemical changes in substrates without themselves being permanently changed in the process; that is, they are catalysts. By the same token, hormones change the chemical properties of their corresponding receptors without themselves being chemically changed in the process; that is, hormones rather than their receptors are behaving like catalysts. Thus, the hormone receptor both recognizes and responds to its conjugate messenger. For ease of writing, this is the collective sense in which receptors will be referred to in this chapter.

Hormones, broadly defined in this way as chemical messengers, can all be characterized by their selectivity and specificity. The selectivity of hormones describes their role in physiological and pathophysiological regulatory processes. The specificity of hormones refers to the evidence that they produce their effects by interacting with identifiable protein receptors. Hormones, then, have drug-like qualities, like a natural, physiological pharmacopoeia. This is the idea that makes hormone–receptor systems so attractive to pharmaceutical researchers. When new-drug researchers use the drug-like qualities of a hormone as the starting point, they are already a long way toward the goal of discovering a protodrug with desirable selectivity and specificity.

The selectivity of a hormone always entails the concepts of *affinity*, the likelihood of hormone and receptor interacting with each other, and *efficacy*, the response-generating power of the hormone that derives from activation of the receptors. These concepts are defined by parameters in classical thermodynamic models of hormone–receptor interactions. As these hormone-defining parameters are not readily accessible, even in radioligand-binding studies, the industrial pharmacologist usually settles for the empirical parameters of dose–response curves—namely, the maximum response and the dose required for half-maximal response. Modern pharmaceutical research based on hormone–receptor interaction is founded on measuring and interpreting dose–response curves. The target is the ability to manipulate hormonal efficacy as implied in dose–response curves. A significant fraction of a contemporary pharmacopoeia is about drugs that mimic, enhance, prolong, or abolish the efficacy of hormones.

9.2   PARTIAL AGONISTS: PROBLEMS IN DETECTING CHANGES IN EFFICACY

The author was introduced to the problems of efficacy and its expression in bioassays within months of starting his first project in pharmaceutical research while using isoprenaline, a fully efficacious analog of the hormones noradrenaline and adrenaline, to drive the rate of beating of the isolated guinea-pig heart (the Langendorff preparation) via activation of β-adrenoreceptors. Soon after beginning the project, the dichloro analog of isoprenaline, DCI, was described as an antagonist of isoprenaline on bronchial muscle. However, in our cardiac preparation, we found that DCI was as efficacious as isoprenaline itself. Subsequently, the Langendorff preparation was replaced with the rate-controlled guinea-pig papillary muscle preparation. On the new preparation, DCI had no agonist activity but was now a competitive antagonist of the catecholamines. The subsequent rapid development of β-adrenoreceptor antagonists was based on this observation. The tissue-dependence of the efficacy of DCI was puzzling, so we were not prepared for a second encounter with the phenomenon.

The second encounter occurred several years later when our laboratory switched interests to histamine antagonists. No *in vitro* assays for studying histamine-stimulated gastric acid secretion were known at that time, so we used the anesthetized rat lumen-perfused stomach preparation (the Ghosh and Schild preparation). The guanidino analog of histamine (IEG) was one of the first compounds tested. For practical purposes, IEG behaved like a fully efficacious agonist. Several frustrating years later, it was found that IEG was not quite as efficacious as histamine. When IEG was dosed during a plateau of a maximal secretory response to histamine, a small degree of inhibition was revealed. The subsequent rapid development of histamine H_2-receptor antagonists was based on this observation. It was eventually found that had the rat isolated uterus preparation been used for the screening bioassay, it would have immediately shown that IEG was much less efficacious than histamine.

Both DCI and IEG are now classified as partial agonists. Partial agonist, by definition, is a comparative description. When substance B is unable to produce as large a maximum response as substance A in a particular tissue, and when they can be shown to be producing their effects by acting on the same population of receptors, then substance B is defined as a partial agonist. This is a very limited definition, however. These initial observations with DCI and IEG are now generally recognized. The expression of partial agonism is tissue-dependent in a very sensitive way. DCI would have been classified as a full agonist as judged by heart-rate changes and as a simple competitive antagonist as judged by papillary muscle contractions. The variations in the expression of efficacy between closely related analogs of a hormone acting on a particular tissue and the variations in the expression of efficacy by a particular analog acting on different tissues have both practical and theoretical implications.

Kenakin and Beek published a beautiful data set comparing the activities of isoprenaline (classified as a full agonist) with prenalterol (classified as a partial agonist) on six different tissues. Across the tissues, the potency of isoprenaline varied by two orders of magnitude: in tissues where the potency of isoprenaline was very high, the efficacy of prenalterol was also very high, nearly the same as isoprenaline. Where the potency of isoprenaline was low, prenalterol had no detectable agonist activity and, indeed, now behaved like a competitive antagonist. From the point of view of pharmaceutical research the implications are clear. Try to find several tissues that will express the activity of the hormone of interest. The relative potencies of the hormone can point to the likelihood that a particular tissue will expose the efficacy of a partial agonist. In pharmaceutical research, it is necessary in the early stages of a hormone-receptor-based project to be able to detect small changes in the efficacy of hormone analogs. An assay without too much amplification is needed. However, in the later stages of the project (for example, when compounds have been discovered that behave like simple competitive antagonists), high-efficacy amplification systems are required to detect signs of residual agonist activity.

From a theoretical point of view, the efficacy of an agonist in the tissue is dependent on the ratio between the well-understood concept of receptor density and the much more opaque concept of "some kind of coupling factor," the intrinsic ability of bound receptor to generate an intracellular stimulus. The possibility that the same class of receptors might have different coupling efficiencies in different tissues cannot be ignored; however, differences in the density of receptor expression between tissues is now well recognized and is the most attractive way of interpreting the tissue dependence of efficacy. The attractiveness of the concept is not just because of its simplicity but also because it points to a way in which the new technology of controlling the expression of cloned receptor genes can be harnessed to generate new systems to detect and measure efficacy. Although these new receptor expression systems are an interesting extension to the range of bioassays, they are in no sense a replacement for traditional bioassays based on intact, isolated tissues *in vitro*.

9.3   THE VALUE OF BIOASSAYS

The essence of using intact-tissue bioassays in a hormone-related pharmaceutical project is that the hormone can be used to light up its population of conjugate receptors in a conceptually simple biomolecular interaction. If the resulting events are dominated by this initial binding interaction, as described by the Hill equation, rectangular hyperbolic dose–response curves are likely. Simple hyperbolic dose–response curves are certainly found in *in vitro* bioassays, but departures from such simplicity are much more common. We are continuing to understand the different events that can lead to complicated dose–response curves. The receptors themselves can be a source of distortion. The dynamics of receptor expression can introduce variation due to internalization or desensitization. However, the most common receptor-mediated complicating factor occurs when the hormone activates more than one population of receptors. Disclosure of receptor heterogeneity is always interesting and challenging. The problem facing the pharmaceutical researcher is what to do about the discovery. The current climate is that we should always be trying to find more and more specific ligands. However, when a hormone activates more than one set of receptors to produce the same end result, albeit by different processes of transduction, it may be practically more prudent to search for highly nonselective ligands. This may be the best way to reach the goal of desirable selectivity.

The hormone itself can introduce complexity into bioassays. Many hormones must now be seen and understood not as chemical entities but as chemical pathways where hormonal activity is distributed across a number of chemical species. The more we learn about the pharmacological properties of members of a pathway, the more we are realizing that each one has a mix of common and unique properties. The practical point is that we must be careful about which "hormone" we choose to drive our bioassays. A hormonal chemical pathway may contain sinks as well as sources. Metabolism and uptake of a hormone can introduce significant distortions into bioassays. All of these factors leave their fingerprints on dose–response curves, and a pharmaceutical researcher developing a new bioassay has to learn to read the signs.

A particularly exciting challenge to industrial pharmacologists occurs when the cells that synthesize the hormone, with or without storage, are found in the same tissue as their conjugate receptors. For example, these cells can be neurons, mast cells, or enterochromaffin cells. Controlled release of synthesized or stored substances can be achieved by either chemical or electrical stimulation. Intact-tissue bioassay in this mode of indirect agonist offers two exciting opportunities. First, tissue architecture constrains and directs the release of substances to particular cellular targets in a manner that may not be achievable by the hormone diffusing into the tissue uniformly from the organ bath compartment. Second, indirect release may be capable of producing a composite of coreleased substances that potentially can interact with each other. Both of these phenomena are clearly recognized now and offer opportunities to the pharmaceutical researcher. Potentiating interactions at the postreceptor level occurring between coreleased substances offer a particularly important opportunity for the future of drug research.

9.4   ARE BIOASSAYS VALUABLE IN PHARMACEUTICAL RESEARCH?

So far, we have reviewed the various ways in which complex dose–response curves in intact-tissue bioassays can be the pharmacological resultant of two or more interacting activities. Now, if all that these bioassays achieved was to blur and obscure the underlying activities, they would have to give way to the newer, analytically simpler assays based on chemistry and biochemistry. However, the beauty of intact-tissue bioassays is that they are analytically tractable; by using families of dose–response curves and appropriate mathematical models, the complexity of intact hormone–receptor systems can, indeed, be interpreted. Bioassay allows them to be studied as systems in ways denied to simple biochemical assays.

Are intact-tissue bioassays capable of being stand-alones, initial technology for discovering new drugs in hormone–receptor-directed pharmaceutical projects? The answer, based on our own experience and much published evidence, must be positive; but without a doubt, *in vitro* bioassays are slow, resource intensive, and expensive, and require skilled investigators. The questions today are about whether we can economize on these bioassays or even eliminate them altogether by using more productive chemical screens. Radioligand-binding assays are an obvious example. They have been widely used in the industry for many years, but we do not know how their use is optimized in relation to bioassay, even after several years of personal experience observing radioligand-binding assays running alongside bioassays for both gastrin and cholecystokinin receptors. Every compound we have made has been evaluated in both kinds of assay. No doubt and not surprisingly, we have obtained much more information about new compounds using bioassay; however, in retrospect, could we have economized on the bioassays by using binding assays to select out inactive compounds? The judgment at this time is that we would have missed some interesting compounds. To some extent, this is a matter of style more than tactics. In the main, all of the compounds made in our program have been designed to try to answer a question about structure–activity relations. Several thousand dollars will have been spent in making each of them. As a result, a trivial biological evaluation of the binary type, 0 or 1, is inappropriate. At issue is the struggle between biologists and chemists to learn to understand and trust each other. It is not too much of a caricature to see that the chemist believes that every molecule he struggles so hard to make will have interesting properties if only the biologist would evaluate it adequately; the biologist, on the other hand, is convinced that his assays will reveal the desired properties of a molecule if only the chemist would make the right compound. Our experience shows it takes at least two years of continuous collaboration before the chemist and biologist really learn mutual trust!

9.5 THE ITERATIVE PROCESS OF DRUG DEVELOPMENT

A medicinal chemist is involved in a new hormone–receptor-targeted drug project right at the start. To get involved, enough of the structure of the hormone needs to be known to allow all the possible shapes of the molecule to be visualized by physical valence-wire models, by space-occupying nuclear models, or, nowadays, by various computerized simulations on a computer. Whatever way is chosen, these chemists, in principle, walk around the molecule in their mind as they carry out imaginative interrogations: What is it about this molecule that interests me as a chemist? Where are the likely sources of noncovalent interactions and the receptor-ionic charges, electron densities on carbonyls and amino groups, pi-electron systems, and so on? Today, chemists may have additional information from the molecular modeler about conformational probabilities. Whatever the input to their imagination, medicinal chemists distill out a single first question, a question that they believe they can try to answer by making a simple analog or derivative of the natural hormone. Of course, the question cannot be answered with surgical precision. Every precise change in the molecule produces many more consequential changes in its conformation, in charge distribution, in electrostatic fields, and so on, which ensure that the chemical question will likely have an opaque biological answer the first time around.

Answers to the chemists' questions are provided by bioassays. Because there are questions to be answered, every biological result, including (even especially) that the new molecule is totally inactive, is full of interest. Whatever the result, a new question is raised, a new inquisitorial compound has to be made, a new biological test has to be carried out. This iterative process is, in principle, at the heart of all traditional hormone–receptor pharmaceutical research programs; however, in practice, the process cannot be driven like this as a single logical cycle. Generally speaking, compounds take longer to synthesize than to evaluate in bioassay. On average, a medicinal chemist will produce 15 target compounds per year, so a team of chemists are usually involved, working in parallel on parceled-out parts of the perceived problem. The molecular modelers, who are also part of the iterative loop, also have to work at a different rhythm from either the synthetic chemists or biological analysts; nevertheless, the principle of the interrogative loop is always in play.

During our lifetime, we have witnessed continuous and extraordinary advances in medicinal chemical technology, chemical analytical methods, and chromatography, but the most spectacular changes seen in about 40 years of pharmaceutical research have been in molecular modeling. The pharmaceutical industry has made a huge investment in this runaway technology. I sense, though, a certain amount of industrial disappointment in the yield from this investment and would agree that molecular modeling has not dramatically shortened the number of iterative loops in going from a hormone to a hormone-based compound with potential clinical utility. However, this is to miss the point. Three features of molecular modeling are no longer in doubt. The technology is allowing us to tackle problems, such as the ubiquitous polypeptide hormones, that would have been logically and imaginatively impossible 20 years ago. The technology continues to advance with breathtaking speed, a speed that would have been impossible without the earlier major investments. The technology is making a greater and greater contribution to the synthetic chemist's imagination. As far as molecular modeling is concerned, this author is a junkie.

9.6   ME-TOOISM

The logical, imaginative, and iterative approach to new drugs based on hormone–receptor systems sketched out above stands in marked contrast to the industrial approach we experienced 40 years ago and to the direction in which the industry is now moving compulsively at hectic speed. In the past, industrial research was criticized for its practice of random screening and for its generation of "me-too" drugs. Of course, the biological screening was not random; far from it, as the screening tests were chosen with great care to reflect identified medical needs. Pharmacologists tried to reflect the importance of meeting medical needs by using experimental pathology paradigms for screening tests. Thus, assays were often based on experimentally induced animal pathology such as sterile inflammatory responses to foreign bodies such as cotton–wool, or turpentine, or arthritis induced by antigen–adjuvant presentation, or stomach ulcers induced by histamine or aspirin, or convulsions induced by leptazol or electricity, and so on. The compounds screened were not chosen at random, either. They were chosen by working one's way, systematically, through the company's accumulated compound collection, its database, or by systematically ringing the changes of substituents in a lead molecule epitomized by "methyl, ethyl, propyl, butyl, futile"! The intellectual sterility of the process was not because of randomness but because of the lack of a necessary connection between the chemistry and bioassay.

In parentheses, the critical charge of me-tooisms was also, I believe, misplaced. To some extent, I can accept the commercial charge of me-tooism. Premium prices have undoubtedly been asked for compounds with clinically insignificant acute differences, but side effects become recognized on a slow, time-dependent basis. Therefore, inevitably, the older drug has accumulated more reports of side effects on its data sheet and the newer me-too drug can be pedaled by marketing manipulators as "just as good but safer." Personally, I do not have such a cynical view of me-tooism, and there are two reasons for this. Me-too drugs establish the image-challenging thought that compounds having quite different chemical structures can nevertheless have congruent pharmacological properties. The concept of such classes of drugs is the basis of pharmacology. Second, while the different chemical structures have one feature in common, they invariably present often usable and important differences in their pharmacokinetic and toxicological profiles.

9.7   SHORT-TERMISM

As indicated, the development of hormone–receptor-based research programs has changed all that. The logical, imaginative, iterative approach that has been painted has been shown to work regularly and reliably. The record is clear. If you follow John Locke's advice of "steadily intending your mind in a given direction," you will succeed; however, the fact is that the number of iterations and years it will take is entirely unpredictable. This has become a significant problem, as the pharmaceutical industry has allowed itself to be pressured into short-termism as an antidote to exponentially escalating costs of research and development, particularly thanks to extensions to the drug regulatory requirements and to development costs. Consequently, the emphasis today is on speed, on what is called *high-throughput screening*. The potential for high-throughput screening is based on the spectacular advances in immunological and molecular biological technology made in the last 10 years or so. A whole range of procedures is now available that includes cloned receptor genes cotransfected with reporter genes in cell lines or, with even greater chemical purity, assays such as the scintillation proximity assays, where the pure chemical receptors are bound to beads that house the scintillant, thus solving the distance problem. All of these new assays can be executed robotically, and all of these new assays have the following features in common. They are ingenious. They are fundamentally chemical and not biological assays. They are highly productive but express the absolute minimum of information (presence or absence, 0 or 1). Fundamentally, these are automated assays. Important questions are not being asked, so intelligent analysis is compromised. Nevertheless, do these productive, automated, assays provide a greater, faster yield of chemical leads?

At this moment, the question has yet to be answered, but a vital complementary question also must still be answered. Where are the compounds to come from to feed the assays, which can consume around 2000 or more chemicals per week? The immediately obvious sources are the in-house compound libraries. The major drug-research-based companies now have anywhere between 0.5 and 1 million compounds in their compound libraries. So a research program that can assay about 2000 compounds per week will be kept occupied for at least a few years just working through its own library. The problem with in-house libraries is that they are not an ensemble of randomly structured organic molecules. The distribution is severely lumpy. By that I mean that many of the synthesized molecules will be in closely related groups, having been synthesized for previous programs, successful as well as unsuccessful. Unless one is irredeemably optimistic, this may not be an ideal pool of molecules to trawl for new leads.

9.8   COMBINATORIAL CHEMISTRY

The hunger at the heart of this new passion for high-throughput screening has to be satisfied from some other generous source of new compounds for screening. Swapping by contract and purchasing by corporate takeover or amalgamation are obvious approaches, but they are very expensive, offer limited strategies, and do not avoid the lumpiness problem. Fortunately, advances in chemistry have been as extraordinary as the advances in molecular and genetic biology. Combinatorial chemistry is the name of the new game.

I have no personal experience with combinatorial chemistry, but the technology for making large numbers of molecules coupled to appropriate chemical selection procedures began with laboratory experiments to study molecular evolution in purely chemical systems. Spiegelman and coworkers started with a bacterial phage, one of whose four genes was a replicase enzyme, to make copies of itself. They showed that repeated exposures *in vitro* of viral RNA, the replicase, and supplies of the four nucleotides led to entirely new RNA sequences with a 15-fold increase in replication rate; the mutations arose from errors in replication. Subsequently, combination of methods to induce mutations in RNA or DNA, plus repeated steps of amplification by PCR (polymerase chain reaction), has led to the ability to generate up to 10^{13} sequences of single-strand DNA. These can then be screened on columns on which are bound an appropriate protein. A high-affinity DNA ligand for thrombin was discovered in this way. When organic chemists took over from molecular biologists, they developed the techniques for generating libraries of 10^6 to 10^7 peptide sequences. The reactions and the assays were carried out on beads. The technology has advanced by introducing control of sequence development plus the ability to tag each sequence for ease of identification.

Synthesis of constrained peptide sequences has now been followed by combinations of nonpeptide molecules. As greater constraints are introduced, the numerical productivity falls, but presumably the proportion of leads increases.

Combinatorial chemistry is now a rapidly developing activity which, as a technology, is attracting the attention of highly ingenious chemists. At this time, it is impossible to predict where this technology will lead us. We do not know whether some of the basic limitations will be overcome. At this time, all the methods are restricted to binary reactions that take place readily. This is in contrast to the problems facing a synthetic chemist who wants to make a specified molecule. Not only are a number of sequential steps needed, but also many of the stages require demanding conditions for the reactions to occur. Thus, it is difficult to see how combinatorial chemistry can, in the near future, be the basis for the iterative, interrogative approach to hormone–receptor-related ligands.

High-throughput screening of databases plus input from combinatorial chemistry is designed to generate leads. As I understand the process, leads will then be developed using more conventional methods. The assumption seems to be that finding leads is the rate-limiting step in the drug discovery process. Now, I am not convinced that this is so. Developing and optimizing leads into clinically testable new chemical entities (NCEs, as they are termed in the industry) is usually a much slower phase. However, the productivity of the industry, as judged by the discovery of completely new drugs, is limited more by the choice of targets than by the discovery of leads. Care in choosing a target is the most critical decision point in pharmaceutical research.

9.9   SELECTING TARGETS FOR DRUG DEVELOPMENT

My personal approach to choosing targets is to seek answers to six questions:

1. Is the project purged of wishful thinking?
2. Is a chemical starting point identified?
3. Are relevant bioassays available?
4. Will it be possible to confirm laboratory-defined specificity in humans?
5. Is a clinical condition relevant to this specificity?
6. Does the project have a champion?

The wishful-thinking criterion is the most important of all. All drug-discovery projects begin with a desire to prevent illness or treat sickness. Wishful thinking refers to the tenuousness of the perceived relationship between that desire and the means proposed to satisfy it. The most common example today is the claim made again and again: once we know the gene product, then we will be able to find new drugs. So far, no one has shown that this will be likely or even possible. Fortunately, most hormone–receptor-directed projects are relatively free of wishful thinking as far as discovering a ligand is concerned, although the potential utility of the ligand might well be fanciful. Fortunately, again, a hormone–receptor project has a chemical starting point, the hormone itself. We are inclined here to an assumption that we cannot prove; namely, that in seeking new ligands based on the chemistry of the hormone we stand a fair chance of retaining the evolutionarily derived selectivity of the hormone. Hormone–receptor targets also score well on the bioassay criterion. Very often the bioassay expresses an important feature of the selectivity of the hormone. Ideally, efficacy detection offers advantages: for example, in having several bioassays including radioligand-binding assays to choose from. Assays based on different species can be very valuable. An important criterion, I believe, is to develop ligands whose activity is not species-dependent— the most reliable predictor for extrapolation to humans.

In choosing a target, it is important to imagine how to investigate the proposed new ligand in humans. Will we be able, in practice as well as in principle, to confirm the selectivity of the ligand as defined in the laboratory experiment? This can be particularly challenging in relation to central nervous system (CNS)-directed compounds. However, most of the hormones, transmitters, and modulators found in the brain are also found in the gut, so perhaps the specificity of a CNS ligand can be evaluated in the periphery. It is also important before choosing a target to imagine what clinical disorder might be explored by the new specific ligand. No commercial judgment should be involved at this point. The only test is feasibility. For drugs with a new, previously unavailable specificity, plenty of evidence shows that prior commercial assessment is rarely valid. When a drug is developed with a specified mode of action, physicians will have the opportunity to explore unanticipated disorders.

The last question usually has an obvious answer: the need for a champion. The need derives from the common experience that drug research programs often go through lengthy periods of stalemate. During these periods, passion and conviction are needed to prevent the faint hearts from quitting.

Index

Printed in the United States
by Baker & Taylor Publisher Services